EXERCISE
ETC. INC.
1-800-244-1344

LIFESTYLE & WEIGHT MANAGEMENT

CONSULTANT MANUAL

Richard T. Cotton

EDITOR

Christine J. Ekeroth

ASSOCIATE EDITOR

AMERICAN
COUNCIL
ON EXERCISE

San Diego, California

Library of Congress Catalog Card Number: 96-085137

ISBN 0-9618161-5-5
Copyright © 1996 American Council on Exercise® (ACE®)
Printed in the United States of America

A B C D E F

Distributed by:
American Council on Exercise
P. O. Box 910449
San Diego, CA 92191-0449
(619) 535-8227
(619) 535-1778 (FAX)
http://www.acefitness.org

Assistant Editor: Holly Yancy
Design: Grace Anne Swanson
Production: Suzan Peterson
Photographer: Rick Starkman
Anatomical Illustrations: James Staunton
Glossary: Karen Nelson
Index: Bonny McLaughlin
Copy Editors/Proofreaders: Christina Gandolfo, Ronale Tucker
Chapter Models: Michael Barton, Sabra Bonelli, Carol Buehler, Bryan Cochran, Dick Cotton,
Mark DePuy, Diane Duray-Stoner, Kristen Edwards, Scott Fischer, Lisa Garrity, JoAnn Larson,
Jenora Lewis, Elizabeth Loeffler, Diane O'Brien, Tony Ordas, Steve Oschmann, Darlene Ravelo,
Christy Rodriguez, Monica Schrader, Anthony Spencer
Cover Models: John Stinson, Grace Swanson
Acknowledgements: To the entire American Council on Exercise staff
for their support and guidance through the process of creating this manual.

Reviewers

Ross E. Andersen, Ph.D., is an assistant professor of medicine at Johns Hopkins University and is the associate director of exercise science for the Johns Hopkins Weight Management Center. He also is a fellow of the American College of Sports Medicine and his work is supported by the National Institutes of Health.

Susan J. Bartlett, Ph.D., is a postdoctoral fellow at the Johns Hopkins School of Medicine, and a clinical psychologist with the Johns Hopkins Weight Management Center in Baltimore, Md. She also served as a member of the ACE Lifestyle and Weight Management Consultant Certification Examination Committee.

Mary Brouillard, Ph.D., received her doctorate in counseling/health psychology from Stanford University. She has a private practice, is the associate professor at the Medical College of Georgia and is the psychological specialist for the Weight For Life Program. She also served on the ACE Lifestyle and Weight Management Certification Examination and Role Delineation committees.

Gary D. Foster, Ph.D., is an assistant professor of psychology and clinical director of the University of Pennsylvania School of Medicine's Weight and Eating Disorders Program.

Andrew Jackson, P.E.D., is a professor in the department of health and human performance at the University of Houston, and adjunct professor of medicine at the Baylor College of Medicine in Houston, Texas.

Joseph P. Kearney, M.A., is the president and chief executive officer of Apple Health Systems in San Marcos, Calif., and the executive director of Wellways International. He is the author of *Defeat D'Fat: The Wellness Challenge for Living Lite*, and *Defeat D'Stress: Techniques for Coping with Life.*

Brian E. Koeberle, J.D., is a sports and entertainment attorney and the director of operations for the Major League Baseball Players Alumni Association. He is the author of *The Legal Aspects of Personal Fitness Training*, and lectures on various sports and fitness and the law.

David L. Montgomery, Ph.D., is an exercise physiologist with research applied to physical training. He also is a professor in the department of physical education at McGill University in Montreal, Canada, and is the director of the Seagram's Sports Science Center as well as the graduate program.

Glen D. Morgan, Ph.D., is the director of Behavioral Sciences at the Wyoming Valley Family Practice Residency Program in Kingston, Pa. He also is the clinical assistant professor in the department of family and community medicine at the Pennsylvania State University College of Medicine, and the clinical assistant professor of the Physician Assistant Program at Kings College.

Laura Munson, M.S., R.D., is a practicing clinical dietitian and health education specialist at Scripps Clinic in La Jolla, Ca. She received a master's degree in nutrition from Loma Linda University, and is currently a correspondence instructor in nutrition at the University of Nevada, Reno.

Bernadine M. Pinto, Ph.D., is an assistant professor (Research) in the department of psychiatry and human behavior for the Brown University School of Medicine, and is the staff psychologist at The Miriam Hospital. She also served on the ACE Lifestyle and Weight Management Consultant Role Delineation Committee.

Peter V. Sacks, M.D., is a physician with the division of internal medicine at Scripps Clinic & Research Foundation. He was formerly the head of the division of preventive medicine and director of the Bariatric (Weight Control) Program.

Barbara Scott, M.P.H., R.D., is an associate professor in the Nutrition Education and Research Program and the department of pediatrics at the University of Nevada School of Medicine in Reno, Nev.

David K. Stotlar, Ed.D., is the director of the school of kinesiology and physical education at the University of Northern Colorado. He is the author of several book chapters on sports and the law and frequently makes presentations at national and international conferences.

Larry S. Verity, Ph.D., F.A.C.S.M., is a professor of exercise physiology for the department of exercise and nutritional sciences at San Diego State University, and is a preventive and rehabilitation exercise specialist certified by the American College of Sports Medicine.

TABLE OF CONTENTS

FOREWORD

It's something many of us have known for a long time, but the public has yet to embrace the concept that diets just don't work. There are endless gimmicks and best-selling books, infomercials by the dozen and self-proclaimed diet gurus telling the American public they can easily lose weight with their product (supplement, exercise equipment, diet plan, etc.). But almost every time someone falls for the latest pitch, the only thing they wind up losing is their money.

The fitness industry hasn't fared much better. Despite promises that aerobics would make the pounds drop like sweat off the body, research confirms that few people succeed in losing weight through exercise alone. The main problem, of course, is that while people aerobicized and lifted weights, they continued to consume too many calories. Many found themselves actually gaining weight, and abandoned their exercise regimens altogether.

So now it seems as though we are back to square one. It's clear the weight-loss industry has failed since currently one out of every three American adults is overweight — that's more than 58 million people. And in many respects this represents the failure of the fitness industry as well — statistics continue to indicate that fewer than 25 percent of Americans are physically active.

Several years ago it became clear to us that the true solution to American's sedentary lifestyles and growing weight problem would require a meeting of the minds — the integration of basic exercise science and nutrition. Successfully losing weight requires a multifaceted approach: sound nutrition, safe and effective physical activity, appropriate lifestyle changes and psychological and emotional support. Despite such an obvious need, a practical means for bringing these disciplines together did not exist. And so we developed the *ACE Lifestyle & Weight Management Consultant Manual* and certification.

Fitness professionals, weight-loss counselors, dietitians and club managers told us this was just what they were looking for. First and foremost, this certification provides a higher standard for those who want to practice lifestyle and weight management consulting, and will help to prevent those with insufficient training and education from practicing. For those already in the fitness industry, this certification represents the opportunity to expand both their scope of practice and client base, increasing the demand for their services. And, for those already in the weight-loss industry, either through health clubs or weight-loss centers, it raises the standard for both knowledge and proficiency in helping clients to successfully manage not only their weight, but their overall health as well.

This manual is the first step in making these opportunities a reality. In addition to being an excellent study guide for the certification exam, it is a comprehensive resource that you will likely refer to again and again. So get on board with the latest thinking in weight management and go beyond gimmicks and single discipline solutions. Be a part of the new standard for weight management consulting and help change the shape of America.

Sheryl Marks Brown
Executive Director
American Council on Exercise

INTRODUCTION

This project began as nothing more than an idea in 1993. The weight-loss industry was under federal scrutiny while the application of exercise to weight management was becoming more valued. The ACE Lifestyle & Weight Management Consultant certification was born out of a desire to give the weight-management consumer a standard by which to choose an appropriate professional to help them make necessary lifestyle changes. With a group of 20 people from the fields of psychology, nutrition and exercise science, we created the exam content outline (Appendix B), which served as the blueprint for our certification exam and, ultimately, this manual.

The *ACE Lifestyle & Weight Management Consultant Manual* presents the most current, complete picture of the knowledge, instructional and counseling techniques and professional responsibilities that lifestyle and weight management consultants need to safely and effectively help clients make appropriate lifestyle changes. It is designed to serve as a comprehensive resource to help you in your day-to-day practice, and as a study aid for candidates preparing for the ACE certification exam.

We developed this manual and certification to meet the growing demand for an integrated approach to weight management. This new credential represents the knowledge required to develop successful weight-management programs that combine physical activity, nutrition and lifestyle change. In developing this manual, we brought together top experts from the fields of psychology, exercise, nutrition and law. Each chapter is a building block of knowledge, arranged logically to give you an understanding of the basic principles and skills inherent to lifestyle and weight management.

The ability to communicate effectively is essential to a lifestyle and weight management consultant. Chapter 1 covers the basics of communication, counseling and group dynamics that will help you listen to and communicate effectively with your clients. You will learn how to build rapport and trust with them, understand their needs and develop suitable action plans. Chapter 2 is an overview of the theories and techniques of health behavior change in general, and moves on to address the analysis and intervention of your clients' health behaviors as they relate to weight management and modification.

In order to effectively help a client lose weight and shift to a healthier lifestyle, you must first assess their readiness to do so. Chapter 3 focuses on the genetic, psychological and physiological factors related to obesity and how they apply to the various approaches to weight management. You also will learn about the risk factors and contributors (e.g., culture, environment, heredity, inactivity, family history) that may have led your clients to become obese in the first place.

The focus of the manual shifts with Chapter 4 to a different aspect of weight management. An accurate assessment of body composition is an integral part of a comprehensive health screening and is recommended for individuals who wish to begin a weight-loss or exercise program. Chapter 4 addresses common methods of estimating body composition, and discusses the use of these assessments to help establish appropriate and realistic weight goals with clients.

Obesity or overweight is a major cause of health risks such as hypertension, hyperlipidemia, osteoarthritis and coronary artery disease. Despite our nation's intense preoccupation with weight and dieting, the percentage of overweight individuals increased from 25 percent to 33 percent between 1976 and 1991. Chapter 5 discusses the factors that have led to this staggering rise in the prevalence of obesity, as well as the physiological aspects of being overweight and the subsequent health risks.

The hallmark of ACE-certified consultants is their ability to work safely and effectively in promoting lifestyle change for a wide variety of individuals. However, not all clients who seek your services *can* or *should* be treated by you. The purpose of Chapter 6 is to assist in screening for potential contraindications to weight-loss treatment, provide a framework for the assessment of potential clients and identify appropriate referral sources.

Because the balance between energy expenditure and energy intake ultimately determines whether an individual will lose, maintain or gain weight, understanding the factors that influence energy balance is essential for anyone who works with weight-management programs. Chapter 7 addresses the exercise component of achieving energy balance, while Chapter 8 presents you with the fundamentals of nutrition, both of which are essential to long-term weight management.

Chapter 9 gives you the nuts and bolts of developing successful lifestyle and weight management programs for your clients with the understanding that each plan should be an integrated, evolving matrix of exercise, nutritional and behavioral elements. It is especially important to recognize the special needs of certain populations, such as those with health or behavioral conditions that might prevent them from participating in a weight-management program. Chapter 10 helps you sort through what is, and what is not, appropriate for you to do, particularly with respect to the care of clients from special populations and with special needs. Finally, Chapter 11 gives you an overview of the legal system and the operation of various laws and legal principles that may have an impact upon your ability to serve your clients.

It is our sincerest desire that the information presented in this manual, as well as our certification, will serve to enhance the quality of service provided by weight management consultants. Ultimately, this will no doubt lead to greater success on the part of those striving to maintain a healthy weight and lifestyle.

Richard T. Cotton
Vice President, Publications

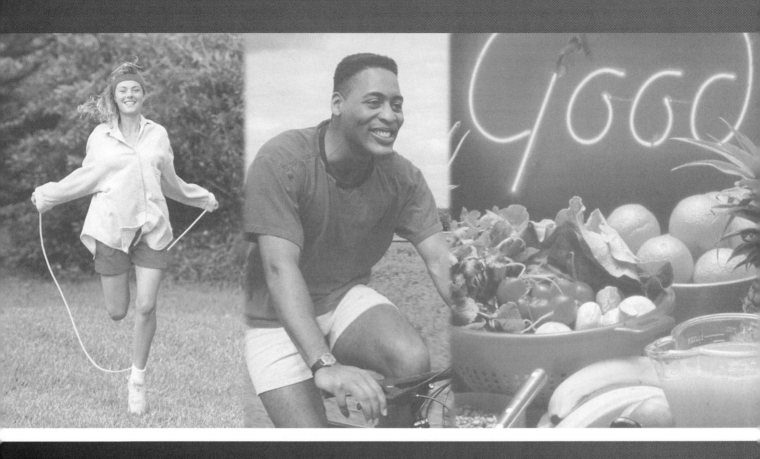

CHAPTER ONE

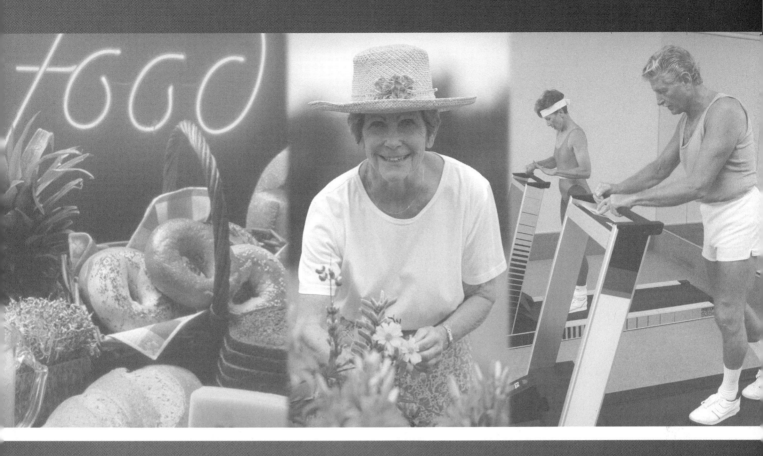

COUNSELING, COMMUNICATION AND Group Dynamics

Susan Bartlett

Susan J. Bartlett, Ph.D., is a post-doctoral fellow at Johns Hopkins School of Medicine, and a clinical psychologist at the Johns Hopkins Weight Management Center in Baltimore, Md. Dr. Bartlett served as a member of the ACE Lifestyle and Weight Management Consultant Certification Examination Committee.

Introduction

Some are born with it, others would rather visit their dentist than attempt it too often. At one time or another in our lives we've all had difficulty with it. Communication is an often elusive, always admirable, ability. It's kind of like charm — difficult to describe but you know it when you see it.

The ability to communicate is not the exclusive domain of individuals with the gift of gab. In fact, communication has more to do with listening and understanding than it does with talking. It's not how well you can convey your knowledge or ideas, but how well you can listen to (not just hear) what others, such as your clients, might be trying to tell you.

Learning the basics of communication is the first step — mastering the areas of counseling and group dynamics is the next. The following chapter will help you in your role as a consultant to listen to and communicate effectively with your clients. Building rapport and trust with clients, understanding their needs and developing an action plan suited to the individual are all a part of effective communication. Whether dealing with clients one-on-one or in a group setting, there are plenty of tools and techniques you can use and master to develop the art of communication. So don't worry if you weren't born with it — you can learn to communicate effectively in any situation.

Client Assessment

A variety of signals — some verbal, others nonverbal — tell your client that you really are listening and do care about them. From the initial handshake to the last words of your meeting, your client is constantly evaluating your knowledge, confidence and credibility. In short, impressions about how helpful you really can be are formed from the first contact. Take the time to make this assessment a positive experience. It will reassure your clients and set the tone for your entire relationship.

Create the Right Atmosphere

The environment in which your meeting is held is an important consideration. Be sure you and your client will be free of distractions and irritants. Consider the room carefully. Is the temperature comfortable and the ventilation adequate? Does it feel private and inviting (rather than like being thrust into a converted storage closet)? Turn off the ringer of the phone and place a "Do Not Disturb" sign on the door to ensure you focus your attention solely on the client. Be sure others are aware that you are unavailable (even for quick questions) when conducting the assessment interview. If possible, face the client directly, or just slightly, to your side

rather than working from behind a desk.

Begin your assessment by briefly introducing yourself and stating your goals for the meeting. Tell your client what you hope to accomplish in this interview in very specific terms. Include details such as the purpose of your meeting, time frame and a brief out- line of how the meeting will progress. Providing these details structures the session and reassures clients that you are comfortable in the role of consultant, helping them to feel less anxious. For example, you might begin something like this:

LWMC: *Mary, my name is _____ and as you know I am a lifestyle and weight management consultant.*

[Add a brief statement about your background here.]

You and I are meeting today so that I can learn something about you, your lifestyle, weight history and eating and exercise patterns. We'll also explore some of the barriers you may have encountered with previous attempts to change your lifestyle. Our meeting will last about __(time)__. At the end of our meeting, I will outline for you my impressions about the factors that are important for both of us to address. We also will set some specific goals to begin working on together. And I hope that in time you will have a chance to know me a little bit better.

Please feel free to stop me any time and ask any questions you may have. Do you have any questions now?

[Address questions.]
Good, then let's begin …

Show You are Listening

Effective communication occurs when clients know they are being heard and feel understood. Communicate interest and caring by maintaining eye contact throughout the meeting. Work toward taking minimal notes during the meeting to maintain eye contact as much as possible when the client is speaking. Frequent breaks in eye contact, such as those that occur when taking detailed notes, are often perceived by clients as disinterest or discomfort with the material being disclosed.

Watch your body posture. Leaning slightly toward the client, maintaining an open posture and appearing relaxed show you are confident and interested. Conversely, a slouched posture or arms folded across your chest can be interpreted as impatience and aloofness.

Watch the client's body posture as well. Look for signs that suggest the client may be uncomfortable with a certain topic such as fidgeting, poor eye

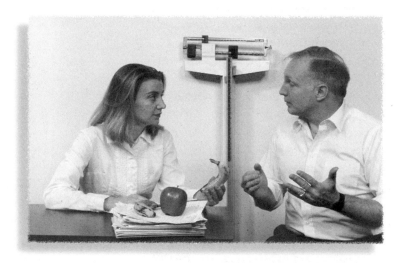

Effective communication occurs when clients know they are being heard and feel understood.

contact and muscle tension. When you notice these non-verbal cues, proceed carefully but don't back down. Be sensitive to the client's discomfort in disclosing personal information and acknowledge their discomfort openly. Statements like "I can see this is difficult to talk about, but it may be very important for me to understand exactly how badly your weight makes you feel about yourself" encourages the client to continue while acknowledging their uneasiness.

It also is important to recognize that how individuals feel about themselves (i.e., self-image) significantly influences both what they are willing to tell you and how it is said. (For a detailed summary of factors that influence an

individual's self-image see Chapter 2.) Watch for incongruities between what is said and how the individual is reacting non-verbally. For instance, clients may provide a brief, superficial answer to questions about their home life then quickly move off the topic. ("Oh, everything is fine. My partner really wants me to lose weight. Don't worry about that.") However, the astute lifestyle and weight management consultant will listen both to what is said and what isn't. Most of us are reluctant to disclose information that we perceive as embarrassing or shameful. Your overweight client may assume you somehow are able to know that their partner says they are supportive but acts differently. They may also downplay the importance of problems in their lives. ("Sure I hate my job, but that's OK.") Remember, these clients are not deliberately withholding information to sabotage their efforts; more likely, they are concerned that you will blame them (or not wish to work with them) if you know about certain aspects of their lives (e.g., a verbally or physically abusive partner).

Certain verbal techniques have been shown to enhance communication. Active listening tells the client that what they are saying is important and worthwhile. Minimal prompts such as "uh-huh" and "yes" reinforce disclosure of pertinent information without interrupting the client's thoughts. Probe for more information (or return the client to a more pertinent topic) as needed. Open-ended questions, which require more than a yes or no response, encourage the conversation to continue. (Tell me more about…")

Periodically, reflect to the client what you have been hearing. Restate what the client has been saying using many of their words and a few of your own. Be careful not to directly parrot responses too frequently, though. Openers like "What I hear you saying…" or

"It sounds like…" are good ways to begin. End the reflection with a summary statement. For example:

LWMC: *Tom, you seem to be saying that while you were in college, you were very active in athletics and extracurricular activities, but since you've been working in the stock exchange, you are more likely to spend your day sitting. That's a big change in your activity level and is likely an important factor in your weight gain.*

Build Rapport

Trusting a stranger with personal details is a difficult task for most of us. As a lifestyle consultant, it is relatively easy to lose sight of how stressful the initial meeting is for most clients. After all, within a few months you will likely feel much more comfortable in the role of consultant. Remember, though, that most of us never feel comfortable taking on the role of the "client" initially.

Carl Rogers, a noted psychologist, identified three core conditions that must be present before clients can fully trust and participate in a counseling relationship: empathy, unconditional positive regard (or respect) and genuineness. Empathy refers to the ability to "enter into the client's phenomenal world — to experience the client's world as if it were your own without ever losing the 'as if' quality" (Rogers, 1961). Empathy refers to a deeper level of understanding in which you come to view the world from the client's frame of reference without judging it. As clients share their thoughts, feelings, beliefs and concerns, you must listen without labeling anything as right or wrong, good or bad. Empathy lays the foundation for honesty and openness in the relationship and will be critical when difficult periods are encountered later in your work together.

Positive regard, or respect, conveys a deep, sincere belief in the client's ability to change. The respectful consultant identifies a client's strengths, allows them to make their own decisions and nurtures self-confidence rather than dependency. Positive regard is conveyed when your attitude says, "I know you can do this. We just need to find the right pathway for you."

Genuineness reflects your ability to be "real" in your interactions with your clients. Instead of hiding behind a professional role, you must respond to the client as an individual rather than a patient or case study. From time to time it may be appropriate to share some of your own experiences with the client. However, do this sparingly. A well-timed, occasional personal disclosure may emphasize your point clearly. On the other hand, consistently referring to your own struggles around weight, for instance, may suggest to the client that you need professional support as much as they do, or may reflect that you might only be able to see them from the perspective of your own experience.

Your relationship with the client begins with the assessment. From the very beginning, the ability to establish a trusting relationship is what can set you apart from peers. Focusing on creating the right atmosphere, demonstrating your ability to listen through effective communication techniques, and building rapport will inspire confidence and trust in your clients. Skilled consultants recognize that efforts in the early stages of the relationship prompt clients to "stick with it" when motivation and morale ebbs on more difficult days.

Developing an Individualized Client Plan

The development of the client plan begins as you and your client identify problematic behaviors and attitudes. Once these have been identified, effective solutions can be developed. You can make this stage an informative and vital step in the process of behavioral change. Conversely, too little time or inadequate attention to problem definition leaves clients feeling confused and uncertain as to how this attempt to change will be any different from all previous endeavors.

Target Behaviors to Change

Identify problematic behaviors by listening carefully to both what clients are saying and what they are not saying. One of the key questions you both need to answer is "What barriers prevented

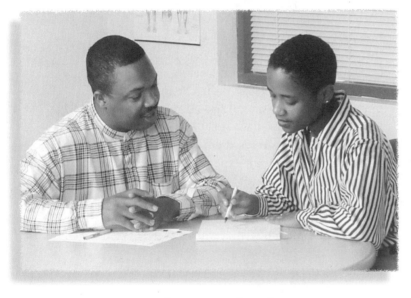

Establishing goals is a highly interactive process between you and your client.

the success of previous attempts to change?" Ask clients to carefully outline previous attempts they have made at dieting, for example. What worked well? For how long? What was going on in their life when motivation and adherence waned? Clients will frequently regard previous attempts to change weight, eating and exercise patterns as failures. In reality, each attempt potentially provides valuable information about what made a difference and what didn't. By drawing on previous strengths and stringing them together, along with identifying barriers to success, you will begin to rough out an

individualized pathway to success for each client.

Establish Goals Together

Once problematic behaviors and attitudes have been identified, you and your client are ready to set goals. Whereas you are required to listen carefully and reflect what is being heard to identify problematic patterns, this stage of the assessment is a highly interactive process between you and your client.

Goal setting is a three-step process:
1. Clarifying problematic patterns
2. Specifying the what, where, when and how to change
3. Committing to the goals outlined

Identifying problematic patterns and attitudes leads naturally to the clarification stage of goal setting. The first step of goal setting involves working with clients to help them clearly spell out their desired lifestyle changes. The tendency is for clients to identify broad, sweeping changes, such as "I need a healthier lifestyle," or "I want to be in better shape." Instead, help them focus on the outcomes they are seeking (e.g., weight loss, improved fitness, better sleep). For example, early in the client assessment interview, Jose stated:

Much has changed since I married and the kids were born. Before, I enjoyed playing pickup basketball two or three nights a week at the gym with the guys. Weekends were pretty active, too, with running or tennis. But since I got married, and especially with the little ones, who has time? My wife is always saying there's a million things to do around the house and it's unfair for me to be out playing around. It's all we can do to keep up with these two preschoolers. I get home from work, we order pizza or pick up some fast food on the way home, get the kids fed, bathed, ready for bed and the night is gone.

With more discussion Jose was able to specify that what he meant by "being in better shape" was losing 25 pounds and being physically active at least three times per week. While clarification of goals may seem redundant, it is vital to obtain explicit agreement from your client about the goals the two of you are working on together.

LWMC: *It seems like a lot of things have changed for you in the last five years. Your job has you sitting in a chair much of the day. Evenings and weekends are devoted to family responsibilities, preventing you from being as active as before. Your food choices have leaned toward convenience items which are higher in fat, sodium and calories. So there have been lots of changes in lifestyle that may have contributed to your weight problem. What specifically would you like to achieve in our work together?*

Jose: *Well, I want to get in better shape. It's time to start a health campaign.*

LWMC: *Tell me more about what you mean by that. What goals do you have for your yourself regarding weight, exercise and eating?*

Jose: *Well, my doctor tells me I should lose the 25 pounds I've gained. And I want to get more exercise. I feel better when I'm more active.*

LWMC: *Okay, I hear two goals. The first goal is that you want to exercise regularly again, but are unsure how to do that with your current schedule. I think that is a very appropriate goal for both of us to work on. The second thing I heard you say was that your doctor thinks it would be helpful to lose weight. Is that what the doctor wants or what you want?*

Jose: *No, no, it's not my doctor saying that ... I mean, it is my goal. I would really like to lose this weight. I carry it mostly around my middle and my clothes don't fit well, and it's harder to get out of the car. It just slows me down. Definitely, that's my other goal. I want to lose 25 pounds.*

LWMC: *Good, we have goal number two. Losing 25 pounds would have important health benefits and seems realistic to me*

given your previous weight history. I think that also is a great goal that we could work on together.

Once outcome goals have been identified, it often is very helpful to record your client's own words verbatim. This is the beginning of the behavioral contract.

The second stage of goal setting involves the specification of concise goals. Here your client maps out a plan of change. While often it is more expeditious to run through specific changes you believe your client must make, having them actively set these goals is ultimately far more helpful. Clients can readily change their behaviors if we help them determine who will change what, to what extent, under which conditions and when. Let's examine how the lifestyle and weight management consultant worked together with Jose to help him outline a plan to meet his goals.

LWMC: *The goals that you want to achieve in our work together are both clear and realistic. In mapping out this plan, we need to consider who will be affected by these goals.*

Jose: *Well, obviously, I will be most affected. I'll need to do things differently, like eat and exercise at a different time. But I guess my wife Helena will be affected, too. After all, we can't have pizza and fast food five nights a week if I'm trying to eat differently. I'll need to talk to her about this. I guess the kids might be affected, too, but not as much.*

LWMC: *So, we have you making most of the changes, and the possibility of asking your wife if she may be able to do some things differently to help you as well. Let's begin with your first goal — becoming more active. Are there any times during the week when you can increase your activity without necessarily taking time away from the family?*

Figure 1.1
Lifestyle Goal
Worksheet.

Lifestyle Goal Worksheet

Date _____   Name _____

1. Activity and Exercise

My intermediate activity and exercise goals:

A _____

B _____

C _____

How I plan to get there:

To increase my lifestyle activity by _____ minutes per day, I will:

_____

_____

_____

To increase my structured activity, I will:

_____	_____ minutes	_____ times per week
_____	_____ minutes	_____ times per week
_____	_____ minutes	_____ times per week
_____	_____ minutes	_____ times per week

2. Weight and Eating Habits:

My target weight is: _____.

In 4 weeks, I would like to weigh _____.

In 8 weeks, I would like to weigh _____.

In 12 weeks, I would like to weigh _____.

To eat healthier and achieve a more reasonable weight, I will:

Add _____   When _____

Add _____   When _____

Add _____   When _____

Add _____   When _____

Substitute _____   For _____

Substitute _____   For _____

Substitute _____   For _____

Substitute _____   For _____

Limit _____   To _____

Limit _____   To _____

Limit _____   To _____

Limit _____   To _____

Figure 1.1 continued

3. Stress Busters:

My overall level of stress is:

1	2	3	4	5	6	7	8	9
Minimal								Maximal

To better manage stress, I can:

A _____   When _____

B _____   When _____

C _____   When _____

4. Counseling and Support:

I plan to meet with my lifestyle and weight management consultant:

_____ Individually _____ times per month

_____ Group _____ times per month

Anticipated absences _____

_____

Other people I can ask for support:

Who? _____   Can help how? _____

Who? _____   Can help how? _____

Who? _____   Can help how? _____

Figure 1.1 continued

5. Additional Goals (sleep, smoking, etc.):

A _____   When _____

B _____   When _____

C _____   When _____

D _____   When _____

E _____   When _____

6. Potential Obstacles and Solutions:

Obstacle   Solution

_____   _____

_____   _____

_____   _____

_____   _____

7. Evaluation of Goals:

We plan to review these goals in _____ weeks on _____.

_____

Client

_____

Lifestyle and Weight Management Consultant

Attainment of Goals

Goals Achieved:

Date   Goal

_____   _____

_____   _____

_____   _____

_____   _____

Additional Goals:

_____

_____

_____

Jose: *Well, sure, I guess at lunch time. There's a group of guys who get together a few times a week at work and run. Sometimes they go over to the court at the gym that's close by — when someone remembers to sign up for it. I've thought about it before, but I always seem too busy or too hungry to join them even though they have asked.*

LWMC: *Getting some activity at lunch time sounds like a great idea. Let's think about what you might need to do differently to allow yourself the time to join with these co-workers. . . .*

Remember, the aim of this step is to help your client state goals in concrete and direct terms. Be certain that all goals specify what behaviors will change, to what extent (i.e., exercise for how long, how many times per week) and under what conditions (every Monday, Wednesday and Friday).

In addition to being very specific, goals must be realistic and achievable. Psychologists have long recognized the importance of shaping behaviors when trying to achieve a goal. Shaping means making small, consistent steps toward a desired goal. Animals are trained over time to perform complex behaviors by first beginning with very small steps that are continuously reinforced. The principle of shaping applies equally to human behavior as well.

Your role in goal setting is to ensure that both the short- and long-term goals are realistic and achievable within a reasonable time frame. For example, Suzanne decided that she would begin jogging to get more exercise, help manage her weight and reduce health risks. She began training to run a marathon as a long-term goal. Realistically, it will take her many months, or possibly even years, to reach that goal (and remember, not everyone can, and should, run a marathon). However, 5K and 10K races may be realistic and achievable within the next few months.

Wrap up this stage of goal setting by recording your client's goals in their own words. A one-page goal setting sheet (Figure 1.1) is often very useful. Have two copies of the goal sheet — one for your client and the other for your files.

The last step in goal setting is to obtain a firm commitment from your client toward achieving the goals you have outlined together. It is at this time that collaboration between the two of you is essential. If you have assumed primary responsibility for both clarifying and specifying the goals, in essence, they remain your goals. The message that is communicated is, "This is what I want you to do. I will make this easy for you by doing the thinking for you." In such situations, the client is often disappointed when the consultant is unable to, in effect, also *do* the work of changing for the client.

Research has shown that people work harder for the goals they have set for themselves. While clients may implicitly or explicitly agree to work on consultant-owned goals, the chances for such goals being met are greatly reduced. Thus, conclude your goal setting with clients by summarizing what you have agreed upon. If you have used a formal goal-setting worksheet, read the entries verbatim (Figure 1.1).

LWMC: *Jose, you have agreed to* [review goals in very specific terms]. *I am here to help. I can best do that by ensuring that your goals are reasonable and achievable, monitoring your progress, providing information and suggestions at times and re-evaluating these goals with you on a regular basis. I think this is a good sound plan that will work for you. Do I have your commitment to work toward achieving these goals?*

[Get a verbal commitment.]

Great. Let's both sign here. We will review these goals and the progress you have made in four weeks.

Implementation and Facilitation of the Client Plan

When behavioral problems have been identified and appropriate goals set, a strong foundation for success is laid. Efforts that you make in these areas will be fruitfully rewarded; conversely, when a client is rushed through the assessment and goal setting phases, the seeds are sown for increased difficulties when trying to implement your client's plan.

Continual review of your client's progress toward achieving goals is essential to long-term success. Clients will be more motivated to keep accurate eating and activity logs when they know you will review these at each session. Encourage ongoing discussion both about what is going well for the client and what is difficult. If all you hear about are the successes, especially beyond the first few weeks, it is likely that your client feels uncomfortable talking about their struggles. Yet your real work together begins as barriers to change are encountered.

How you interact with clients who are working toward their goals can strongly influence their motivation and determination. By focusing on positive changes, building incentives into the program, providing well-timed feedback, **modeling** appropriate behaviors and anticipating and working through obstacles you can help bolster waning enthusiasm and morale.

Focus on Positive Changes

It can be overwhelming for clients to think about losing large amounts of weight (i.e., more than 15 pounds) or converting from a couch potato to a more active lifestyle. Clients often harbor feelings that the way to motivate change within themselves is through

ongoing shame. For example, Barbara has attempted to lose weight many times, but never seems to get past the first 10 pounds:

Whenever I let myself feel good about my weight loss, it goes to my head. Then I begin rewarding myself with food, and that's the beginning of the end. So I need to keep telling myself how disgusting I look, and that 10 pounds is nothing when I have 30 more to go.

The downfall of this motivational approach is that it rarely succeeds. Help your clients take credit for every behavioral change they accomplish. Redirect the focus to specific behavioral changes that have already been made and the consequences of these changes.

Barbara: *I can't think about the fact that I've lost 10 pounds. I'm still fat. Look at me.*
LWMC: *While it is true that you do have more weight that you want to lose, I see a lot of positive changes in your behavior in the last few weeks. Let's review how your lifestyle has changed since we began working together. On our first walk together, we covered about half a mile in 15 minutes. How long have your walks averaged in the past week, and what distances are you covering?*
Barbara: *Well, that's very true. Now I walk at least 2 miles and do it in half an hour a minimum of three days per week. And I don't huff and puff the whole way up the stairs like I used to. It used to be embarrassing at work. I would arrive at the third floor and be too out of breath to talk for a minute or two.*
LWMC: *That's impressive and represents an important change in your fitness level. What other changes have you noticed?*

Build Incentives into the Program

Two methods have proven consistently useful in helping people change behaviors: records and rewards. Have your clients keep detailed records of the new

AMERICAN COUNCIL ON EXERCISE

13

CHAPTER ONE

COUNSELING,
COMMUNICATION
AND GROUP
DYNAMICS

behaviors they are shaping. Reviewing them regularly with you provides incentive and motivation. Help your clients devise regular rewards for achieving short-term goals. Small rewards for frequent achievements are best initially. Later, as behaviors become more habitual, these incentives can be gradually reduced. Rewards can involve anything that is meaningful for your client from a piece of new exercise clothing to concert tickets. However, it is best to avoid rewards that are specifically related to eating. Rewards like dinner at a special restaurant are rather like having a cigarette to celebrate quitting smoking. Brainstorm with your clients to arrive at creative and novel approaches.

Provide Feedback

Providing your clients with feedback lets them know how well they are progressing toward achieving their goals. Constructive feedback offers support to your clients but also gently challenges them when needed. Egan (1990) identified three types of feedback:

✔ Confirmatory feedback lets clients know when they are on course; that is, moving successfully toward achieving their goals.

✔ Corrective feedback provides information on how to get back on course if they have strayed.

✔ Motivating feedback points out the consequences of both adequate and inadequate movement toward achieving goals and includes suggestions for improving performance.

When providing feedback to your clients, be especially sensitive about how you word suggestions. Keep the tone positive and gentle with a brief message that is to the point. Avoid accusations or inferring motives (e.g., "It seems you didn't do well with your eating changes because you weren't interested enough to bother planning").

Provide feedback sparingly. A little can go a long way, but too much can overwhelm your clients and cause them to abandon their efforts to change. Focus primarily on positive behavioral changes that your clients have made between visits. Initially, these changes may seem to come easily — the honeymoon stage of behavior change. It is relatively easy for most of us to change our behavior for brief periods of time but persistence is the key to long-term success.

Anticipate Obstacles

Work with any client long enough (i.e., at least three months) and they are likely to encounter obstacles that impede lifestyle change. Typically, motivation and enthusiasm to change wanes as obstacles are encountered. Your goal is to support your clients through difficult times, helping them to regain their confidence and motivation.

A skilled consultant will begin talking with clients about potential obstacles to change from the start of their work together. Some clients, for instance, are information gatherers. They actively seek out the best consultant, read everything available and ask their healthcare providers for the most appropriate methods to change. However, once they have gathered this information, they find themselves unable to act on it. Instead, they continue to read, ask questions and seek assistance. The tools are there but are never utilized.

Kirschenbaum (1987) has investigated the phenomenon of giving up and has identified several important factors including:

1. Low initial commitment to change
2. Diminished sense of **self-efficacy** (belief in one's ability to change)
3. Use of self-punishment rather

than self-reward strategies

4. Depressive or pessimistic thinking patterns
5. Lack of consistent self-monitoring
6. Difficulty coping with initial setbacks
7. Failure to use effective habit-changing techniques
8. Paying attention to the wrong things (for example, how unfair it is that there is a box of donuts at work every day rather than how I am failing to cope with tempting foods in my environment).

When you identify any of these factors with your clients, talk openly about them. Most clients you will work with have already made attempts to change their lifestyle. Attempts often begin with enthusiasm and commitment that diminishes considerably over time. From the beginning, stress the importance of making changes in lifestyle that can be sustained — not only initially, when enthusiasm is high, but also down the road when priorities change.

Model and Rehearse Lifestyle Changes

It has been said that we are more than half of who we are through imitation. In other words, we often observe and imitate the behaviors of others — a process known as modeling. You have a unique opportunity to both describe and model a healthier lifestyle for your clients. Models are most effective when their behaviors match their words. Follow the lifestyle that you advocate for your clients. Eat regularly scheduled meals, pack a lunch for work and include some activity in your own day. Remember, your clients are watching your actions both in and out of consulting sessions.

It often is helpful to include role-playing sessions from time to time in your work together. For instance, when clients are concerned about not overeating at a family function (e.g., picnic, wedding, celebration), help them work through the scenario with you as a "dress rehearsal." Ask them to share their thoughts about how they will feel when they see a sideboard of tempting foods. Encourage them to rehearse with you how to handle prompts from others to "just go ahead" and enjoy themselves at the buffet.

Encourage clients to find appropriate role models in their lives as well. Models who are likely to be most effective are friends, co-workers, family and other associates the client has ongoing opportunities to observe on a regular basis. You may even want to create a short list of biographies you have read that detail the lifestyle changes of athletes or other celebrities.

Group vs. Individual Consulting

Group approaches to consulting have become increasingly popular in recent years. Clearly, there are financial incentives for both you and your client, but other factors may be even more potent. While one-on-one time with you is reduced, the opportunities for support, motivation, energy and learning are limitless.

Irvin Yalom, a psychiatrist at Stanford University, has devoted much of his professional career to the study of what makes groups helpful. He has identified several factors, among them the instillation of hope, sense of support and similarity, sharing of information and the ability to learn from each other.

Early Preparation

Running effective lifestyle and weight management groups involves more than simply placing several clients in a room and consulting with each individual. A skilled group leader will spend considerable time planning before the group begins. It is helpful to meet individually with each prospective member to assess their interest and suitability for group consultation. Positive signs to look for in potential group members include a commitment to the same meeting time each week, an ability to both listen and share in their meeting with you, and an interest in being with and providing support to others. Some nervousness from your clients is to be expected, but consider carefully whether to include clients who are vocal about their dislike of groups.

In your initial meeting or screening of potential group members, it is important to review the potential benefits of group sessions, where and when to meet, what to expect in the meetings and your policies regarding absences and payment of fees. Explore your client's expectations of what a group session will be like and address any concerns that are raised, such as "Will I be weighed in front of everyone?" and "How much do I have to tell about myself?"

Development of the Group

Groups that function as a cohesive support unit, like any trusting relationship, take time to develop. Initially, it is important for you to provide structure and a sense of security for new members. The first meeting is filled with some anxiety for everyone. Review the goals of the group and the expectations of group members. For example, outline agreements such as the expectation that group members arrive on time, are prepared for each meeting (by completing homework or readings between sessions), share the space and support each other. State the goals of the group in concrete, behavioral terms, much as you would when goal setting with individual clients. Setting a positive

tone, outlining what will occur during the first meeting and subsequent sessions and helping members to find commonalities with each other will make everyone feel more comfortable and confident.

Any group that meets for more than a few sessions will move through fairly predictable stages. Initial goals and objectives for the group involve helping the members to get to know and become interested in each other, and creating a feeling of involvement or belonging. This is usually accomplished within the first session or two. At the same time, you need to nurture an atmosphere which facilitates interaction among members, and the sharing, listening and acceptance of other's ideas.

As the group matures, help members to assume increasing responsibility for problem identification and problem-solving approaches. At this stage, rather than continuing as the "expert," encourage the members to share their thoughts and experiences to help each other. In a trusting and supportive atmosphere, members can enhance their ability to make decisions and receive feedback on positive behavioral changes that have been accomplished. Often, when difficulties are encountered, the same suggestion coming from a group member who has first-hand experience will carry more weight than the best "pearl of wisdom" provided by the group leader.

Finally, groups will conclude by supporting each member to continue the positive behavioral changes they have begun and commit toward future goals in the absence of group support. This often is a difficult time for group members as they question how well they can function without the structure and support of the group. The transfer from group to individual responsibility, however, is essential for long-term success. While some members will attempt to postpone the ending of the group, it is important to help them make this shift toward assuming more individual responsibility. Encourage your clients to talk about their future plans and even begin to emotionally disengage from the group in the last few sessions.

Dealing with Difficult Situations

Despite your best efforts at screening, it is inevitable that, from time to time, difficulties will arise in the group. Behavioral problems will emerge very early on. For example, silent or withdrawn members, or those who arrive

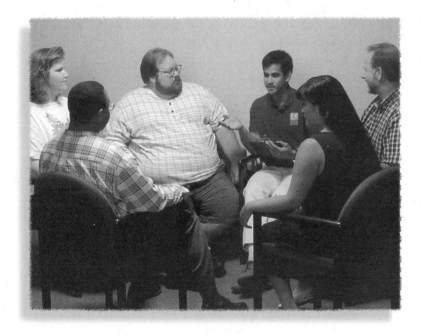

Groups that function as a cohesive support unit take time to develop.

consistently late, are at increased risk of dropping out and may eventually irritate the rest of the group. Try to meet individually with the person just before the group begins to help draw them out or address any fears they may have about talking. Keep the meeting brief and positive, and ask permission to call on them at some point during the group for their views.

On the other hand, overly talkative individuals may be just as problematic. Their talkativeness may stem from anxiety — when there is any sort of silence, they feel that it needs to be filled. Use

non-verbal behavior such as breaking eye contact and looking at other members when the dialogue has continued beyond a comfortable limit. Look for a natural breaking point in the conversation and redirect. For example, "Elaine, that's a good point you are making. Sophie, I'm wondering what your thoughts are about this." It also can be helpful to gently remind such individuals that "the details are really not that important. What you seem to be saying is ..." Always do this with respect, gentleness and in a non-judgmental tone.

Chronic "yes — but'ers" also will tax the patience of the group. When individuals consistently blame others or make excuses, ask the group members for their thoughts. This must be done tactfully and with sensitivity and respect for the individual. Here again, gentle confrontation from other group members can be remarkably effective.

Conducting effective, enjoyable groups is a learned skill. Initially, it is helpful to have a co-leader with you to help share the responsibility. You may wish to have another lifestyle and weight management consultant, or someone with skills in a very specific area. For instance, a lifestyle and weight management consultant and a dietician can approach dietary counseling from both behavioral and nutritional perspectives; on the other hand, an exercise specialist can enhance the focus on activity programming while you concentrate on behavior change. When leading groups alone, consider asking professionals from other disciplines to "guest lecture" and add some variety to your group program.

The preceding section highlighted some of the issues to address when running groups. However, you will want to do some additional reading from the Suggested Reading list included at the end of the chapter for comprehensive coverage of group issues.

Professional Responsibility

Your role as a lifestyle and weight management consultant is a privileged one, and as such, you have a personal and professional obligation to act in a responsible manner. Many lifestyle and weight management consultants also are credentialed in other disciplines (e.g., exercise specialist, registered dietitian, social worker, counseling professional, registered nurse) and are obligated to know and follow the ethical standards of their professional boards.

Know Your Scope of Practice

You have an obligation to be knowledgeable in a wide variety of areas including nutrition, psychology, behavior change, exercise programming and counseling. Over time, as clients feel comfortable and trust you, they will seek advice on an increasingly broad range of topics. For example, joint or muscular injury is common among active individuals; however, only a physician is qualified to diagnose an injury and thus provide treatment advice. Lifestyle and weight management consultants are not equipped to deal with psychological or psychiatric illnesses such as eating disorders (e.g., anorexia and bulimia nervosa) or depression. Also, while general nutritional recommendations related to decreasing fat consumption and eating more complex carbohydrates do not violate laws, prescribing a specific diet with food, vitamin and calorie consumption may be regulated by the state and require the license of a registered dietitian or nutritionist. Laws vary from state to state. You must know the scope and limits of your practice and refrain from areas for which you have no formal training.

Establish Referral Networks

A skilled consultant will establish a network of professionals in related disciplines to refer to. For example, referrals to physicians for general medical care and exercise clearance, orthopedic surgeons for joint and back difficulties, registered dietitians for specific nutritional counseling, psychologists or other mental health professionals for psychological or personal difficulties may be warranted. By working directly with referral sources you know and trust, your clients are more likely to receive continuity of care. Additionally, these related professionals often will serve as invaluable referral sources to you as well.

Protect Client Confidentiality

Lifestyle and weight management consultants have both a legal and moral obligation to protect the confidentiality of all information their clients provide them with. In essence, this means you are obligated to keep private the names, records and information related to all of your clients. The concept of confidentiality is not difficult to understand; clients will feel able to be open and honest about themselves and their lifestyles to the extent that they believe this information will remain private. More importantly, however, all clients have a right to expect that what they discuss will be kept private except where a legal statute dictates otherwise or when they have provided explicit written consent authorizing the consultant to disclose information to another specified individual.

Most breaches of confidentiality are not deliberate acts — rather, they occur inadvertently. For example, Jennifer, a lifestyle and weight management consultant, works part-time at a local fitness center. When at the center, she uses a spare office that is used by personal trainers in the evening. Typically, she sees eight clients, two days per week. At the beginning of the day, she pulls each of her client's files and puts them on her desk. *Potential breach of confidentiality:* The names of all clients may now be seen by others who visit her office that day. Client names are privileged information and must be kept confidential.

Jennifer keeps client files in a cabinet next to her desk. While the filing cabinet is unlocked, it is usual practice of the fitness club that the room is locked. *Potential breach of confidentiality:* On days when Jennifer is not at the club, she has no knowledge of who actually uses the room and for what reasons. Her client files are not adequately protected. Files must be kept in a locked cabinet with restricted access.

Establish a network of professionals in related disciplines to refer to.

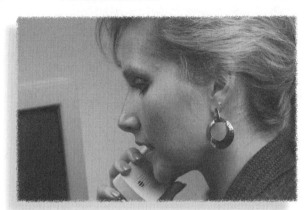

Keep Accurate Records

Many professionals have specific mandates about what constitutes appropriate record keeping. Keep a record of each meeting you have with a client (and of meetings which are scheduled but canceled for any reason). It is good practice to carefully document the initial assessment and goals, planned interventions, medical history and exercise clearance and any contact with relevant healthcare providers (e.g., physician, dietitian, etc.). All counseling sessions must be briefly documented including the date, length of session, topics discussed and goals established. You may wish to keep your client's food and activity records on file as well. It is prudent

to avoid writing very detailed notes, however, to protect confidentiality.

Know Yourself

Lifestyle and weight management consultants, like everyone, have their own personal biases and preferences. Age, gender, ethnic and personal differences abound in an increasingly diverse culture. Sensitivity to individual differences, as well as knowledge of practices and philosophies of other cultures, is required. (For an excellent review of issues and techniques of cross-cultural counseling see Sue & Sue, 1990). What distinguishes an effective consultant from an ineffective one is the extent to which these biases influence and interfere with the best interests of the client.

A clear example of a possibly detrimental personal bias is the passionate belief that aerobic exercise is the key to weight loss. While clearly this type of exercise will benefit many clients, it also may be inappropriate for others, such as those individuals with a history of knee, back or foot problems. Also, current research suggests that lifestyle activity (e.g., walking, gardening, short bouts of activity throughout the day) also may be effective in managing weight and improving risk profiles. The consultant who rigidly prescribes the same exercise (aerobics) for all clients is doing a disservice to many. Creative consultants will look for the best fit between activity and individual preferences and lifestyle.

A more subtle example of personal bias may involve the consultant who is currently experiencing a major life stressor, such as finding out their partner has been diagnosed with a serious illness. The consultant may feel powerless in their own life and that of their loved one. Sometimes, inadvertently, the need to regain control can be shifted to the counseling arena. For example, in the need to feel more powerful and competent, the consultant may present themselves as having all the answers to a client's problems. Sessions may become didactic in tone with the consultant constantly providing advice and trying to direct the client's life. This dynamic can become especially problematic because once the consultant assumes responsibility for the client, the likelihood of real change occurring or being maintained is greatly reduced.

Lifestyle and weight management consulting can be an emotionally taxing profession. Therefore, you must seek to constantly examine factors in your own life which may interfere with your ability to function effectively. If there is any question, it often is helpful to consult with a colleague to review whether personal issues may be creating blind spots or clouding your ability to counsel effectively. Regular peer supervision will enhance your ability to work effectively with clients. At times, clinical supervision from another professional, such as a social worker or psychologist, can provide valuable insight into overlooked areas.

Stay Current

As a lifestyle and weight management consultant, you reflect a blending of many disciplines into a behavioral and lifestyle specialist. To become certified, a broad area of knowledge from many disciplines is required. However, certification as a lifestyle and weight management consultant is just the beginning. Ongoing professional development and education is essential to remain in touch with accurate, up-to-date information. The area of exercise science provides a classic example. The American College of Sports Medicine (1991) recently revised its position statement on exercise. Individuals who received their training prior to 1990 were steeped in the classical exercise threshold model (e.g., exercise at 70 percent to

85 percent VO_2 max, three to five times per week, for a minimum of 30 minutes). While this prescription can optimize athletic performance, recent investigations have found that significantly lower intensity, duration and frequency of exercise also can improve fitness and health. Similarly, in the early 1990s, research findings seemed to suggest that monitoring fat grams was more effective than counting calories for weight control. What a boon that was for dieters who were tired of keeping food logs. It seemed that all that was necessary was to focus on consuming low-fat or no-fat foods, and one could avoid the tedium of calorie counting. However, more controlled studies over longer periods now show that keeping fat grams low is not enough — an

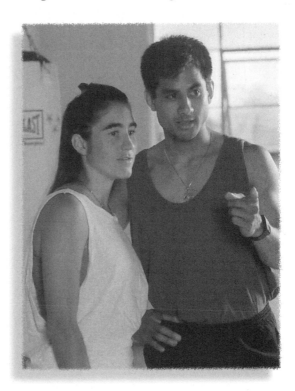

You have both a legal and moral obligation to keep private the names, records and information related to all of your clients.

emphasis on both fat and calorie control is needed for sustained weight loss. With hormones, medications and genetic therapy for weight control in the news nearly every week, you must stay current through professional training, workshops, readings and conferences.

Summary

Our current lifestyle, with its emphasis on high-stress workplaces, increasing responsibility, diminishing resources and social strife, is conducive to developing problems in living and well-being. You have a unique capacity to help individuals change the patterns that result in health risks, disease, weight gain and often unhappiness in their lives. Specific skills are required in communication, building rapport, developing safe and effective goals, and implementing and facilitating your client's plan. Professional responsibilities accompany the trust your clients place in you. Knowledge of, and proficiency in, effective counseling and communication techniques may well account for the considerable differences among consultants in their success rates and overall career satisfaction.

References

American College of Sports Medicine. (1991). *Guidelines for Exercise Testing and Prescription.* Philadelphia: Lea & Febiger.

Egan, G. (1990). *The Skilled Helper.* Belmont, CA: Wadsworth.

Kirschenbaum, D.S. (1987). Self-Regulatory failure: A review with clinical implications. *Clinical Psychology Review,* 7, 77-104.

Rogers, C. R. (1961). *On Becoming a Person.* Boston: Houghton Mifflin.

Yalom, I.D. (1985). *The Theory and Practice of Group Psychotherapy.* New York: Plenum.

Suggested Reading

Andersen, R. E., Brownell, K. D. & Haskell, W. L. (1992). *The Health and Fitness Club Leader's Guide: Administering A Weight Management Program.* Dallas: American Health.

Brownell, K. D. (1994). *The LEARN Program for Weight Control.* (6th ed.) Dallas: American Health.

Brownell, K. D. & Fairburn, C. G. (1995). *Comprehensive Textbook of Eating Disorders and Obesity.* New York: Guilford.

Brownell, K. D. & Rodin, J. (1990). *The Weight Maintenance Survival Guide.* Dallas: American Health.

Carkhuff, R. R. (1987). *The Art of Helping.* (6th ed.) Amherst: Human Resource Development.

Corey, G. (1981). *Theory and Practice of Group Counseling.* Monterey: Brooks/Cole.

Jasper, J. (1992). The Challenge of Weight Control: A Personal View. In T.A. Wadden & T.B. Van Itallie (Eds.), *Treatment of the Seriously Obese Patient.* (pp.411-434). New York: Guilford.

Merritt, R. E. & Walley, D. D. (1977). *The Group Leader's Handbook: Resources, Techniques, and Survival Skills.* Champaign: Research Press.

Sue, D. W. & Sue, D. (1990). *Counseling The Culturally Different: Theory and Practice.* New York: Wiley & Sons.

Stunkard, A. J. (1976). *The Pain of Obesity.* Palo Alto: Bull Publishing.

Stunkard, A.J. (1993). Talking with Patients. In A.J. Stunkard & T.A. Wadden (Eds.), *Obesity: Theory and Therapy.* (pp. 355-363). New York: Raven.

Yalom, I. D. (1985). *The Theory and Practice of Group Psychotherapy.* New York: Plenum.

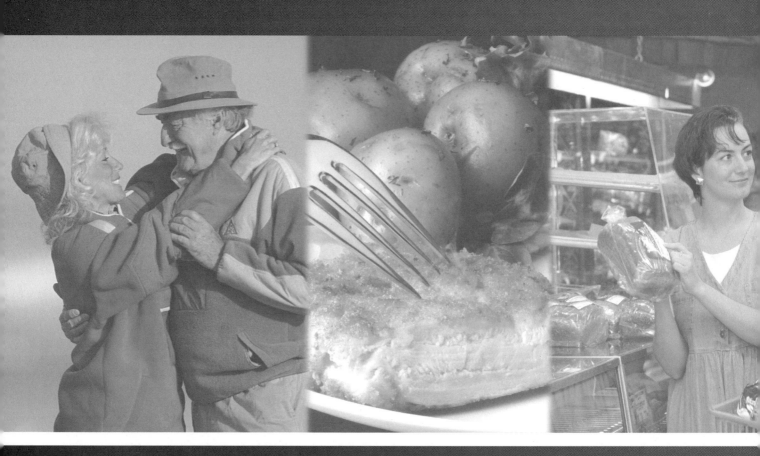

CHAPTER TWO

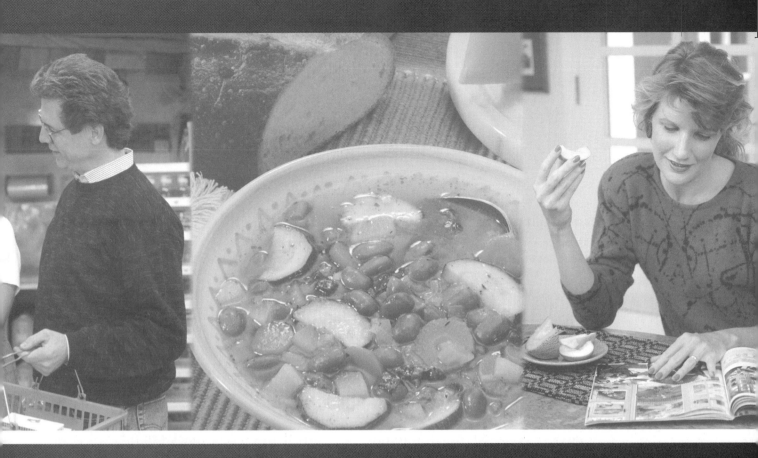

HEALTH BEHAVIOR Psychology

Glen D. Morgan

*Glen D. Morgan, Ph.D., is the director of Behavioral Sciences
at the Wyoming Valley Family Practice Residency Program in
Kingston, Pennsylvania. He also serves as the clinical assistant
professor in the Department of Family and Community Medicine
at the Pennsylvania State University College of Medicine and in
the Physician Assistant Program at Kings College.*

Introduction

Health Psychology is concerned with psychology's contribution to the promotion and maintenance of health, the prevention and treatment of illness, as well as the identification and evaluation of the factors that optimize health. It developed as a result of a growing body of research that pointed to the interdependency of psychological and behavioral processes with health. This chapter will address analysis and intervention with health behaviors, specifically those related to weight management and modification.

The last 20 years have witnessed a dramatic evolution in the conceptualization of disease, health and behavior. Advances in public health and pharmacology have largely eliminated or controlled diseases that were the leading causes of death through the early part of this century. Instead of pneumonia, influenza tuberculosis and smallpox,

Table 2.1

**Health Behavior Changes Frequently Recommended
with Diagnosis of Common Diseases and Conditions**

Disease or Condition	Health Behavior Frequently Recommended				
	Weight Loss	Diet Adherence	Physical Activity	Smoking Cessation	Stress Reduction
Hypertension	X	X	X	X	X
Post-myocardial Infarction	X	X	X	X	X
Coronary Heart Disease	X	X	X	X	X
Diabetes	X	X	X		X
Gallstones	X	X			
Hyperlipidemia	X	X			
Asthma				X	X
Rheumatoid Arthritis	X .				X
Colon Cancer		X			
Lung Cancer				X	
Breast Cancer		X			
Low Back Pain	X		X		X
Tension Headache			X		X
Chronic Bronchitis	X		X	X	
Emphysema	X		X	X	
Surgery	X	X	X	X	X

Adapted from *Behavioral Counseling in Medicine: Strategies for Modifying At-Risk Behavior.* Reprinted with permission of Oxford University Press.

citizens of Western nations are now more likely to die of cancer and cardiovascular disease (Hammonds & Scheirer, 1984). Lifestyle factors, in fact, significantly contribute to more than half of the annual deaths in the United States (Goldstein, Guise, Ruggiero, Raciti & Abrams, 1990). It is important to note that these diseases are significantly influenced by behavior and lifestyle factors such as diet, weight and tobacco use. Thus, modification of behavioral risk factors may serve to prevent or reduce the symptoms of many diseases. Health behavior changes are frequently recommended for reducing symptoms or arresting further progression of disease (Table 2.1).

Scientists are not the only ones to recognize the link between health and behavior. In the last two decades, the public's interest in, and demand for, information on health, wellness, risk factors and disease prevention has been unparalleled in history. Not only are health articles regular features in daily newspapers and popular magazines, books on health and health behaviors often top the best seller lists. Books about diets and weight loss probably have the broadest appeal among nonfiction titles.

The evolving landscape of healthcare also is changing how each American looks at health and lifestyle. Healthcare reform not only involves medical care, it is an economic, political and social phenomenon. Increasingly, Health Maintenance Organizations (HMOs) are dominating the healthcare marketplace. The prevailing motivating factor in this change is healthcare cost control. Managed care systems operate on the premise that keeping enrollees healthy will reduce medical visits, hospital admissions and medication use. Consequently, many programs provide incentives both to practitioners (to encourage risk-factor reduction) and to enrollees (to stay healthy by adopting healthier lifestyles).

These converging factors of healthcare reform, growing public awareness of health issues and desire to maintain health, and the economics of healthcare have provided new opportunities for development of cost-effective weight management programs. An irony of HMOs is that primary care health practitioners are expected to see more patients in less time, while simultaneously providing the additional services of preventive care. Consequently, patient education and lifestyle change counseling is becoming increasingly difficult during medical visits. It is now imperative to look beyond physicians, psychologists and other healthcare professionals to provide these services. Lifestyle and weight management consultants have a unique opportunity in this emerging marketplace to play an important role in assisting clients change health behaviors.

Determinants of Behavior

Most behaviors have multiple, intertwined determinants. Cigarette smoking provides an example of the interaction of psychological, social, economic and biological factors. Most individuals begin smoking at the urging of a close friend; nicotine is not only highly addictive, it is known to have psychoactive effects; the billions spent yearly on marketing cigarettes induce teens to initiate smoking and influence established smokers to switch brands; finally, recent research shows genetic predisposition to nicotine dependence (Fisher,

Haire-Joshu, Morgan, et al., 1990). Being overweight or eating improperly is no less complex. Heredity has a strong influence upon body size and shape. An individual's eating patterns are usually the result of several variables: learned behavior, available foods, moods, habits, social and environmental triggers, and hunger. Furthermore, these factors can influence each other. Being overweight may contribute to a poor self-image that, in turn, leads to negative predictions of one's ability to change their eating habits. For example, a stressed, tired individual may grab some fast food on the way home from work, then feel guilty about their food choice. Later, seeing a television commercial about pizza might trigger an urge to eat even more. Finally, resignation about being overweight combined with a day of failed efforts might provoke them to eat several bowls of ice cream.

Health Belief Model

The **Health Belief Model** provides an explanation of health-related behaviors (Becker, 1974). This model suggests that an individual's decision to adopt (or to not adopt) healthy behaviors is based largely upon their appraisal of their susceptibility to an illness combined with their perception of the probable severity of the consequences of having the illness. A second part of this model is the person's view of the benefits of the behavior change as opposed to the costs of changing. The final section of the model refers to internal, environmental and social cues to action (Feuerstein, Labbe & Kuczmierczyk, 1986). For example, a client is not likely to try losing weight or exercising when they do not feel prone to disease (susceptibility) or perceive the consequences of disease as minor (severity) or see behavioral change as too difficult (costs).

Social Factors

Social factors play a significant role in the acquisition, maintenance and cessation of behaviors. Family members and friends can be sources of assistance and support as well as stress or sabotage. For example, overweight individuals whose social network is comprised of others who are overweight may feel less social pressure to modify their weight. They also are less likely to be exposed to good examples of healthier eating or exercise patterns. The opposite is also true. If one's social network is full of thinner individuals, there may be more social influences to modify eating habits. Encouragement (not nagging) and reinforcement from friends, family and co-workers can be powerful incentives for initiating and maintaining behavior change (Morgan, Ashenberg & Fisher, 1985).

Stages of Change

An individual's motivation or readiness for change is an important factor in determining whether or not they will make the effort to change. Change does not occur as a single event; rather, it is a process that develops over time. The **stages-of-change model** is useful for understanding lifestyle modification (Prochaska & Goldstein, 1991). According to this model, people go through distinct, predictable stages when making lifestyle changes. These stages are: precontemplation, contemplation, preparation, action and maintenance. The process is not linear; individuals may move back and forth between stages (Prochaska, DiClemente, & Norcross, 1992).

Precontemplation is a stage where the individual does not intend to change anytime soon (that is, within six months). Clients in the precontemplation stage may be unaware of, or denying, the need for lifestyle change. They might be pessimistic about either their ability to change or about the effectiveness of change methods. In this stage, they are likely to selectively filter information that justifies their decision to maintain their unhealthy lifestyle. Smokers who deny the health risks and refuse to consider stopping are obvious precontemplaters.

Contemplation represents a period when the client weighs the costs (effort, treatment effectiveness, finances, time) and benefits of lifestyle modification. They may, for example, be considering joining a fitness or weight-loss program in the near future. This stage is often characterized by ambivalence about changing. Individuals can remain in this stage for months or years, wavering between approaching readiness to make an effort at change or distancing themselves from it.

Individuals who have decided to initiate an effort to change within a month's time are in the preparation stage. They are making observable efforts to begin the change process. Clients in this stage may have set up an appointment with a nutritionist, have started to limit their consumption of high-fat foods or exercise periodically.

Individuals in the action stage are in the process of changing their behavior: they are walking regularly for exercise, planning meals, reducing caloric consumption and keeping a diet record. During this stage, individuals are at greatest risk for relapse.

Maintenance represents the stage of successful, sustained lifestyle modification. While the individual may no longer be experiencing a *change* in behavior, they continue to actively utilize methods to monitor and control their behavior. Additionally, they might modify or engineer their environments to reduce the probability of slips or relapse. The individual seeking to maintain health-related behavioral change may periodically check their weight, blood pressure and resting pulse.

Principles of Behavior Change

Habits are stable behaviors formed by constant repetition of the same pattern over time, to the point where they are automatic and may even be unconscious. Horace Mann, a well known educator, once said that "Habits are like a cable. We weave a strand of it every day and soon it cannot be broken." Though most behaviorists might disagree with Mann (habits *can* be broken), there is no refuting the strength of habits and the difficulty of changing them. Habits can be so ingrained in

Antecedents, such as an ad for cigarettes, are triggers that lead to a particular behavior or consequence, such as smoking.

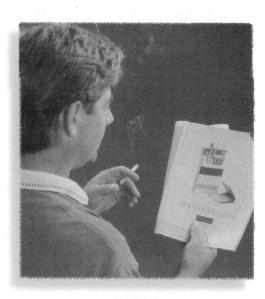

daily life that they become automatic. Just as habits are formed by learning processes, changing them requires learning as well. Though "breaking" is a common term regarding changing habits, the process may be more akin to "unweaving."

Behavioral scientists view behavior as following certain orderly or lawful relationships; this is particularly true for an individual's relationship with their environment. There are several basic principles of behavioral psychology that are important to understand to effectively help others change their unhealthy habits.

Antecedents

Behaviors have **antecedents** (stimuli that precede the behavior) and **consequences** (stimuli that follow the behavior). Antecedents are the stimuli that lead to given behaviors. They are sometimes referred to as cues or triggers. Antecedents can be events, situations, thoughts or feelings. A ringing phone, anxiety or finishing a meal are all examples of potential antecedents for smoking a cigarette. Initially, these cues are neutral — they elicit no behaviors when encountered. The desire to smoke or eat or other behavioral response comes only after repeatedly pairing the specific behavior with the environmental stimulus over time. If people habitually eat popcorn at movies, for example, they will want popcorn even if they have just finished a substantial meal.

Consequences

Consequences may be either positive or negative. Positive consequences tend to increase the probability of the behavior recurring in a similar situation in the future, while negative consequences have the opposite effect. Examples of positive consequences are praise, money, affection, dessert or gifts. Negative consequences might be rejection, guilt, ridicule, injury or a hangover.

Antecedents and consequences become tied to the behavior with each successive repetition (Taylor, Ureda & Denham, 1982). Going to a restaurant (antecedent), trying a burrito for the first time (behavior) and getting a stomachache (consequence) could likely decrease the probability of eating burritos (or even trying new foods). In contrast, having a wonderful dinner out with friends is a positive reinforcer and strengthens the chances of going out on future occasions. Habits become stronger with each repetition of the antecedent-behavior-consequence cycle.

Behavior Chains

It is not unusual for behaviors to be preceded by a series of other behaviors, each one connected to a preceding behavior in some way. Skipping lunch, for example, may lead to buying donuts on the way home from work. This, in turn, may be followed by feelings of guilt or self-reproach for straying from a diet. Subsequent irritability may lead to an argument with a significant other, and then eating two bowls of ice cream. This series of connections is often referred to as a **behavioral chain**, and highlights the complexity of most behaviors. Along with explaining the behavior, it provides useful information for changing it. The terminal behavior will not occur if any links in the chain are broken. It is usually easier to alter behavior earlier rather than later in the chain. Buying cheesecake at a bakery on Tuesday may be an initial link in a chain that ends with binging on four pieces of it on Thursday. Intervening links might include: a trying day at work, fatigue and frustration. Not buying cheesecake in the first place would be an easier link to break than battling an urge to binge when feeling frustrated and tired.

Shaping

Shaping behavior is the reinforcement of successive approximations until a desired goal is reached. This principle is used daily by teachers. When children learn to print their name, they are first taught to hold a pencil, then to form the outline of the first letter, and then they practice. Each behavioral repetition brings them closer to their final goal. This principle has applications for setting step-wise objectives leading to the final goal.

Observational Learning

The social environment provides models for behavior that can affect a client's behavior (Glanz, Lewis & Rimer, 1990). Seeing others exercise can serve as both an example and a prompt to change behavior. A positive model for health behaviors is more effective if the person shares similarities with the client. You might consider encouraging clients to seek out friends or family who model the goal behavior to help support them in their efforts.

Cognitions and Behavior

The previous examples illustrate how behavior may also be influenced by current thoughts (**cognitions**) or feelings. Cognitions can function either as antecedents or consequences for overt behaviors, influencing the person's actions in a manner similar to environmental events. Feeling lonely, for example, may trigger eating episodes that can lead to guilt.

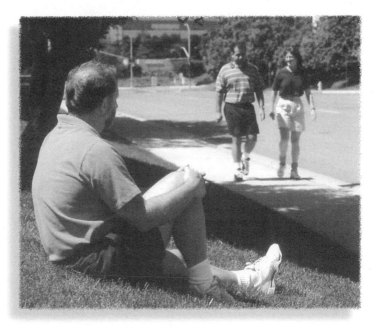

Behavioral Strategies

Several principles of behavioral change are significant in weight control and lifestyle management interventions. Some strategies (such as self-monitoring) have dual functions as both an assessment tool and as a

Watching others enjoying the benefits of exercise can serve as both an example and a prompt for an individual to change their behavior.

Table 2.2
Behavioral Strategies

Stimulus Control Methods

Substitution of Incompatible Behavior

Behavioral Contracts

Rewards

Cognitive Methods

Self-monitoring

behavior-change vehicle. Decisions regarding appropriate strategies should be based on behavioral-change objectives as well as client variables (Table 2.2).

Stimulus Control Methods

Stimulus control methods, sometimes called "cue extinction" are a means to break the connection between events or other stimuli and behavior. For the overeater, this might involve limiting the locations in the house or times when eating takes place. Over time, the triggers lose their power and the target behavior "extinguishes." Initially, this can be quite difficult. Clients should be reassured that the urges to eat will eventually weaken.

Substitution of Incompatible Behavior

One behavioral management method is to substitute an alternative behavior for an undesired one. Instead of watching TV (which may be an antecedent for snacking) the client could take a walk, read a book, write a letter or perform any other activity that is not associated, or is incompatible, with eating.

Contracts

Many clients respond well to written agreements specifying the target behavior, the frequency and timeline. Called **behavioral or contingency contracts**, they also can identify a consequence should the conditions of the contract be met (or fail to be met). Contracts should be signed by the client and the consultant.

Rewards

Rewards from a significant other can be powerful reinforcers of a client's efforts at behavioral change. Rewards are positive consequences, such as those mentioned earlier: praise, money, affection, dessert or gifts. It also is reasonable for clients to plan their own self-rewards to coincide with reaching objectives in the program. Not only can rewards have extrinsic value, they are symbolic of making progress. The acknowledgment from others in the form of a reward often is more influential than the reward itself.

Cognitive Methods

Cognitive behavior therapy proposes that emotional reactions are not direct responses to environmental events but are mediated by thoughts (cognitions). That is, instead of an event leading directly to an emotion, an event leads to a thought which, in turn, leads to an emotion. Seeing a dog may produce fear in people who say to themselves, "Dogs are dangerous." Seeing the same animal may not produce fear in a dog owner, who might think, "That dog looks just like mine." After eating a high-calorie dessert (event), thinking, "That was delicious. What a perfect compliment to a fine meal," versus "I ate too much again. I am fat and have no willpower," will lead to two entirely different emotional reactions.

"Cognitive quicksand" is irrational or overly negative thinking that causes emotional distress. Cognitions concerning events play a large role in determining reactions to those events (past, present or future). These are the "shoulds," the "musts," and the "have to's." They can lead to guilt, anxiety and worry. A specific example of such negative cognitions is dichotomous or "light-switch" thinking. This is when one looks at events as being all positive or all negative — there is no neutral ground. When clients view events in this manner (they are either fat or thin, smart or stupid, successful or a failure), they may be perfectionistic, high-strung, miserable to others and on an emotional roller coaster. This type of thinking usually takes place when people exclusively link their self-worth to their achievements.

As a consultant, you should assist your clients in identifying and altering maladaptive, unrealistic or extreme thinking patterns. For the exceedingly self-critical client, it helps to ask them if they would be as judgmental of their best friends if they behaved similarly. Eating a piece of cake is probably just a minor diversion from the perfect diet — it will not contribute to the decay of societal morals or cause global warming. It is not unusual for the piece of cake to be seen as not just a piece of cake, but as representative of no motivation, predictive of continued failure and as leading to a 1- to 2-pound weight gain.

Implementing Behavioral Change

Health behavior psychology techniques have been predominantly used by health psychologists and clinical psychologists. The last ten years, though, have witnessed a broadening of the applications of scientific findings in health psychology. Physicians, nurses and other health providers are using health psychology techniques and scientific findings in patient education and in primary and secondary prevention interventions. Interventions, across disciplines, may be directed at an individual, a group or an entire community

Table 2.3
Variables for Assessment

Stage of Change
Expectations
Health Beliefs
Previous Behavior Change Attempts
Exercise History
Family History
Mood
History of Psychological Difficulties

(for example, through a televised health awareness and screening program).

Basic Teaching Method

The basic teaching method was developed to be straight-forward, useful across a range of lifestyle health behaviors and applicable in both clinical and non-clinical settings. There are three fundamental steps: assessment, teaching and evaluation. It is grounded in the principle that a major determinant of health lifestyles is learned behavior and that the principle method in fostering behavioral change is teaching. The term "teaching" is preferable to intervention, which generally occurs in healthcare settings.

Assessment

Assessment of client characteristics is essential to developing appropriate, effective intervention plans. A general rule of thumb is that more useful and valid information can be acquired when a greater variety of assessment methods (interview, self-monitoring, questionnaires, significant other inquiry) are employed. Comprehensive assessment will review demographic, health and behavioral variables (Table 2.3).

Initial assessments usually begin with an interview. It is more efficient to gather information using questionnaires, and then clarify and focus upon specific

Self-monitoring is an excellent way for your client to identify both positive and negative behaviors, as well as the thoughts and moods related to them.

points during the interview. When interviewing a client, you should review the following variables associated with the target behavior: when it began (onset), how it has varied over time (course), the situations it occurs in and the patient's impression of its seriousness and amenability to modification. It also is useful to find out if there is a

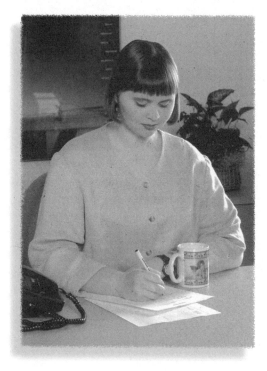

family history of the same problem. Along with providing information about positive or negative models, this can lead into questions about family support and general social support.

A basic behavioral assessment tool is self-monitoring. Here, clients record the date, time, place, situation and specific features of the target behavior. Thoughts and mood may be recorded as well. For weight management, it is important to record the food and portion sizes. It may be useful to record exercise, especially if that is part of the comprehensive treatment plan.

It is important for you to find out about your clients' previous attempts to change target behaviors. They often dismiss previous attempts as being "unsuc-

cessful," but it is rare to find that there was not some useful technique or temporary success. People often criticize past programs that may have worked well initially, but they were unable to maintain the change over the long term. It is then useful to reflect to the patient that the same strategies may be worth revisiting, with more focus upon maintenance strategies and relapse prevention. Success in changing other health or lifestyle habits also may predict success and suggest strategies.

Determining your clients' readiness to change is essential. Precontemplators will not be amenable to developing a behavioral-change plan. If they do, it is unlikely to be successful. Generally, people in this stage of change won't even make it to an assessment session. They often attend only at the urging of their doctor or spouse. This gives you an opportunity to explain health risks of the target behavior and briefly describe treatment techniques, emphasizing their effectiveness. The client should then be instructed to wait until they are ready to change before returning. Beginning treatment with an insufficiently motivated client increases the probability of poor outcome and scapegoating of the program. Determining your clients' health beliefs (belief in disease susceptibility) may provide another view of variables affecting motivation.

Finally, it is important to assess client expectations for the program. Are their predictions or hopes for outcome reasonable? Do they anticipate an amount of effort and time for change that is consistent with the program requirements? Unrealistic expectations will either cause your client to feel like a failure or see the program as ineffective. It is time well spent to compare client expectations with program requirements to clarify a realistic outcome.

Careful, comprehensive assessment is the cornerstone in lifestyle management programming. It is critical for developing strategies that are tailored to the client's specific background, needs and psychosocial features. When carefully done, it will guide you to optimal programming and favorable outcomes.

Teaching

Teaching and learning are dynamic, interdependent processes. During this interaction, the client is constantly integrating information and beginning behavioral change. You must continuously modify your client's instructions based on observation and verbal feedback. This process is not linear, but goes back and forth in a cyclical manner (from assessment to teaching to evaluation back to teaching).

The first step in the teaching process is to set goals. It is important to have realistic, attainable expectations for both short-, moderate- and long-term goals. It is common for clients to wish to achieve more in less time and with less effort than is feasible. You might consider cutting your client's goals by half or a third to ensure success. It is important to separate the ideal from the real. It helps to explain that, since most behaviors are learned over time, it takes time to change them. Ideally, goals should include behavioral, psychological, physical and physiological measures. It is typical that progress will be seen in different spheres at different times. Having more than one focus may keep your client from becoming discouraged about their progress in one area.

Development of the behavioral plan should be a collaborative effort by both you and your client. The plan must require enough effort to cause behavioral change but not so much as to excessively tax your client's resources. A program that is the central focus of your client's

life will be difficult to maintain in both the short and long terms. Negotiation may be necessary to come to a mutually agreed upon plan and set of goals, which will more likely lead to satisfying outcomes.

Previous assessment will reveal a variety of potential behaviors that should be addressed during programming. The initial step in program development is to identify those goals and objectives that will be addressed. The plan should be systematic, progressive (step by step), concrete and cohesive. Assessment for weight management may reveal targets such as food shopping, habits, exercise, food choices, portion control, emotions, timing of meals and snacking. Strategies could include meal scheduling, limiting places to eat,

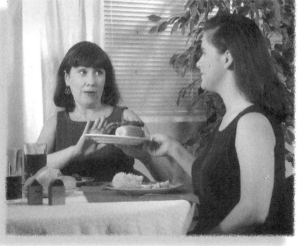

nutrition education and stress management techniques. Once triggers or cues for eating have been identified, stimulus control or substitution of alternative activities can be employed. Initially, it may be useful to focus on one or two behaviors or strategies. As these new behaviors become integrated into the client's repertoire, new target behaviors or strategies can be added. The idea is not to make the program painful or difficult but easily adaptable to your client's daily routine.

Teaching your client to realize when they've had enough to satisfy their hunger will help them say "no" to second helpings and stick to their weight-management program.

In the 80s, behavioral management research for health risk factor modification focused upon developing more powerful programs that would increase outcome rates. Most sought to achieve this by combining strategies that had been successful when used alone. A review of these studies suggests that these multicomponent programs often did not have substantially better results than more simple approaches. Clients might reach a saturation point regarding the number of strategies they can effectively employ. A parallel interpretation is that adherence decreases with increasing program demands. Thus, this research raised the point that focused, rather than broad, programming might yield better outcomes. Consequently, you must be attuned to your client's saturation point and remember that adding program requirements may backfire. This, of course, may vary over the course of treatment, based on normal expected fluctuations, environmental stressors or time constraints. It is better to keep program demands flexible, in tune with your client's time and energy constraints. It is critical to involve the client as an equal participant in programming adjustment.

It is useful, however, to use a variety of methods to prevent boredom. New strategies can be introduced as "experiments" for your clients to "try out" to see if they are effective for them. Since the strategies are meant to change behavior, they interrupt daily patterns and will be moderately difficult at first. For example, most clients who have tried self-monitoring perceive it as an imposition. When challenged on how much time they actually spend on self-monitoring, they admit that it is probably less than a total of 10 minutes per day. Clients generally agree that this is not unreasonable, given their goals. You can also inform them that self-monitoring, by itself, causes significant

behavior change.

Behavior change is difficult, requiring substantial effort. People would not seek out help if they had been successful on their own. As a consultant, you may play the role of an educator, a guide and a coach, but not drill sergeant. Reassurance about your clients' progress, and praise for their efforts are powerful positive reinforcers. When a strategy or objective appears out of reach for a client, you might remember the principle of shaping. It works best when the final objective can be reduced to component parts where the client can address them one step at a time. The metaphor of walking to the top of a stairway is a useful way to explain this process. Often, clients feel they must simply change all at once. They may see their failure to change as reflective of poor motivation or insufficient ability. This is akin to leaping to the top of the stairs in a single bound. Poorly conditioned clients, as an illustration, should not begin running a mile or two daily. Instead, they should begin their exercise program by walking 10 to 15 minutes, gradually increasing their pace and distance over time. This, then, is congruent with taking the stairs step by step. While the final objective is the same, the means to reach the objective differs, leading to success.

Social Support. During behavioral change efforts, the client should be encouraged to ask significant others for help. Avoiding high-calorie snacks is much easier when other family members agree to keep them out of the home. Clients will exercise more regularly when they have a buddy to accompany them. When others are sources of stress or sabotage, you might suggest ways for your client to respond to or cope with them. They may be able to conveniently avoid the others. If this is not realistic, it may be possible to talk to the others and politely, but firmly, explain the impact of their behavior and ask them to change.

Self-help and support groups have played a prominent role in many health-related and lifestyle management programs. Social support from formalized groups or from the individual's social network can be powerful. Being part of a group that shares a problem can combat isolation, increase optimism about personal change and enhance motivation. It may also be a source of useful information regarding effective change techniques. Conversely, there may be risks associated with some self-help programs. They may provide instruction and information that is not based on scientific evidence that can be either useless or even dangerous. Clients occasionally substitute them for necessary professional treatment. Consequently, you might consider evaluating these groups carefully before suggesting client participation.

Friends, family and coworkers can encourage clients to stay on track, compliment them on their efforts and remark on their success. Alternatively, they can be sources of sabotage, discouragement and frustration. People can differ regarding their perceptions of helpful actions by others. The question, "How are you doing on your weight loss program?" may be supportive to one person and irritating to another. It often is useful to involve significant others in the plans for behavioral change to solicit their help as well as to provide suggestions.

Cognitive Strategies. It is not unusual to observe clients engaging in light-switch thinking when they are setting objectives or are frustrated with their progress. First, you might inquire if they would be so critical of a close friend having a similar experience (rarely would they be). This clearly illustrates a more realistic way of evaluating their behavior. You then might ask them to

identify those components of the program they have successfully completed. This keeps them from viewing several bad days, or a difficult time with one task, as indicative of their entire effort. This process helps develop a more realistic appraisal of the process of behavioral change and the progress that has been made. This, combined with your review of progress, usually is sufficient to reassure your client.

You must try to be objective and accurate or your client might view you as patronizing. Also, your client may be addressing real problems that might require refinement of the lifestyle management plan. Sometimes, clients are

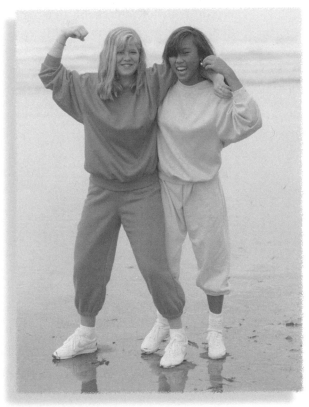

People tend to exercise more regularly when they have a friend to accompany them.

putting in less effort than they are capable of. Recognition of this on their part is essential to getting back on track. It is up to both you and your client to jointly review progress and agree upon a plan or resolution.

Independent Practice. Individuals must practice a behavior in order to change a behavior. Often, people wait for inspiration or motivation before trying a new behavior. Simply meeting with a consultant and thinking about changing is not sufficient to alter behavioral patterns. Breaking old habits and establishing new ones requires both planning and repetitive practice. This concept can be communicated to your clients by the following statement: "It is easier to act yourself into a new way of feeling rather than feel yourself into a new way of acting." The misconception that behavior change is accomplished only through talking can be addressed by assigning homework tasks at each session. It also clarifies that behavior change is not your responsibility but the responsibility of your client. Independent practice can take many different

Outside pressures, such as work and family, may make it especially difficult for some clients to adhere to their programs.

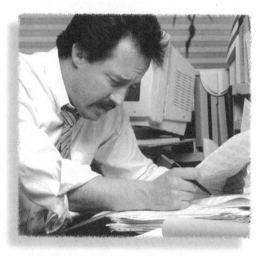

forms, from generating objectives to keeping a log of efforts. Self-monitoring is an effective, standard assignment because it provides continuous feedback and the opportunity for self-correction. Other assignments to consider are: experimenting with new strategies, writing down objectives for specific behaviors, clarifying expectations, finding sources of social support, brainstorming alternative behaviors for particularly difficult situations, generating a plan for how the standard plan could be altered for special occasions, or making a list of

personal rewards for reaching short-term goals.

Evaluation

Evaluation is a continuous process. Throughout the program, you should continuously monitor the effectiveness of the strategies, your client's level of effort, compliance with behavioral tasks and degree of satisfaction. This ongoing tracking of progress is referred to as **formative evaluation.**

Using multiple assessment methods provides advantages over single method assessment. There is greater accuracy when behavioral, psychological, physical and physiological measures are utilized. For weight management these might include: client satisfaction, feedback from significant others, weight change, change in clothing size or measurements, subjective reports of "feeling better," fitness measures, blood pressure changes, changes in medication needs (weight loss can lead to less need for diabetes or hypertension medications) and changes in eating patterns. Smoking cessation objectives can include: situations where smoking has been eliminated, completing an action plan for handling urges, days since last cigarette, ratio of days cigarette free to those with slips, measures of carbon monoxide in expired air (a physiologic measure of smoking), fitness measures and changes in frequency of urges for cigarettes following cessation.

Self-monitoring, in addition to being an excellent initial assessment method, is a useful formative evaluation tool. It provides you with feedback regarding your client's adherence to the treatment plan and enhances their awareness of their behavior by providing immediate feedback. As such, it often provokes behavior change.

At the conclusion of the program, it is important to reiterate maintenance issues, review progress and critical lessons learned, and to discuss early identification of relapse warning signs. It also is helpful to elicit comments regarding both the most and least helpful elements of the program. This information will allow you to refine their application of behavioral management principles. The evaluative process that occurs at program end and during follow-up is referred to as **summative evaluation.**

Follow-up. Follow-up is useful for several different reasons. First, you may learn how well your client has been able to maintain their behavior change. It also gives you the opportunity to make simple suggestions regarding staying on track, as well as provide you with outcome data for the effectiveness of the program. Finally, follow-up communicates to your client that you are committed to helping them. Follow-up often serves as a prompt for the client to recommit themselves to the behavior change effort and may result in their requesting several booster sessions. Though face-to-face meetings are most useful, contact by phone or mail also can be valuable. Frequency of follow-up is best individualized to the needs of the client. Most clinical research programs evaluate outcome at six- and 12-month periods. Earlier follow-ups, though, might help catch clients before they begin to slip.

Relapse Prevention. Relapse is the mirror image of maintenance, and generally refers to a return to baseline behavior. It is not unusual for clients to drift off track a bit. This is sometimes referred to as a slip or a lapse. During behavioral change efforts, fluctuations are normal and should be expected. Your role is to encourage and redirect the client. Relapses should be viewed as an opportunity for fine tuning. Clients may experience some frustration or disappointment that they are not doing better. They may perceive themselves as

a failure and be ready to give up. This is an opportunity to explain that learning is a process that does not usually occur at a constant rate and direction. Slips are normal, not reflections of failing, and should be viewed as learning opportunities. There are two metaphors that might prove useful when discussing the challenges of behavior change. One is of a baby learning to walk. They need a lot of help, and they fall a lot. Their efforts, though, are consistently and hugely reinforced. No one would think of telling the child, "Forget it — you will never walk." Another metaphor that nicely illustrates the process of behavioral change is that of a football game. All football teams experience gains and losses in yardage during a game. The short-term goal may be to get a first down; the moderate — to score; the long-term — to win the game. Giving up after a few slips in a behavioral change effort would be like a football team leaving the field in the first quarter after losing yardage. It is fairly obvious that slips are occasions for you to address some of the cognitive quicksand issues that inevitably arise during lifestyle modification efforts utilizing the cognitive approaches outlined earlier.

Compliance Difficulties. It is common in medical practices for patients to take medicines inappropriately, or inadequately follow their physician's advice. Estimates of noncompliance range from 4 percent to 92 percent, and average from 30 percent to 35 percent for medical therapies. A difficulty with the term noncompliance is that it suggests that all the fault lies with the patient, and that it is reflective of poor motivation or laziness. Failure to follow a physician's advice (even this phrase blames the patient) is, as this chapter has illustrated, the result of an equation of intertwined determinants. Your task is to evaluate adherence issues utilizing multiple assessment techniques and address the following questions:

✔ Are there specific situations or times where behavior occurs or does not occur?
✔ Can antecedents and consequences be identified?
✔ What are the barriers to change?
✔ Is the patient overloaded?
✔ Do they feel there is not enough time?
✔ Do they perceive themselves as failing and that it is their fault?
✔ Have they lost their confidence in their ability to change?
✔ Are they frustrated?
✔ Are the benefits of behavior change outweighed by the costs of that behavior change?

There are two important guidelines when addressing adherence issues. First, always attend to those things your client is doing well (not just the problem areas). Second, be sure that both you and your client have realistic expectations. Less than optimal adherence is an opportunity to further refine and tailor the treatment program to fit your client. Your primary objective is to optimize your client's chance for a successful experience.

When to Ask for Help

One of the most disconcerting circumstances for anyone to be in is the sudden recognition of "being in over your head." Everyone has limitations to their abilities, regardless of the endeavor. Awareness of personal limitations and the development of a protocol for consultation or referral is essential to conducting a safe lifestyle management program.

It is prudent to either consult or correspond with your client's family physician when initiating a lifestyle

management program. Some health behavior problems may be reflective of underlying medical issues. Overeating can be due to depression or a medical condition (for example, hyperthyroidism). Poor diet is a reason to screen for diabetes, hypertension (high blood pressure), or **hyperlipidemia** (high cholesterol). A history of coronary or pulmonary problems could affect the direction of programming, particularly with respect to the exercise component. In addition to addressing the above issues, communication with physicians can provide a valuable perspective on the client's motivation and readiness to change their lifestyle. Collaborative efforts with health professionals enhance the opportunity to design optimal programming for the client.

Clients should always consult with their physician or other health professional if their health status changes. In the case of significant or sudden changes, suspension of treatment should be considered until medical clearance is obtained.

Psychological disorders or conditions may prevent your client from participating successfully in a lifestyle-management program. Although this topic is addressed in Chapter 6, it bears mention here since these difficulties may surface after treatment has begun. If psychological problems are suspected, it is important to consider consulting a psychologist, psychiatrist or family physician. There are several problem areas that the consultant may encounter. Eating disorders (anorexia nervosa and bulimia nervosa) affect between 1 percent to 4 percent of young women, and are marked by the following features:

✔ body-image disorder (they see themselves as much fatter than others do)
✔ marked (overly rapid or severe) weight loss
✔ excessive concern with weight

and appearance
✔ extreme fear of gaining weight
✔ compulsive exercising
✔ purging (vomiting, laxative or diuretic use to control weight)

Low self-esteem is common in eating disorders, but can be a sufficient barrier to behavioral change by itself. Here, clients may exhibit persistent dissatisfaction with their efforts and progress, be excessively self-critical and very resistant to your suggestions of alternative interpretation. Similarly, distorted or unrealistic thinking that endures and interferes with adherence to the program is reason for referral.

Distorted thinking, especially self-criticism, helplessness and hopelessness are common in depression. Other features of depression include loss of interest in people or activities, fatigue, energy loss, insomnia, sadness, guilt and irritability. Anxiety is also common in today's society. Symptoms of anxiety disorders include irritability, fears, panic attacks (palpitations, dizziness, fear of dying or going crazy, trembling, chest pain and shortness of breath), muscle tension, restlessness, apprehensiveness, concentration difficulties and difficulty falling asleep. The clinical features, prevalence and diagnostic criteria for the above disorders are thoroughly described in the *Diagnostic and Statistical Manual of Mental Disorders - IV* (American Psychiatric Association, 1994).

A change in your client's adherence or satisfaction with the program may be indicative of psychological distress. You should gently inquire about concerns, thoughts and feelings. If you suspect the possibility of a psychological difficulty, express your concern and ask your client if they would consider talking to their physician or a psychologist. This sensitive and personal area is best dealt with in a direct and compassionate manner.

Your feelings often are an effective tool for working with clients. If you feel uneasy or think that your client's needs might exceed your expertise, this is reason enough to evaluate your concern further. In short, if you feel you are in over your head, you probably are. You also must carefully attend to the impression that you are exerting greater effort than your client. This is often a reflection of poor motivation or perhaps your client has reverted to a stage of contemplation rather than action. In this case, the rule could be: "If you are working harder than the client — you are probably working too hard." It also is an opportunity to review your client's plan and evaluate if there is an opportunity to improve its tailoring, or fit, to the client.

When there are concerns about a client's progress or suspicions of significant problems, begin by carefully reviewing the assessment data. This may yield directions for modification. It is then useful to discuss the circumstances with a colleague. They may suggest different approaches or reinforce a decision for consultation or referral with a health professional.

Marketing Lifestyle Management Programs

Development of lifestyle management programs also should utilize marketing principles. Winett (1995) developed a comprehensive framework for health behavior change that capitalizes upon social marketing strategies and concepts. Successful effective programming will address the product (the program itself), costs (both financial and time requirements), promotion (advertising) and incentives and location (site and accessibility). Even excellent lifestyle management programs have failed because of inadequate promotion or costs that were out of reach of the consumer.

Summary

Health psychology provides guiding principles and scientific support for lifestyle management programming. Lifestyle management programming must be grounded in the science of health psychology, and utilize a variety of strategies tailored to a client's individual needs. Health behaviors are complex and have multiple determinants. This chapter presented a three-step protocol for behavioral management/lifestyle management consulting: Assessment, Teaching and Evaluation. Assessment is essential for thorough understanding and guidance in planning programming. Teaching encompasses objective and goal development, identification of behavioral strategies and management plan implementation. Evaluation is an ongoing process throughout the program, which allows revision and refinement, as well as periodic follow-ups after program termination. Finally, evaluation yields data regarding program effectiveness and provides directions for program improvement.

References and Suggested Reading

American Psychiatric Association. (1994). *Diagnostic and Statistical Manual of Mental Disorders.* (4th ed.) Washington, DC: American Psychiatric Association.

Becker, M.H. (1974). The Health Belief Model and Personal Health Behavior. *Health Education Monographs,* 2, 324-473.

Feuerstein, M., Labbe, E.E. & Kuczmierczyk, A.R. (1986). *Health Psychology: A Psychobiological Perspective.* New York: Plenum Press.

Fisher, E.B., Jr., Haire-Joshu, D., Morgan, G.D., Rehberg, H. & Rost, K. (1990). State of the art: smoking and smoking cessation. *American Review of Respiratory Diseases,* 142: 702-720.

Glanz, K., Lewis, F.M. & Rimer, B.K. (1990). *Health Behavior and Health Education.* San Francisco: Jossey-Bass.

Goldstein, M.G., Guise, B.J., Ruggiero, L., Raciti, M.A. & Abrams, D.B. (1990). *Behavioral Medicine for Medical Patients.* In: Stroudmire, A. (ed.) *Clinical Psychiatry for Medical Students.* Philadelphia: Lippencott.

Hammonds, B.L. & Scheirer, C.J. (1984). *Psychology and Health.* Washington, DC: American Psychological Association.

Morgan, G.D., Ashenberg, Z.S. & Fisher, E.B., Jr. (1988). Abstinence from smoking and the social environment. *Journal of Clinical and Consulting Psychology,* 56, 298-301.

Prochaska, J.O., DiClemete, C.C. & Norcross, J.C. (1992). In search of how people change: Applications to addictive behaviors. *American Psychologist,* 47, 1102-1114.

Prochaska, J.O. & Goldstein, M.G. (1991). Process of smoking cessation. *Clinics in Chest Medicine,* 12, 727-735.

Taylor, R.B., Ureda, J.R. & Denham, J.W. (1982). *Health Promotion: Principles and Clinical Applications.* Norwalk: Prentice-Hall.

Winett, R. (1995). A Framework for Health Promotion and Disease Prevention Programs. *American Psychologist,* 50, 341-350.

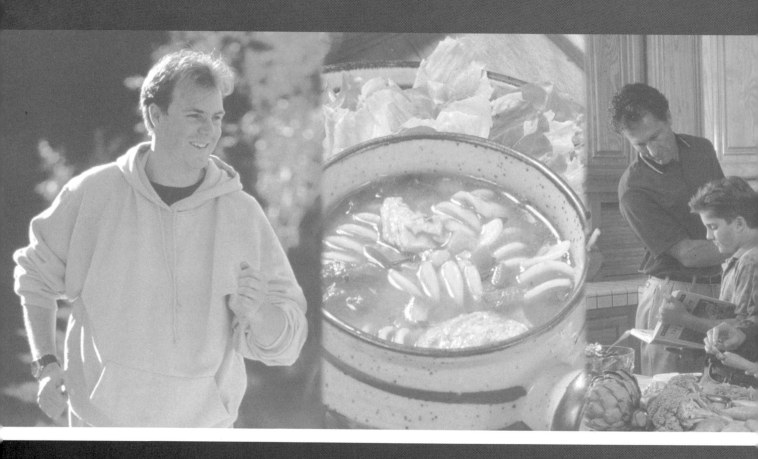

CHAPTER THREE

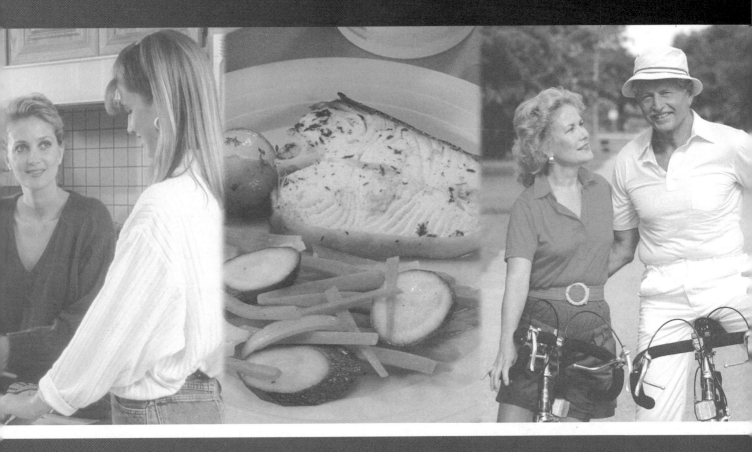

THE PSYCHOLOGY OF WEIGHT MANAGEMENT AND Obesity

Marian B. Tanofsky

Marian B. Tanofsky, B.A., is a research associate at the Yale Center for Eating and Weight Disorders in the Department of Psychology at Yale University. The focus of her research is on eating disorders, stress-related eating and gender differences in eating disordered patients. She will be pursuing a doctorate in clinical psychology.

Denise E. Wilfley

Denise E. Wilfley, Ph.D., is assistant professor in the San Diego State University/University of California - San Diego Joint Doctoral Training Program in Clinical Psychology. Previously, she was co-director of the Yale Center for Eating and Weight Disorders, and research scientist and lecturer in the Department of Psychology at Yale University. Internationally recognized for her research in eating disorders and short-term group psychotherapy, Dr. Wilfley continues to conduct research on the etiology, maintenance and treatment of eating disorders.

Introduction

Consumers spend billions of dollars each year on weight-loss products. As a lifestyle and weight management consultant, it is your responsibility to understand not only the psychology behind these efforts, but how you can best help your clients attain their weight-loss goals in a reasonable and realistic manner. Most individuals' efforts to lose weight are fueled more by concerns about their appearance than their health. In some cases, individuals use extreme weight-control techniques and develop eating disorders as they vacillate between out-of-control overeating episodes and weight-loss attempts. Some believe body dissatisfaction and chronic dieting problems are now the norm in our culture, as individuals of all backgrounds, race, gender and strata are seeking weight-loss treatment. As a lifestyle and weight management consultant, you must gain a full understanding of overweight individuals and the broad risk and contributing factors that clients may present you with. In addition, you will need to know about the issues and problems that may arise throughout treatment.

A primary goal of this chapter is to offer lifestyle and weight management consultants an understanding of what may cause people to become overweight, and explain how to best work with each client to execute an individualized weight-loss plan and support them throughout its duration.

While many of the clients you work with will not be extremely obese, most of them will be overweight to some degree. An individual is classified as mildly, moderately or severely overweight based on their Body Mass Index (BMI) (see Chapter 4). You will be working primarily with mildly or moderately overweight individuals. You will rarely work with severely overweight clients, since their weight level requires treatment from a specialist.

Prevalence and Heterogeneity of Overweight

Overweight individuals are very difficult to categorize, as they comprise a **heterogeneous population** that is not consistently associated with any distinct psychological or behavioral syndrome. As a lifestyle and weight management consultant, it is important for you to be aware of not only the high prevalence of overweight individuals in the U.S., but also of which races, minorities and groups are at higher risk for carrying excess weight. Table 3.1 outlines the prevalence of overweight in the U.S. and the mean Body Mass Indices (BMI) of overweight individuals. Table 3.2 illustrates the prevalence of overweight and BMIs in different cultures (Kuczmarski, 1994). While your clients may differ, they tend to share a

Table 3.1

Prevalence of Overweight in Males and Females in the U.S. in 1994

	Percentage of Overweight in Population	Mean BMI*
Males	31.4%	26.3
Females	35.3%	28.3
Total	33.4%	28.3

*BMI = Weight in kilograms per height in meters.

Source: Table adapted from Kuczmarski, A. (1994). Increasing prevalence of overweight among U.S. adults. *JAMA*, 272, 205-211.

commonality of being predisposed to gaining and maintaining additional body weight. This predisposition is characterized by biological, societal and psychological contributions. Additionally, the activity level of these individuals, as well as the onset of their overweight, are likely to contribute to their excess weight (Kuczmarski, 1994).

Biological Contribution to Overweight/Obesity

The primary determinant of our body shape and weight is the genes we are born with. If our parents and their parents had large builds or the tendency to carry extra weight, the chances are high that we will have the same predisposition. Similarly, our **resting metabolic rate (RMR)**, the amount of energy that the body consumes in a given period of time in a resting state, also is a result of our biological make-up. While RMR can be increased (for example, through exercise) or decreased (it has been suggested through weight cycling), the metabolic rate with which we are born is not under our control. It is important to remember that many overweight individuals have a genetic disposition to be heavy and/or have a lower RMR than people who are not overweight (Stunkard & Sobal, 1995).

Table 3.2

1994 Percentages of Overweight Across Various Races and Ethnic Groups

	Males		Females	
	% of Overweight	Mean BMI	% of Overweight	Mean BMI
Caucasian	32.3%	28.4	32.9%	26.0
African-American	30.9%	26.4	48.6%	28.3
Mexican-American	35.5%	26.8	46.7%	27.6
Cuban-American	28.5%	10.3%	31.9%	6.9%

*BMI = Weight in kilograms per height in meters.

Source: Table adapted from Kuczmarski, A. (1994).
Increasing prevalence of overweight among U.S. adults. JAMA, 272, 205-211.

See Chapter 5 for more information on RMR.

Societal Contribution to Overweight/Obesity

Various social influences play a role in determining the body weight norms of individuals and of the culture as a whole. Because these influences also help to formulate what is considered the ideal body in every society, it is important to understand how a client has formulated what body weight they feel is appropriate.

Body weight is first influenced by the nuclear family. Parents influence their children's weight by upholding what body size standards they think are appropriate, based on their own genetics and social upbringing, and by the types of foods they serve at mealtime. Organizations such as the workplace and schools also establish norms for appropriate food portions to eat, how often it is eaten and appropriate body size (most likely based on the majority of people).

Broader societal issues are important as well. For example, in less-developed countries where food may not be abundant, a lower body weight may be more common, and a higher body weight might be considered more desirable.

Our society's idea of an aesthetic body weight has been influenced through the mass media. Most of the population can be reached through television, computers, magazines and other mediums, and receive the message that the ideal body should be lean and fit (Sobal, 1995, Wilfley & Rodin, 1995).

Cultural/Environmental Factors Influencing Overweight/Obesity

An individual's body size also is based on their race, ethnic background and cultural environment. Some races are genetically predisposed for larger or smaller body builds. For example, while Asians tend to have smaller, slender physiques, most African-Americans carry more weight and have larger bone structures.

Body size may also be determined by an individual's environment. If part of their culture is to eat certain types and amounts of foods based on their ethnic background, their body size will be influenced (Kumanyika, 1995). If an individual was raised eating rich or fatty foods, they may carry extra weight as a result of consuming more calories while growing up and, most likely, during adulthood. Therefore, it is important to be aware that each client has a distinct background that may affect how much

Table 3.3

Health Risks of Obesity

Diabetes Mellitus	Type II (non-insulin dependent) is highly correlated with obesity, the more severely obese and the longer time being obese as determinants.
Hypertension	Rises in weight in obese individuals increases prevalence of high blood pressure.
Stroke	Due to an increase in blood pressure, an increased risk for stroke.
Dyslipidemia	Two abnormalities of circulating lipids: elevation of triglyceride levels and depression of high-density lipoprotein cholesterol (HDL) levels.
Cardiovascular Disease	Angina pectoris, nonfatal myocardial infarction, and sudden death occur more frequently in obese individuals.
Gallbladder Disease	Changes that occur in obese people predispose them to gallstone formation.
Respiratory Disease	Increased weight in the chest leads to poor respiratory motion and decreased compliance of the respiratory system. As a result, sleep apnea may occur.
Some Cancers	In women, increased rates of endometrial, gallbladder, cervical, ovarian cancer and in post menopausal women, breast cancer; in men, higher incidence of colorectal and prostate cancer.
Arthritis and Gout	Increased stress on weight-bearing joints is common in the obese; gout is often prevalent in those with excess fat.

Source: Pi-Sunyer, F.X., (1995). Medical complications of obesity. In K.D. Brownell & C.G. Fairburn (Eds.) *Eating Disorders and Obesity: A Comprehensive Handbook*, (pp. 401-405), New York: Guilford Press.

weight they can lose and what type of plan will work better for them.

Psychological Contribution to Overweight/Obesity

Because much of the psychological distress that overweight individuals experience is due to an unrealistic body image, it is important for you to understand the upsetting feelings that clients may be experiencing. The media conveys the message that if we just undertake the right diet, exercise enough and have enough willpower, we can have the perfect body. Because many people are not born with the biology to have a lean and fit body, there is widespread discontent among those who cannot attain the cultural ideal. Many individuals turn to dieting, exercise, surgery or any type of "magic pill" that promises to change

their bodies. This conflict between the "real" body and the "fantasy" body causes a tremendous number of people of all sizes to suffer from body-image distress and dissatisfaction. People continue to view their bodies as "works in progress" and, since there is always room for improvement, they are constantly experiencing some level of disappointment. Some sense of dissatisfaction can be normal and lead people to try to improve themselves, but it is important for you to be aware that some overweight clients may experience more severe psychological distress than those who have less weight to lose.

Body Image Distress in Overweight/Obese Individuals

Overweight men and women usually suffer from more severe body image distress than normal-weight individuals because they are even further from the aesthetic ideal. Disapproving feelings about their bodies and appearances often cause them to feel negatively about other aspects of their lives as well. In addition, research has found that individuals often perceive their bodies as much larger and more unattractive than is objectively the case. They also will subjectively observe other people as leaner, more fit and more attractive than may be realistic. With such low self-perception, it makes sense that overweight individuals frequently suffer from low self-esteem and feelings of worthlessness. This is compounded by a society that tends to look down on overweight people. They live in a world that is consistently reinforcing a dissenting message that they are "no good" and are failures (Stunkard & Sobal). Most of your clients will suffer from this stigma. Our current culture seems to regard obesity as a moral problem. Overweight people receive a message that they have no willpower, and that they are indulgent, lazy or stupid. This bias has been confirmed by studies in which children tend to describe their overweight peers as lazy and "not wanting to be friends with them," further reinforcing the negative attitude. Besides a judgmental society, overweight individuals must also deal with pressure to lose weight from family, partners and peers (Wadden & Wingate, 1995).

Health Risks of Obesity

Overweight and obese individuals carry a greater risk for developing the various health problems and diseases outlined in Table 3.3 as a result of their extra body weight. To stress the significance of these physical conditions, it is important to note that (outside of cancer, AIDS and violence), diabetes mellitus, hypertension, strokes, hypercholesterolemia and cardiovascular disease are the leading causes of morbidity and mortality in the developed world. You must be aware of these conditions and be able to recognize when an individual is at a level of overweight that increases health risks significantly. In such cases, a medical referral may be in order (Pi-Sunyer, 1995). See Chapter 6 for more information on referrals.

When the biological, social and psychological influences are incorporated with the health risks of being overweight, it becomes clear that treating severely overweight individuals is a complex task. Your work with overweight clients needs to be approached with compassion and sensitivity to body image problems and psychological distress, the social stigma that the overweight bear and the concerns that they may have about their physical health. With these considerations in mind, you will be able to introduce your clients to the concept of exercise as a core component in attaining weight loss and weight management.

The Role of Physical Activity and Exercise in Weight Loss

Exercise aids in weight maintenance in normal weight individuals and in weight loss in overweight persons. By facilitating weight maintenance, exercise plays a critical role in weight loss, as keeping weight off is often a much greater challenge than the initial weight loss. For those trying to lose weight, even minimal increases in lifestyle activities (such as taking the opportunity to walk instead of ride) can bolster energy expenditure. Exercise plays a critical role not only in our body size and its regulation (as it can alter weight through burning calories), but also in our appetite, basal metabolism and body composition. Additionally, exercise has been shown to produce several health and psychological benefits. Table 3.4 indicates some of the possible links between exercise and weight control.

In addition to expending energy, several studies have shown that exercise can be effective in regulating appetite. By moderately increasing physical activity, food intake and appetite tend to decrease. Moreover, many individuals have found it useful to use exercise as a deterrent during times when they may otherwise overeat (Wilfley, Grilo & Brownell, 1994). See Chapters 5 and 7 for more information on the role of exercise in weight control.

The Role of Exercise in Conjunction with Dieting. While dieting is a clear part of the weight-loss process, exercise may be an even more critical component. A shortcoming of dieting in the absence of exercise is that when weight is lost, it is not solely due to the loss of body fat. As much as 25 percent of weight lost by dieting alone is lean body mass. However, when dieting is combined with exercise, the loss of lean body mass is decreased. In fact, studies have shown that regular exercise, even in the absence of dietary restriction, can produce significant body-fat loss with minimal deprivation of lean tissue. Since increasing lean body mass and decreasing body fat may increase RMR, exercise may be the most important component for lasting weight loss (Wilfley, Grilo & Brownell, 1994).

Health Benefits of Exercise. Physical activity also has been associated with good physical health. Studies have shown that even modest levels of exercise can have a beneficial effect, as physically fit individuals frequently have lower mortality rates than those who do not exercise (Blair, 1989). These findings counter the notion that only vigorous exercise can produce health benefits.

Table 3.4
Possible Links Between Exercise and Weight Control

✔ expends energy

✔ may decrease appetite

✔ may enhance metabolic rate

✔ may preserve lean body tissue

✔ may limit preference for dietary fat

✔ enhances health

✔ improves risk factors associated with overweight

Has positive psychologic effects:

✔ improves self-esteem and psychologic well-being

✔ decreases mild stress and anxiety

✔ increases confidence

✔ may enhance dietary adherence

Source: Table reprinted with permission from Grilo, C.M., Brownell, K.D. and Stunkard, A.J. (1993). The metabolic and psychological importance of exercise in weight control. In A.J. Stunkard & T. Wadden (Eds.) *Obesity: Theory and Therapy*, 2nd Ed., (pp. 253-273), New York: Raven Press.

Those overweight individuals for whom adherence is difficult will find this information especially promising. Exercise, with or without dieting, has also been shown to offset or improve medical conditions such as high blood pressure, elevated cholesterol and diabetes (Wilfley, Grilo & Brownell, 1994).

Psychological Benefits of Exercise. In terms of emotional well-being, exercise is often associated with improved mood and self-concept, and decreases in depression, anxiety and stress. Physical activity also has been shown to increase dietary adherence which, in turn, evokes feelings of mastery. Such positive psychological correlates may enhance self-efficacy, self-determination and self-esteem, which ultimately increases the dieter's chances of permanently managing their weight (Wilfley, Grilo & Brownell, 1994).

Exercise in the Overweight/Obese

While more individuals are exercising these days than in the past, many still remain sedentary and do not attain the physical and emotional rewards of exercise. A number of people who begin an exercise program are unable to adhere to the regimen and quit before they have achieved their goals. Because of this, it is important to pay close attention to the physical and psychological barriers that are preventing overweight individuals from engaging in regular exercise. Poor fitness and excess weight may cause exercise to be painful and fatiguing, and the prospect of exercising may heighten already painful feelings of body-image dissatisfaction (Wilfley, Grilo & Brownell, 1994). Overweight individuals may associate exercise with negative experiences such as being teased as a child or in adulthood. The embarrassment and shame of being observed may be a barrier to exercise, as might a lack of confidence, knowledge or experience. As a lifestyle and weight management consultant, be prepared to work with your clients to overcome their negative feelings toward physical activity, and to develop exercise plans that are reasonable and fit well into their lifestyles.

Client Assessment

When first meeting with a potential client, it is crucial to establish an environment that facilitates clear communication, understanding and acceptance, regardless of a person's body weight, shape or dieting and exercise history. It is critical to continue this atmosphere of consistent support throughout the entire program. This is especially important for obese individuals who may feel embarrassed since they are most likely approaching treatment after many previously failed attempts at losing weight. Set your client at ease by acknowledging their frustration and pain in being scrutinized by an unyielding society, and openly discussing the worries and anxiety of initiating another weight-loss treatment. Most importantly, begin the process of helping your client recognize that their self-worth is independent of body weight. This idea should be encouraged throughout the duration of their program.

Establishing Rapport

Begin by encouraging clients to talk about their feelings regarding weight loss, obesity (if applicable), their past experiences and what they hope to gain from treatment with you. Listen carefully to each client, as the individual reasons for their overweight will likely be distinct. Actively involving clients in discussions about their goals and decisions about their treatment plan will not only foster autonomy, but it also will help them to embrace weight control and take responsibility for their own accomplishments. It is critical to treat your clients with respect regarding their reported food intake, eating patterns and exercise, especially if the amounts are inconsistent with changes in their weight. At times, your client will feel frustrated and disappointed with their progress. It is important to discuss the notion of "two steps forward and one step back;" that is, progress will not always be consistent and change is gradual. Encourage an atmosphere conducive to sharing feelings of both disappointment and success.

Assessing Client History

In order to develop a treatment plan, it is essential to learn about the dieting and exercise history of your client. Explore if your client was overweight as a child, or if the excess weight was put on in adulthood (for example, after pregnancy, menopause, or a physical or emotional trauma), as an individual who has struggled with their weight throughout life may have a harder time with treatment than one who has put on weight due to a specific event. While accurately measuring an individual's resting metabolic rate is a complicated process and not accessible to many lifestyle and weight management consultants, by learning more about eating patterns and weight gains and losses, you can frequently estimate if your client has a slower or faster RMR. To further adapt an appropriate plan, you will want to take into consideration your client's past and present emotional state — are they depressed, anxious, or is there evidence of psychological problems warranting a referral? Additionally, their social history in relation to shape and weight will need to be obtained as well as an understanding of what social and interpersonal changes your client is anticipating as a result of losing weight. Finally, assess whether your client is at risk for any health concerns. Once this information is consolidated, you can determine if your client is an appropriate candidate for weight loss, (or if a referral is in order) and begin setting up a treatment plan. (See Chapter 6 for more information on assessment.)

Assessing Dieting and Weight History

In obtaining an accurate dieting and weight-loss history, the first step will involve gaining a broad picture of the types of programs that have been attempted. Have your clients self-restrained their food intake? Have they participated in commercial programs or liquid fasts? Have they had surgery to reduce weight? Additionally, you will want to know if they are weight cyclers or if only one or two substantial weight losses have been part of their past. After assessing the number and frequency of each diet, it is important to explore how

your client views this history. Do they feel as though they have been successful at weight loss (regardless of any weight put back on)? Or, has their perception (or reality) been that of many failures? If the latter is the case, it will be necessary to estimate the level of your client's skepticism and pessimism and to adapt the treatment to address such feelings. You will also want to learn what parts of each program fit well with their lifestyle, and how each program was difficult for

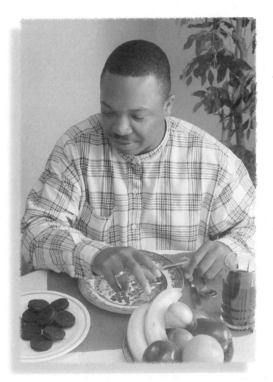

them to follow. For example, if your client tried a liquid fast and lost a large amount of weight, only to gain all of it back, you will want to find out how they viewed the weight loss and how it fit into their lifestyle. At this point you may want to review with your client their ultimate goal and discuss how previous attempts, and perhaps their outlook on them, have helped or hindered the process of attaining that goal. With this particular individual, you might want to recommend a slower, more reasonable weight-loss plan that allows room for some setbacks in order to attain lasting

Your client's dieting and weight history can help you understand why their past attempts at weight loss were or were not successful.

weight loss.

Finally, you will want to assess what types of feedback and messages from family members, significant others, friends, co-workers and the media your client has received as a result of attempted or repeated efforts with dieting. Has this individual generally been supported in their efforts? Or have they been berated for unsuccessful repeated attempts? You will want to use this critical information when developing your client's treatment plan.

What is your client's exercise history? Determine what factors led them to give up on their attempts to exercise in the past.

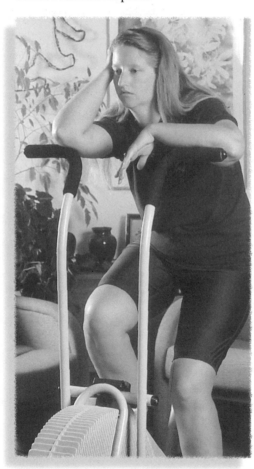

Assessing Exercise History

Assessing your client's previous experience with exercise is the next step. Has exercise been part of their lifestyle in the past? Or, will beginning any type of physical activity be a novel, and perhaps overwhelming, experience? For example, it will be necessary to fully explore your client's history to determine

whether exercise has been a positive or negative experience for them. Did this individual play on sports teams as a child and teenager? Or were they the last chosen to play in gym class? In using this information to tailor the treatment plan, take into consideration your client's job and responsibilities (for example, are they sedentary during much of the day or very active?) and the frequency of physical movement they do every day. It will also be important to take into account each individual's age, gender and amount of overweight when setting up an exercise plan for weight loss.

Assessing Psychological History

Psychological history and coping ability are important areas to assess when developing a weight-loss program or determining if a client is currently an appropriate candidate for weight loss. If an individual is suffering from a psychiatric problem, the condition may interfere with the success of the program. For example, if a potential client appears very depressed, losing weight may be ill-advised, since it is not an appropriate treatment for clinical depression. If your client's depression is considerable, make an appropriate referral to a mental healthcare specialist who can assess and treat the psychological problem. People may try to lose weight while they are under the care of a therapist for another problem. Under this circumstance, obtain permission to contact their therapist to discuss whether this is an appropriate time to initiate weight-loss treatment.

Recognizing your client's level of stress and how they cope with stressful situations also will indicate whether weight loss is presently appropriate and, if it is, how it can be best approached. Does this individual eat more, less or the same under stressful situations? Do different types of stress (e.g., anger, sadness) affect their eating? Information about how this person handles setbacks, disappointments or frustration may help to explain seemingly inexplicable setbacks during weight loss. Your best preparation for supporting a client during stressful times is to have a clear understanding of the client's high-risk situations by being well informed of both current and past psychological problems. For example, if feelings of failure bring about depressive symptoms, warn your client about potential feelings of sadness if a plateau or lapse is encountered.

Assessing Psychosocial History

In learning about your client's psychosocial history, you will be able to gain an understanding of how weight has affected their social functioning with family, significant others, peers, friends and co-workers. By understanding the relationship between weight and social experience, you will learn what your client is anticipating as a result of weight loss. Does it mean better friendships or more intimacy in relationships? Enhanced satisfaction with work? Greater involvement with hobbies and interests? The ability to achieve current life goals and challenges? If your client is counting on weight loss to improve on or change any of these variables, clarify that weight loss, even when successful, is unlikely to alter anyone's entire life. Clients' expectations should be discussed openly and honestly before beginning a program.

Assessing Health and Medical History

Finally, when developing a treatment plan, learn about and take into consideration any health problems your client has or has had in the past. If an individual suffers from any of the health risks previously discussed (i.e., diabetes, hypertension, stroke, hypercholestero-

lemia and cardiovascular disease), it is your responsibility to contact the healthcare provider to discuss your client's treatment plan. Additionally, confirm that the healthcare provider is monitoring and/or treating the condition. Similarly, if this client has suffered health problems in the past, maintain contact with a nurse practitioner or physician to ensure that there is no current health risk. Be familiar with the types of signs or symptoms both you and your client should be aware of in case of a relapse of the previous condition. Even if there is no evidence of current health problems, any client who is considerably overweight (for example, on the heavier end of the "moderately overweight" category) should also be monitored conjointly by a healthcare provider. Finally, you should be knowledgeable of the types of physical health and psychological risks that can arise from chronic dieting, eating disorders and obesity so that you can either adjust your treatment plan appropriately or refer a client to a specialist.

Identifying Client's Current Eating and Exercise Patterns

After taking into consideration a client's history with weight, dieting and exercise, the next step is to develop a picture of the individual's current patterns. You will want to clarify what their eating and exercise habits are like and assess how difficult they are going to be to change. Does this person eat three meals? Are they a grazer (picking at food all day long)? Is starving all day and bingeing in the evening their pattern? If it is hard for them to recall, suggest they begin monitoring their food intake before implementing a plan. Learning about a client's eating habits may not only give you insight into how the weight problem has developed and been maintained, but it will also give you the groundwork to identify where changes can be made. Similarly, you will need to gain an understanding of your client's current exercise patterns. Are they a person who already engages in physical activity or has exercise been avoided throughout their life? Is the level and amount of exercise too much or too little for healthy weight loss? Again, answering these types of questions will help you to begin to formulate a plan that is appropriate for this individual. During this process, it is very

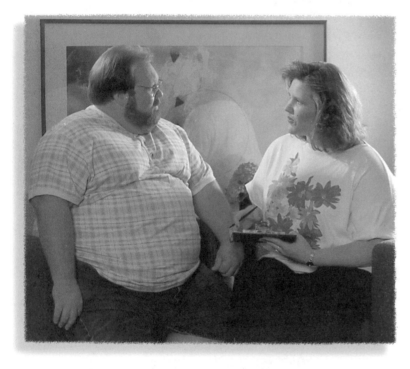

It is crucial that your client understand the idea of reasonable weight loss. An initial goal of 5 percent to 10 percent of body weight is considered reasonable since it is easier to lose and keep off.

helpful to your client if you are clear about what their strengths and weaknesses are, and which parts of their current patterns are working and which are not. In this way, you are including your client in developing their own treatment plan and proposing some of the positive aspects of their current patterns, while also addressing the ones that need work.

Consolidating Your Assessment

Take some time with the client at the end of your first or second meeting to clearly consolidate the information you have collected. Explain how past

expectations, patterns and thinking may have contributed to either the success or failure of past or current weight problems. Address your client's own body image issues, and stress that weight loss is not a panacea.

Why Now?

In assessing if the time is right to begin a program, the first question that needs to be answered is "why now?" Is it because of poor physical health? Feelings of depression? Pressure from co-workers, spouse or friends? Or is this person seeking to lose weight with the hope that their social life will improve, or a promotion at work will come about? Once you learn why a person has chosen the present time to attempt weight loss, you can help them determine if now is, indeed, the best period to begin the rigors of treatment. For example, if your client is currently under a lot of stress at work, they may want to wait until they have more time to focus on a weight-loss program. The guidelines listed in Table 3.5 should help you in deciding whether or not your client is ready to begin treatment (Foster, 1995).

The most crucial understanding to establish with your client is the idea of reasonable weight loss. While you do not want to diminish any person's hopes of becoming more fit and healthy, stress losing a sensible amount of weight as opposed to an ideal amount. Five percent to 10 percent of body weight is considered reasonable since it is easier to lose and keep off.

In addition to the medical benefits of losing moderate amounts of weight, there also are many psychological and behavioral advantages involved. People can more easily lose smaller amounts of weight than larger amounts. By achieving the initial weight loss, an individual will be rewarded with a greater sense of self-efficacy, motivating them to set another reasonable goal. With

Table 3.5

Areas to Consider When Assessing if Timing is Right for Weight Loss

Client's Attitude	How motivated is this person?
Client's Goals	Is your client considering reasonable weight loss and exercise goals? Will their goals fit reasonably into their current lifestyle?
Hunger and Eating Cues	What makes your client responsive to eating cues? Do they eat out of hunger, because food is available, out of habit, or for some other psychological need?
Control Over Eating	Do external pressures to eat threaten your client's control over eating?
Emotional Eating	Does your client eat based on response to emotions?
Exercise Attitudes and Patterns	It is important to understand how your client thinks about physical activity, as exercise is the best known way to keep off lost weight.

Source: Brownell, K.D. (1994). *The LEARN Program for Weight Control*, Sixth Ed. Dallas: American Health Publishing Company.

continued success, your clients are more likely to remain committed to their program and to changing their lifestyles permanently.

Make it clear that while weight loss will be gradual, it will be a true loss of fat. This is different from the "fast and easy" diets that result in rapid water loss rather than actual weight loss. Your client should also be aware that you will be working with them on maintenance from the very beginning by developing comfortable changes in the behaviors and attitudes that affect eating and activity.

Is Your Client Ready to Change?

Weighing the benefits and sacrifices of engaging in a weight-loss program is a crucial part of assessing a client's readiness. If a person views the sacrifices they will make as minor when compared to the benefits of losing weight, it may be a good time to initiate a program. You and your client should outline what changes will need to be made (e.g., limiting intake of fatty foods, free time lost to exercise) as part of the program, and what will be gained (e.g., feeling and looking better). In this way, you and your client can determine if the balance is in favor of moving forward (Brownell, 1994).

Keep in mind that individuals often begin a program with a burst of enthusiasm that may fade once the rigors of the program set in. Weight cycling, feelings of failure, decreased self-esteem and frustration are some of the problems that may be perpetuated if an individual is not ready to make a commitment to weight loss. The information in Table 3.5 will help you to determine if your client is ready to begin a weight-loss program.

Reviewing Client Goals

Once a decision to begin a program has been made, suggest programming goals and review them with your client. Get their feedback and find out how

Table 3.6

Short-term and Long-term Psychological Goals

Short Term	Long Term
Weekly goals for problem areas	Improved self-esteem
Praise or tangibles for meeting weekly goals	Improved problem-solving abilities
Keeping records of emotions before and after eating	An understanding of the connection between emotions and problem eating
Practice assertive requests, setting limits and sharing feelings	Ability to communicate to family, friends and co-workers regarding weight control needs
Engage in activities that have been avoided due to weight or negative body image	Engaging in a variety of activities without feeling negatively towards their own body

Source: Brownell, K.D. (1994). *The LEARN Program for Weight Control,* Sixth Ed. Dallas: American Health Publishing Company.

they envision attaining those goals. Be sure to cover the following areas in your discussion:

✔ How do genetics play a role in this individual's weight?
✔ How will current eating and exercise patterns make weight loss easier or more difficult?

Based on this information, there may be several attitude or outlook goals that your client can set. Some of these goals will be attained more quickly than others, and it is important for you and your client to review what they can expect. Table 3.6 outlines some of the short-term and long-term psychological goals that have often been associated with losing weight.

Establishing Treatment Guidelines

Discussing the logistics of the program will establish a mutual understanding between you and your client about how weight loss will be approached. Talk about the frequency of sessions, how often a client will be weighed and by whom (e.g., during visits with you or at the client's home), and whether food diaries will be reviewed. Contract together what kind of rules should be set if your client cannot make an appointment; for example, how far in advance do they need to contact you and is there a late cancellation fee? You may find this suggestion especially helpful when clients who feel that they are not doing well avoid coming to meetings. Stress that this is exactly the time to come so that you can both learn from the difficult periods of the weight-loss process. The program agenda, in terms of number of sessions (or whether the program will be open-ended), should be discussed.

The Weight-loss and Exercise Plan

As every individual differs, so will every treatment plan that you adapt. For the specifics of designing the plan, refer to Chapter 9. There are, however, a few guidelines that are standard in maintaining a healthy body.

AMERICAN COUNCIL ON EXERCISE

57

CHAPTER THREE

PSYCHOLOGY
OF WEIGHT
MANAGEMENT
AND OBESITY

Table 3.7

Behavioral Weight-loss Principles Described in Five Leading Treatment Manuals

1. Stimulus Control
   A. Shopping
      1. Shop for food after eating.
      2. Shop from a list.
      3. Avoid ready-to-eat foods.
      4. Don't carry more cash than is needed for shopping list.

   B. Plans
      1. Plan to limit food intake.
      2. Substitute exercise for snacking.
      3. Eat meals and snacks at scheduled times.
      4. Don't accept food offered by others.

   C. Activities
      1. Store food out of sight.
      2. Eat all food in the same place.
      3. Remove food from inappropriate storage areas in the house.
      4. Keep serving dishes off the table.
      5. Use smaller dishes and utensils.
      6. Avoid being the food server.
      7. Leave the table immediately after eating.
      8. Don't save leftovers.

   D. Holidays and Parties
      1. Drink fewer alcoholic beverages.
      2. Plan eating habits before parties.
      3. Eat a low-calorie snack before parties.
      4. Practice polite ways to decline food.
      5. Don't get discouraged by an occasional setback.

2. Eating Behavior
   1. Put fork down between mouthfuls.
   2. Chew thoroughly before swallowing.
   3. Prepare foods one portion at a time.
   4. Leave some food on the plate.
   5. Pause in the middle of the meal.
   6. Do nothing else while eating (read, watch television).

3. Reward
   1. Solicit help from family and friends.
   2. Help family and friends provide this support in the form of praise and material rewards.
   3. Utilize self-monitoring records as basis for rewards.
   4. Plan specific rewards for specific behaviors (behavioral contracts).

4. Self-monitoring
   Keep a diet diary that includes:
   1. Time and place of eating.
   2. Type and amount of food.
   3. Who is present/how you feel.

5. Nutrition Education
   1. Use diet diary to identify problem areas.
   2. Make small changes that you can continue.
   3. Learn nutritional values of foods.
   4. Decrease fat intake; increase complex carbohydrates.

6. Physical Activity
   A. Routine Activity
      1. Increase routine activity.
      2. Increase use of stairs.
      3. Keep a record of distance walked each day.

   B. Exercise
      1. Begin a very mild exercise program.
      2. Keep a record of daily exercise.
      3. Increase the exercise very gradually.

7. Cognitive Restructuring
   1. Avoid setting unreasonable goals.
   2. Think about progress, not shortcomings.
   3. Avoid imperatives like "always" and "never".
   4. Counter negative thoughts with rational restatements.
   5. Set weight goals.

Source: Table reprinted with permission from Stunkard, A.J. & Berthold, H.C. (1985). What is behavior therapy? A very short description of behavioral weight control. *American Journal of Clinical Nutrition*, 41, 821-823.

They include: eating a variety of foods; eating foods that are low in fat, saturated fat and cholesterol; eating plenty of vegetables, fruits and grains; using sugar, salt and alcohol in moderation; and incorporating regular physical activity into daily routines. In addition, Table 3.7 offers many behavioral weight-loss principles and methods for achieving them (Stunkard, 1985). Your clients may find it helpful to experiment with these principles and incorporate as many of them into their lifestyles as possible.

Table 3.8
Recommendations for Maximizing Exercise Adherence in Obese Persons

General Principles

✔ Be sensitive to psychologic and physical barriers.

✔ Increase focus on enhanced self-efficacy.

✔ Focus on reasonable exercise goals by emphasizing consistency and enjoyment, not amount and type.

✔ Begin at a person's fitness level.

✔ Encourage clients to define routine activities as "exercise."

✔ Focus on compliance as the priority.

✔ Consider what physical activity is appropriate based on stage of life, gender, and prior experience with exercise.

✔ Evaluate social support network.

Specific interventions
Prescription

✔ Provide clear information about the importance of exercise.

✔ Define daily activities as exercise.

✔ Maximize walking and use of stairs.

✔ Incorporate a programmed activity that is enjoyable, fits with lifestyle, and is feasible as client's fitness improves.

Behavioral

✔ Introduce self-monitoring, feedback, and goal-setting techniques.

✔ Identify other benefits outside of weight loss, including physical changes, increased mobility, and lowered heart rate.

✔ Recommend exercise for soothing emotional distress when risk for overeating is high.

Source: Table reprinted with permission from Grilo, C.M., Brownell, K.D. & Stunkard, A.J. (1993). The metabolic and psychological importance of exercise in weight control. In A.J. Stunkard & T. Wadden (Eds.) *Obesity: Theory and Therapy,* 2nd Ed, (pp. 253-273). New York: Raven Press.

Self-monitoring by Record Keeping

A key component of the weight-loss process listed in Table 3.8 is self-monitoring by record keeping. This is an area in which you will need to work closely with your clients, as the food and exercise diaries that they keep can tell you a great deal about them. Record keeping not only assures you and your client that they are adhering to the program, but it helps both of you to learn about what works (i.e., eating three meals keeps them from snacking all day), and what does not (i.e., your client has the tendency to skip exercising if they plan to work out in the morning), and you will be able to review how their efforts can be improved. Finally, by completing exercise and food diaries, your client will feel responsible for their progress and experience a sense of empowerment.

Increasing Program Adherence

Probably the most critical component in increasing adherence to a weight-loss program comes from how you and your client approach your work together. The program should be viewed as a "change in lifestyle," as opposed to a "diet" or "exercise regimen" that will be terminated once the desired weight is lost. Most of your clients will have a history of trying diets that entailed excessive changes in their usual eating and exercise patterns, and demanding guidelines that were burdensome to follow. Changing the habits that have caused weight gain, and developing healthier, personalized patterns that sensibly fit into your client's daily life will increase adherence substantially. Adapt a plan to their individual lifestyles. For example, a full-time working parent (who may need to consider time constraints and stress reduction) will need to adopt a different exercise plan than a retired woman who may have never incorporated physical activity into her life, but is now focusing on its health benefits. Table 3.8 outlines an approach that may be useful in maximizing exercise adherence in overweight and obese persons (Wilfley, Grilo & Brownell, 1994).

Monitoring the Effectiveness of the Plan

Once the program has been initiated, you and your client must take the time to continuously review it and its effectiveness in order to keep it on track. How is the program fitting into your client's lifestyle? Are they perceiving the changes in eating and exercising patterns positively or negatively? Overall, how is your client feeling about your work together? These questions should be addressed frequently to assess the effectiveness of the program and to recognize what areas may need to be altered (Brownell, 1994).

Dealing with Potential Setbacks

As weight loss is a difficult endeavor for any individual, you will inevitably encounter clients who are not experiencing the level of success that they would like. This may be the result of intentional or unintentional noncompliance with the program, or it may be the result of a biological link — genetically, this individual may be unable to lose weight by using methods that have worked for others. If you are noticing that your client's weight loss results are not matching what they are reporting, it is critical that you approach them with compassion. By understanding the shame involved in this person's inability to comply with treatment, you can help your client address why the program is difficult and work on making it more realistic. Keep in mind that if a client is misrepresenting their efforts, they may

Table 3.9

Risk Factors for Lapses or Relapses During Weight Loss

✔ Negative Emotional States

✔ Motivational Level

✔ Response to Treatment

✔ Coping Skills

✔ Social Support

Source: Brownell, K.D., Marlatt, G.A., Lichtenstein, E. & Wilson, G.T. (1986). Understanding and preventing relapse. *American Psychologist*, 42, 765-782.

be unaware of how to measure food portions or how to judge their level of exercise. In any of these cases, when addressing the contradicting results, acknowledge the client's frustration without accusation. Suggest working on the areas that they can control. By carefully reviewing portion sizes, calorie intake and time exercised, you may be able to pinpoint where the problem in following the program exists.

In some cases, your client will openly admit to not adhering to the program. It is your job to help this individual get back on track. Again, acknowledge their frustration without being accusatory. It may be helpful to suggest exploring the circumstances of this person's overeating, such as mood, social interactions and their feelings about you and their program.

You also may encounter a situation in which you are confident of a client's adherence, yet the results are still disappointing. Focus on the successful changes that they have made to maintain their motivation. Using this approach when setbacks occur will not only safeguard your rapport, but it will increase your client's trust and confidence in you and your commitment to helping them lose weight (Wadden & Wingate, 1995).

Preparation for Lapses

Lapses are an inevitable part of the weight-loss process. Prepare clients for lapses and help them understand that lapses are useful learning opportunities. It is critical that you help your client review in detail what happened prior to a lapse in an effort to illuminate the factors that led up to it. Actively plan with your client how to deal with future high-risk situations.

Take time to explain the difference between lapses and relapses to clients. Lapses should be viewed as expected slips, mistakes or events that are part of the process of developing a new healthy

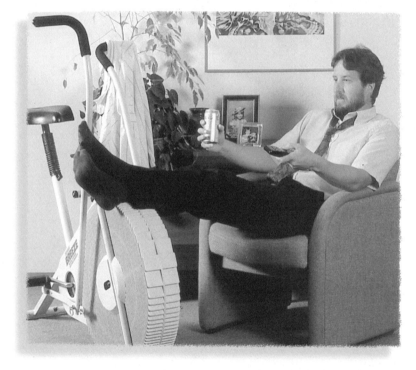

While most relapses are due to situational factors, they also may result from personal negative emotional states, such as depression.

lifestyle. An example of this might be when an individual overeats as a result of feeling angry. By self-monitoring and keeping records of their feelings when the lapse occurs, the client may learn that feelings of anger are a risk for overeating.

A **relapse**, on the other hand, happens when so many lapses have occurred that the outcome is a return of the original problem on a consistent basis. Inform your client that while a relapse

is frustrating, it can have some positive purposes. First, like lapses, relapses can teach your client more about their strengths and weaknesses. Second, several failures may push an individual to seek needed professional help or, in some cases, more intensive treatment. Finally, the relapsed client will realize that it often takes several attempts at weight loss to achieve success.

Anticipating Your Client's Potential Lapse/Relapse

There are several factors that contribute to the occurrence of lapses and relapses that can be monitored during the program. By understanding the risk factors for each individual (outlined in Table 3.9), you can better prepare your client to cope with these setbacks.

While lapses usually occur as a result of situational factors (e.g., seeing an ex-partner with a new person), relapses can result from personal negative emotional states, such as depression.

It is important to review a client's initial reaction to the program, as it can indicate how well, or how poorly, it will proceed. In some cases, it is those who adhere "perfectly" when beginning a program that are at greater risk for relapse. Individuals who allow themselves some initial lapses and allow their weight loss to become part of their lifestyle may do better in the long term. Try to observe a client's coping skills in order to determine if they are at risk for a lapse. Those who anticipate that they might regain small amounts of weight from time to time are less likely to consider themselves failures and may be less likely to relapse. Reviewing a client's support system (family, friends, co-workers) also will allow you to gain some insight into the likelihood of lapses or relapse since this support has been linked to long-term success in weight management (Brownell, Marlatt, Lichtenstein & Wilson, 1986).

Sample Client Profile and Treatment Plan

The following sections offer an illustration of a sample client profile and the considerations a lifestyle and weight management consultant might focus on when developing an appropriate plan.

Client Profile

Carolyn is a 40-year-old female, caucasian secretary who is 5'5", weighs approximately 185 pounds, and has a BMI of 31, placing her in the moderately overweight category. She wants to lose about 60 pounds. While she has never weighed as much as 185 pounds, Carolyn has always carried more weight than other women her height (she has a stature similar to her mother, who also has a large body build). She has weighed between 140 and 150 pounds since her late teens and early twenties.

Carolyn grew up in a traditional Italian household where mealtime, which included eating rich foods, was a special time for the family. She has always been quite conscious of her excess weight, feeling, at times, as though she doesn't "measure up" to others because of it. For this reason, she always hated gym class in school and, while she enjoyed swimming, she was too uncomfortable to wear a bathing suit in public. As a result, Carolyn would frequently restrict her food intake by counting calories or trying different diets that she would hear about from friends or read about in magazines. She would develop rules to eliminate all fattening foods from her diet, and restrict herself to limited amounts of "good" foods. While her efforts would work initially, Carolyn would frequently go off her diet and give up before reaching her goal. Inevitably, her weight would always climb back to the same 140 to 150 pounds.

Before becoming pregnant with her first child, Carolyn joined a commercial diet program that helped her monitor her food intake and offered her a place to weigh herself weekly. She also was obligated to purchase prepackaged foods and special vitamins and supplements. Although she never reached her goal of losing 40 pounds, she did lose 15 pounds (getting down to 135) on this program. After giving birth to her son, her weight climbed to 160 and she was unable to stay on a diet. After giving birth to her second son, she gained an additional 10 pounds.

Two years ago, Carolyn's father died. Although she had been very close with him, she had been so busy with work and parenting in the past few years, that she hadn't spent as much time with him as she would have liked. She experienced feelings of sadness and guilt surrounding his death, and noticed that she found herself eating more frequently during stressful times. In the past six months, there has been friction between her and her older teenage son, and she has been eating more and making poorer food choices than ever. Her weight has climbed to 185 pounds. Carolyn rarely exercises due to the discomfort of her body size and a lack of motivation. She almost never weighs herself because she fears she has gained weight. Carolyn is becoming increasingly concerned about her weight and how it may be affecting her health since her mother has been suffering from diabetes mellitus for the past several years.

Client Plan

The following offers an illustration of how you, as a lifestyle and weight management consultant, might talk with Carolyn.

✔ *Review with Carolyn how her genes and physiology likely contribute to her weight problem. Since Carolyn's body type is similar to her mother's, she has inherited a* tendency to carry extra weight. *Explain to her that part of her excess weight is not a result of her own habits or efforts, but rather part of her biology, which cannot be changed.* Goal: Help Carolyn recognize that part of her weight problem is NOT her own fault, and that while she will be able to lose some of her excess weight, her goal of 125 pounds may be unreasonable based on her genes.

✔ *Due to her current physiology, Carolyn may burn fat and calories more slowly than other individuals.* Goal: To speed up how quickly Carolyn burns calories by including physical activity in her plan. Because Carolyn does not exercise regularly, physical activity must be consistent and should be one that she enjoys (i.e., swimming).

✔ *Review the societal, cultural and environmental factors that have contributed to her weight problem. Carolyn's upbringing has clearly contributed to her excess weight. Given that she was brought up in a home in which mealtime was important to the family, and where rich, heavy foods were served, it makes sense that she considers meals a priority and has a preference for fattening foods.* Goal: Help Carolyn see the connection between her upbringing and her weight problem. Let her know that you are going to help her find other activities that may come to hold more significance than mealtime. Also, explain to Carolyn that, unlike diets she has tried in the past, she will not completely eliminate any foods. Rather, her plan will incorporate a variety of foods, including moderate amounts of more fattening foods.

✔ *Discuss how improving her body image will enhance weight loss. Carolyn's body size has made her feel as though she doesn't "measure up." Let her know that*

while you understand how she feels, her goal is unrealistic and has most likely hindered her past weight-loss efforts. Goal: Explain to Carolyn how many women, as they grow older, tend to gain weight (particularly at certain developmental points such as pregnancy and menopause), and that the majority of women do not have slim figures like those portrayed in the media. It will take time, but try to convince her that her idea of how much she should weigh is distorted (trying to weigh 120 when her natural weight for most of her life has been between 140 to 150). Explain how this has caused her to become frustrated and abandon her weight-loss efforts because she hasn't reached her goal weight. It also is worthwhile to spend some time discussing the other important areas that define her self-worth (i.e., parenting or career) to see how she achieves the goals she sets in those areas.

✔ *Talk about the health risks that Carolyn should be aware of. Carolyn may not be experiencing any health problems yet, but her years of overeating, poor food choices and lack of exercise may make her susceptible to health risks. Also, Carolyn is likely to have a predisposition for diabetes mellitus since her mother suffers from it.* Goal: Review some of the health problems that Carolyn is at risk for due to her excess weight. Stress that her concern regarding diabetes is justified, and that she should have a physical (if she hasn't had one in awhile), and inform her treating physician of her family's medical history. Once you have confirmed that she does not currently have any health problems that need immediate attention, discuss with Carolyn how even modest weight loss and exercise will decrease the health risks related to overweight.

✔ *Review the role of physical activity in her weight-loss plan. Since Carolyn has had negative experiences with exercise due to her weight, incorporate a plan that not only fits into her lifestyle, but that also is pleasurable. She has indicated that she has enjoyed swimming, so you have a good place to start.* Goal: Encourage Carolyn to seek out swimming programs for overweight adults at local community centers or YMCAs (or comparable organizations that might have swimming pools). Or she could find times when the pool is less crowded. If she still feels uncomfortable, suggest that she make a greater effort to increase physical activity in her daily life. Carolyn may be able to start feeling better, and lose some initial weight so she feels ready to put on a bathing suit, simply by walking more. Recommend that she take the stairs instead of the elevator to her office, or park her car further from her destination. Brainstorm with her about ways she could make exercise an integral and regular part of her lifestyle, and incorporate her ideas and recommendations into her program. Carolyn will feel that she has ownership of her plan, empowering her to take action.

✔ *Assess Carolyn's motivation level and readiness to approach weight loss. Because Carolyn has reached her highest weight ever, and is aware that her health could become compromised because of it, she may be more motivated to lose weight now than at other times in her life. She does, however, have a pattern of losing and regaining weight and, at times, of not reaching her weight-loss goals.* Goal: Talk about Carolyn's commitment to her health and weight loss. Talk about her lifestyle and how she must broaden the types of foods that she eats (incorporating foods that are lower in fat than she is used to),

and add physical activity to her life. Make sure that she is willing to make the time to put in this effort. Talk about developing reasonable weight-loss goals based on her age, height and bone structure. Stress that she may be more successful if she begins with a smaller, more attainable goal of losing 10 pounds, then trying to lose additional weight after she has achieved that loss. Additionally, you'll want to discuss how her eating patterns under stress may cause her to lapse. The two of you can come up with strategies to prepare for and curb setbacks. For example, Carolyn may find it useful to monitor her feelings when she is overeating. If she realizes that she is experiencing stress, she may be better able to consciously find an activity (perhaps taking a relaxing bath) other than eating to alleviate her upsetting emotions.

✔ *Discuss the guidelines for treatment. Though Carolyn has not given any indication of whether or not she will be committed to following a program, it is important to set up guidelines for working together.* Goal: Set a weekly meeting day and time that will not conflict with any of Carolyn's other responsibilities. Determine the cost of treatment and a payment schedule based on her financial situation. You may suggest that since Carolyn no longer weighs herself, this may be something you can do at your meetings so you can discuss the implications of her weight loss or gain. Talk about her feelings at that time. Finally, you might want to consider setting up a cancellation policy. For example, outside of extenuating circumstances, Carolyn will need to call you at least 24 hours in advance to cancel an appointment, or she will be charged for the meeting.

Special Issues and Considerations

It is essential to discuss what to do if you are unsure if an individual is an appropriate candidate for weight loss. If there is clear evidence of an eating disorder, prominent health risks that need active medical attention, or if a person is clearly out of a relatively normal weight range (morbid obesity or

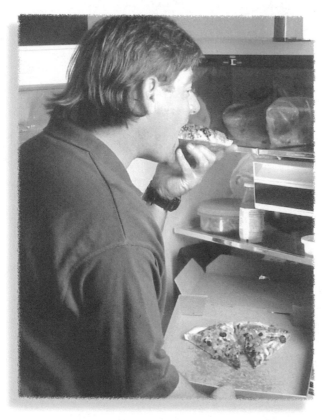

Individuals with binge eating disorder (BED) experience a loss of control during recurrent episodes of binge eating. Individuals with this or any other eating disorder must be referred to a healthcare professional who specializes in their treatment.

"severely" overweight), you should discuss an appropriate referral for this individual. Frequently, however, a potential client's readiness for weight loss is more ambiguous. If this is the case, you may need to consult with other professionals before making a definitive decision. Whether you are giving someone a referral or requesting time for further assessment, be sensitive when explaining your reasons for not immediately taking them on as a client. Explain that while weight loss may be a good idea in the future, right now there

may be other, more imperative problems to overcome before weight loss can be successful. There is a continuum of problems that clients may come to you with. You will need to be aware of the signs in order to make an appropriate referral.

Chronic Dieters

Chronic dieters perpetually try to restrict their food intake to lose weight. These individuals tend not to be successful, though, because they frequently counterregulate by overeating when they stray at all from their diet. As a result, their body weight fluctuates. Chronic dieters tend to suffer from much of the same type of psychological distress as obese individuals. You are certainly equipped to work with chronic dieters, as most of their behavior does not become pathological. You should focus on helping these clients approach weight loss as a lifestyle change, as opposed to going on and off a program. Keep in mind that a small percentage of chronic dieters may be at risk for more severe problems such as eating disorders (Polivy & Herman, 1995).

Eating Disorders

As a lifestyle and weight management consultant, it is critical to have a knowledge of eating disorders so you can recognize a client struggling with a problem that requires specialized attention. You should understand the physical and psychological symptoms of eating disorders, as well as the consequences if they go untreated.

The three primary eating disorders are anorexia nervosa (AN), bulimia nervosa (BN) and, in both younger and older adults, binge eating disorder (BED). While patients with AN and BN are primarily female (up to 90 percent of those receiving treatment), it is estimated that three females to every two males suffer from BED. Table 3.10

Table 3.10

DSM-IV Criteria for Eating Disorders

Anorexia Nervosa	Bulimia Nervosa	Binge Eating Disorder
Body weight abnormally low — 15% below expected	Recurrent episodes of binge eating	Recurrent episodes of binge eating
Intense fear of gaining weight or becoming fat, even though underweight	A sense of loss of control during these episodes	A sense of loss of control during these episodes
In postmenarcheal women, amenorrhea - missing at least three periods	Recurrent use of compensatory behavior designed to prevent weight gain, such as self-induced vomiting, laxative abuse, strict dieting, fasting or vigorous exercise	The absence of regular use of compensatory behavior to prevent weight gain
Disturbance in the way in which one's body is experienced	Self evaluation is unduly influenced by body shape and weight	Self evaluation is unduly influenced by body shape and weight
	A minimum of two binge episodes a week for at least three months	A minimum of two binge episodes a week for at least six months

Subtypes

Restricting —
no bingeing or purging

Bingeing or purging —
engaged regularly in
such behavior

Source: *Diagnostic and Statistical Manual of Mental Disorders.*

outlines the criteria indicated in the *Diagnostic and Statistical Manual of Mental Disorders, IV (DSM-IV)* for diagnosing individuals with AN, BN and BED (APA, 1994).

Symptoms of Anorexia Nervosa

The most evident indication of an individual with AN is that their body weight is 15 percent below the normal weight for their height. For example, a woman who is 5'5" and weighs 95 pounds may be suffering from AN. Common symptoms include **amenorrhea** (absence of menstrual period), constipation, abdominal pain, cold intolerance, lethargy, anxious energy, fatigue

and headaches. Other signs of AN may include hypertension, low body temperature, dry skin, lanugo-like hair, **bradycardia** and swelling. Additionally, individuals suffering from AN often do not recognize, or tend to minimize, the dangers of their physical state. If a potential client is significantly underweight and experiences any of the aforementioned symptoms, refer them to a physician, nurse practitioner and/or an eating disorders specialist (Wilfley & Grilo, 1994).

Symptoms of Bulimia Nervosa

Individuals with BN tend to be of average weight or, in some cases, fluctuate 10 pounds above or below the normal weight for their height. Symptoms include irregular menses, abdominal pain, lethargy, fatigue, headaches, depression, swelling of the hands and feet and bloating. People with BN often appear healthy, but some signs of the disorder can be parotid gland enlargement and enamel erosion on the teeth. If a potential client describes eating large amounts of food, and then purging (either by vomiting, or overusing laxatives or diuretics), refer them to an eating disorders specialist (Wilfley & Grilo, 1994).

Detecting Binge Eating Disorder

While men and women suffering from BED are most often overweight, there are few visibly discernible signs of the disorder. Therefore, if you suspect that someone is struggling with BED, ask the following questions:

1. Are there times during the day when you could not have stopped eating, even if you had wanted to?

2. Do you ever find yourself eating unusually large amounts of food in a short period of time?

3. Do you ever feel extremely guilty or depressed after eating?

4. Do you ever feel even more determined to diet or to eat healthier after that eating episode?

If an individual answers affirmatively to these questions, they may be suffering from BED and should be referred to an eating disorders specialist (Bruce, & Wilfley, 1995).

Referrals for Clients with Eating Disorders

Individuals suffering from any of these three disorders tend to suffer from other psychological disorders, such as depression and anxiety. If a client appears to be struggling with either BN or BED, it is essential that a referral be made to a healthcare worker who specializes in the treatment of eating disorders (this can include psychologists, social workers, medical doctors and nurse practitioners), as this individual is most likely not currently an appropriate candidate for weight loss. Similarly, if you believe someone is suffering from AN, a referral to a specialist is in order. However, because patients with AN have dangerously low body weights, immediate medical attention may be necessary.

Exercise Abuse

Before concluding this section, it is important to make mention of exercise abuse. While it is clear that exercise is a healthy and positive endeavor, it can become compulsive when approached in the pursuit of extreme thinness. When screening a client for exercise abuse, it is helpful to assess the following areas:

1. Are they unable to stop thinking about exercise?

2. Do they feel anxious when an exercise session is missed, and that it must be made up or else weight will be gained?

3. Do they exercise despite being advised against it (i.e., because of an exercise-induced injury)?

4. Is exercise increased after overeating?

5. Do they focus on the amount of fat or calories being burned while exercising?

If an individual endorses any of these questions, they may be overexercising and should be referred to an eating disorders specialist (Wilfley, Grilo & Brownell, 1994).

Summary

Weight control is pursued by many individuals in the U.S. who hope to transform their bodies into the ideal. Because this goal is frequently unrealistic, efforts to reach it can be taken to extremes, even to the point of emotional distress or psychological problems such as eating disorders. As a lifestyle and weight management consultant, you need to be aware of the many problems that potential clients may present. You must have an understanding of, and compassion for, each client's unique issues regarding weight loss and psychological distress. Exploring an individual's readiness for weight loss and working closely with them throughout the weight-loss process will encourage trust and understanding between you and your client. Normalizing lapses and helping people to learn from both lapses and relapses will further promote a positive weight-loss experience. Remember, the most significant way to help any individual is to be patient and understanding, and to acknowledge each person's unique concerns throughout your work.

References

American Psychiatric Association. (1994). *Diagnostic and Statistical Manual of Mental Disorders.* (4th ed.) Washington, DC.

Blair, S.N., Kohl, H.W., Paffenbarger, R.S., Clark, D.G., Cooper, K.H. & Gibbons, L.W. (1989). Physical fitness and all-cause mortality. *Journal of the American Medical Association,* 262, 2395-2400.

Brownell, K.D. (1994). *The LEARN program for weight control.* (6th ed.) Dallas: American Health Publishing Company.

Brownell, K.D., Marlatt, G.A., Lichtenstein, E. & Wilson, G.T. (1986). Understanding and preventing relapse. *American Psychologist,* 42, 765-782.

Brownell, K.D. & Wadden, T.A. (1992). Etiology and treatment of obesity: understanding a serious, prevalent, and refractory disorder. *Journal of Consulting and Clinical Psychology,* 60, 505-517.

Bruce, B. & Wilfley, D.E. (1995). Binge eating among the overweight population: A serious and prevalent problem. *Journal of the American Dietetic Association,* 96, 1-8.

Foster, G.D. (1995). Reasonable weights: Determinants, definitions, and directions. In: F.X. Pi-Sunyer & D.B. Allison (Eds.) *Obesity Treatment: Establishing Goals, Improving Outcomes, and Reviewing the Research Agenda.* (pp. 35-44). New York: Plenum Press.

Grilo, C.M., Brownell, K.D. & Stunkard, A.J. (1993). The metabolic and psychological importance of exercise in weight control. In: A.J. Stunkard & T. Wadden (Eds.) *Obesity: Theory and Therapy,* (2nd ed.) (pp. 253-273). New York: Raven Press.

Kuczmarski, A. (1994). Increasing prevalence of overweight among U.S. adults. *Journal of the American Medical Association,* 272, 205-211.

Kumanyika, S.K. (1995). Obesity in minority populations. In: K.D. Brownell & C.G. Fairburn (Eds.) *Eating Disorders and Obesity: A Comprehensive Handbook.* (pp.73-77). New York: Guilford Press.

Pi-Sunyer, F.X. (1995). Medical complications of obesity. In: K.D. Brownell & C.G. Fairburn (Eds.) *Eating Disorders and Obesity: A Comprehensive Handbook.* (pp. 401-405). New York: Guilford Press.

Polivy, J. & Herman, C.P. (1995). Dieting and its relation to eating disorders. In: K.D. Brownell & Fairburn (Eds.) *Eating Disorders and Obesity: A Comprehensive Handbook.* (pp. 83-86). New York: Guilford Press.

Rodin, J. (1992). *Body Traps.* New York: William Morrow & Company.

Sobal, J. (1995). Social influences on body weight. In: K.D. Brownell & C.G. Fairburn (Eds.) *Eating Disorders and Obesity: A Comprehensive Handbook.* (pp.73-77). New York: Guilford Press.

Stunkard, A.J. & Sobal, J. (1995). Psychosocial consequences of obesity. In: K.D. Brownell & C.G. Fairburn (Eds.) *Eating Disorders and Obesity: A Comprehensive Handbook.* (pp. 417-421). New York: Guilford Press.

Stunkard, A.J. (1992). An Overview of current treatments for obesity. In: Thomas A. Wadden & Theodore B. Zanltallie (Eds.) *Treatment of the Seriously Obese Patient.* (pp.33-43). New York: Gilbert Press.

Stunkard, A.J. & Berthold, H.C. (1985). What is behavior therapy? A very short description of behavioral weight control. *American Journal of Clinical Nutrition,* 41, 821-823.

U.S. Department of Agriculture & U.S. Department of Health and Human Services. (1990). *Dietary Guidelines for Americans.* (3rd ed.)

Wadden, T.A. & Wingate, B.J. (1995). Compassionate treatment of the obese individual. In: K.D. Brownell & C.G. Fairburn (Eds.) *Eating Disorders and Obesity: A Comprehensive Handbook.* (pp. 564-571). New York: Guilford Press.

Wilfley, D.E. & Grilo, C.M. (1994). Eating disorders: A women's health problem in primary care. *Nurse Practitioner Forum,* 5, 34-45.

Wilfley, D.E., Grilo, C.M. & Brownell, K.D. (1994). Exercise and Regulation of Body Weight. In: M. Shangold & Mirkin, G. (Eds.) *Women and Exercise: Physiology and Sports Medicine,* (2nd ed.) (pp. 27-59). Philadelphia: F.A. Davis Company.

Wilfley, D.E. & Rodin, J. (1995). Cultural influences on eating disorders. In: K.D. Brownell & C.G. Fairburn (Eds.) *Eating Disorders and Obesity: A Comprehensive Handbook.* New York: Guilford Press.

Suggested Reading

American Dietetic Association. (1994). Position of the American Dietetic Association: Nutrition intervention in the treatment of anorexia nervosa, bulimia nervosa, and binge eating. *ADA Report,* 94, 902-907.

Brownell, K.D. & Fairburn, C.G. (1995). *Eating Disorders and Obesity: A Comprehensive Handbook.* New York: Guilford Press.

Brownell, K.D. (1994). *The LEARN Program for Weight Control.* (6th ed.) Dallas: American Health Publishing Company.

Rodin, J. (1992). *Body Traps.* New York: William Morrow & Company.

Rodin, J. & Brownell, K.D. (1995). *The Weight Maintenance Survival Guide.*

Stunkard, A.J. (1959). *The Pain of Obesity.*

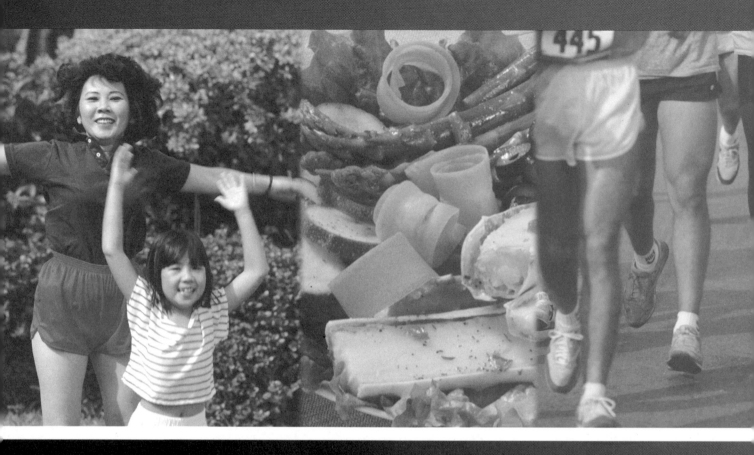

CHAPTER FOUR

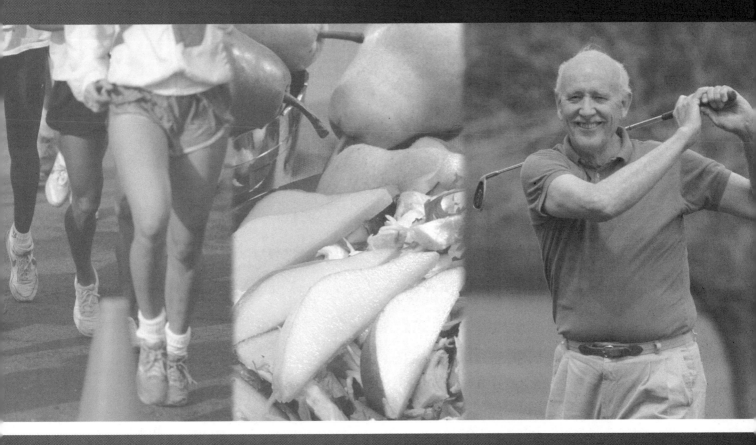

BODY COMPOSITION Assessment

Ross E. Andersen

Ross E. Andersen, Ph.D., is an assistant professor of medicine at Johns Hopkins University, and focuses on the treatment of obesity. His research areas include the changes in resting metabolism, body composition and fitness that accompany weight-loss and exercise programs. His work is supported by the National Institutes of Health, and his articles have appeared in Redbook and Reader's Digest as well as other publications.

Introduction

An accurate assessment of body composition is an integral part of a comprehensive health screening and is recommended for individuals who wish to begin a weight-loss or exercise program. The evaluation of body composition can quantify the body's major structural components: muscle, fat and bone.

Height–Weight tables are the reference most individuals use to assess the appropriateness of their weight. Unfortunately, these tables are only a guideline and provide no information on relative body composition. This is important because research has demonstrated that it is excess body fat — not weight — that is associated with health risks.

In the last decade, the recognition of this important link between health and body fat has led to a rise in the number of techniques for estimating body composition. For example, near infrared interactance (NIR) **body composition** analyzers (such as Futrex™) can be purchased through mail-order catalogs or fitness magazines for less than $100, and have even been offered as a service at health-food stores. Plastic skinfold calipers are now being sold as part of a comprehensive weight-loss program on popular television infomercials.

Body composition assessment is central to helping overweight people lose and ultimately manage their weight. A thorough understanding of the accuracy of available body composition assessments is critical for you as a lifestyle and weight management consultant. Methods of assessment vary in expense, precision and bias. Furthermore, the interpretation of body composition information requires sophistication and expertise. This chapter addresses common methods of estimating body composition, including weight measurement, **anthropometric** techniques, bioelectric impedance (BIA) and NIR. The sophisticated, highly accurate methods used in clinical and research settings, such as **densitometry**, total body water and imaging techniques, also are reviewed. The use of body composition to help establish appropriate and realistic weight goals with clients is discussed.

Estimating Body Composition

The most accurate method of assessing body composition is dissection during post-mortem examinations. Indeed, much of what we know about body composition has come from the early work of anatomists and anthropometrists who, through dissection, were able to make assumptions and examine properties of the various body tissues. While dissection is the most precise method to measure body composition,

Table 4.1

Validation Levels for Different Techniques Used to Estimate Body Fat

Validation Level	Technique
Level I - Direct	Dissection
Level II - Indirect *(based upon quantitative assumptions)*	Densitometry Total Body Water Dual Energy X-ray Absorptiometry (DEXA)
Level III - *Doubly Indirect (calibrated against a Level II method)*	Anthropometry Skinfolds Impedance NIR

Source: Adapted from Martin & Drinkwater (1991).

it also is the only way to directly measure it.

Since there are no direct methods of assessing body composition in living human beings, all body composition assessments are indirect and based upon the assumptions of various properties of the body. Martin and Drinkwater (1991) proposed three levels of validation or accuracy for body composition assessment (Table 4.1). The first level is direct assessment and involves dissection. The second level is indirect and measures a parameter other than fat, and the calculation of relative body-fat percentage is based upon the relationship between the measured component and body fat. For example, densitometry (i.e., underwater weighing) assumes that both fat and fat-free tissue have constant densities, and estimates are based on a series of calculations that measures the density of the whole body. This type of assessment is indirect. For example, the assessment of total body water (TBW) assumes that fat-free tissue has a constant fraction of water and that fat has little or no water. Third-level techniques are doubly

Table 4.2

Metropolitan Height–Weight Tables, 1983 (pounds)

Men					Women				
Height		Frame			Height		Frame		
Feet	Inches	Small	Medium	Large	Feet	Inches	Small	Medium	Large
5	2	128-134	131-141	138-150	4	10	102-111	109-121	118-131
5	3	130-136	133-143	140-153	4	11	103-113	111-123	120-134
5	4	132-138	135-145	142-156	5	0	104-115	113-126	122-137
5	5	134-140	137-146	144-160	5	1	106-118	115-129	123-140
5	6	136-142	139-151	140-164	5	2	108-121	118-132	128-143
5	7	138-145	142-154	149-168	5	3	111-124	121-135	131-147
5	8	140-148	145-157	152-172	5	4	114-127	124-138	134-151
5	9	142-151	148-160	155-176	5	5	117-130	127-141	137-155
5	10	144-154	151-163	156-180	5	6	120-133	130-144	140-159
5	11	146-157	154-166	161-184	5	7	123-136	133-147	143-163
6	0	149-160	157-170	164-188	5	8	126-139	136-150	146-167
6	1	152-164	160-174	168-192	5	9	129-142	139-153	149-170
6	2	155-168	164-178	172-197	5	10	132-145	142-156	152-173
6	3	158-172	167-182	176-202	5	11	132-148	145-159	155-176
6	4	162-176	171-187	181-207	6	0	138-151	148-162	158-179

Weight according to frame (ages 25 to 59) for men wearing indoor clothing weighing 5 lbs.; for women wearing indoor clothing weighing 3 lbs.
Source: Reprinted with permission from the Metropolitan Life Insurance Company, New York.

Figure 4.1

Breadth of elbow measurement.

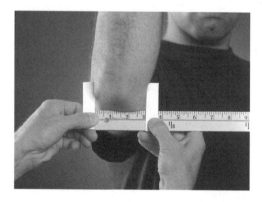

indirect since predictions are based upon Level II estimates.

Assessing Body Composition From Body Weight

Overweight or obesity is an excess of adipose tissue resulting in increased body weight. Body weight is easily measured and can provide useful information when the weight is adjusted for height or stature. You should always measure body weight directly since self-reports tend to be inaccurate. (Many clients will not weigh themselves for several months or even years, and may provide verbal reports of very outdated weights.)

Measuring Body Weight and Height. Accurate balance-beam scales or digital scales designed for commercial use provide the best measures of weight. Scales should be placed on a flat surface. If the floor is carpeted, the scale should be placed on a one-half-inch piece of plywood. Scales need to be calibrated frequently (i.e., weekly). Weight should be measured without footwear and in light clothing (shorts and T-shirt). If you routinely work with clients weighing more than 300 pounds, you may need to purchase a special scale that can precisely measure their weight. It is embarrassing for these clients when their weight cannot be assessed on a typical balance-beam scale. (Worse still, and much less reliable, is to ask the client to stand on two scales simultaneously to measure weight.)

Height is best measured using a wall-mounted stadiometer. The metal sliding stadiometer on the back of most commercial balance-beam scales also can provide reasonable assessments of height.

Height-Weight Tables. Height-Weight tables are widely available and can serve as an initial reference point to assess degree of overweight. Best known and most widely used are the 1983 Metropolitan Life Insurance Company Height-Weight Tables (Table 4.2), which were developed from statistics associated with the lowest risk of **mortality**. Recently, these tables have excluded the words "ideal" or "desirable" due to misinterpretations of their meaning. However, the client's weight can be compared with the suggested weight from the table and expressed as a percentage of the reference weight.

Estimating Frame Size. The 1983 Height–Weight tables also include an adjustment for frame size. The client's frame size can be accurately assessed by measuring the breadth of the elbow. To do this, ask your client to flex their elbow at a 90-degree angle with the upper arm parallel to the floor (Figure 4.1). Measure the distance between the epicondyles (inside and outside projections of the elbow bone) of the humerus. Ideally, this is done with a broad-faced sliding caliper. Smaller-framed persons can be assessed using a good skinfold caliper. If the proper caliper is not available, elbow breadth can be

Table 4.3
Frame Size Determined from
Height and Elbow Breadth

Height	Frame Size Small	Medium	Large
Males			
61-62	<2½	2½ - 2⅞	>2⅞
63-66	<2⅝	2⅝ - 2⅞	>2⅞
67-70	<2¾	2¾ - 3	>3
71-74	<2¾	2¾ - 3⅛	>3⅛
75	<2⅞	2⅞ - 3¼	>3¼
Females			
57-58	<2¼	2¼ - 2½	>2½
59-62	<2¼	2¼ - 2½	>2½
63-66	<2⅜	2⅜ - 2⅝	>2⅝
67-70	<2⅜	2⅜ - 2⅝	>2⅝
71	<2½	2½ - 2¾	>2¾

Height is given in inches, without shoes.

Adapted from Metropolitan Life Insurance Company (1983).

estimated using a metric ruler. Place the thumb and the index finger on the outside of each epicondyle and measure the distance between them with the ruler. Once the elbow breadth has been determined, frame size can be determined from Table 4.3.

Calculating Percent of Ideal Weight. Researchers may use a given percentage of ideal weight as criteria for entry into a study. For example, if we wanted to calculate Becky's percent of ideal weight, we could go to the charts with the following data:

Becky's Current Weight: 175 lbs
Becky's Reference Weight
(Based on a medium frame): 140 lbs

Percent Ideal
$$\frac{(\text{Current Weight} - \text{Reference Weight})}{\text{Current Weight}}$$

$$\frac{175 \text{ lbs} - 140}{175} = 20 \text{ percent above reference weight}$$

Table 4.4
Body Mass Index

Height (inches)	19	20	21	22	23	24	25	26	27	28	29	30	35	40
								Weight (pounds)						
58	91	95	100	105	110	115	119	124	129	134	138	143	167	191
59	94	99	104	109	114	119	124	128	133	138	143	148	173	198
60	97	102	107	112	118	123	128	133	138	143	148	153	179	204
61	100	106	111	116	121	127	132	137	143	148	153	158	185	211
62	104	109	115	120	125	131	136	142	147	153	158	164	191	218
63	107	113	118	124	130	135	141	146	152	158	163	169	197	225
64	110	116	122	128	134	140	145	151	157	163	169	174	203	233
65	114	120	126	132	138	144	150	156	162	168	174	180	210	240
66	117	124	130	136	142	148	155	161	167	173	179	185	216	247
67	121	127	134	140	147	153	159	166	172	178	185	191	223	255
68	125	131	138	144	151	158	164	171	177	184	190	197	230	263
69	128	135	142	149	155	162	169	176	182	189	196	203	237	270
70	132	139	146	153	160	167	174	181	188	195	202	209	243	278
71	136	143	150	157	165	172	179	186	193	200	207	215	250	286
72	140	147	155	162	169	177	184	191	199	206	213	221	258	294
73	144	151	159	166	174	182	189	197	204	212	219	227	265	303
74	148	155	163	171	179	187	194	202	210	218	225	233	272	311
75	152	160	168	176	184	192	200	208	216	224	232	240	279	319
76	156	164	172	180	189	197	205	213	221	230	238	246	287	328

Body Mass Index. More useful estimates of body composition can be obtained by adjusting weight for height or stature and calculating a height-normalized index. The most commonly used index is the **Body Mass Index (BMI)** or Quetlet index, which is calculated as follows:

$$BMI = \frac{Weight\ (kg)}{Height\ (m^2)}$$

Example: Weight = 95.2 kg
Height = 1.72 m

$$BMI = \frac{95.2}{(1.72)^2} = 32.2$$

Use Table 4.4 to determine body mass index. Find your client's height in the far left column, and move across the row to the weight that is closest to their own. Their body mass index will be at the top of that column.

People in a normal weight range usually have a BMI between 19 and 25. Individuals who are considered mildly overweight make up approximately 90 percent of the overweight population, are 20 percent to 40 percent above their normal weight and tend to have BMIs between 27 and 30. Moderately overweight people make up 9.5 percent of the overweight population, are considered 41 percent to 100 percent

Table 4.5
BMI Reference Chart

Weight Category	BMI Range	Percent Above Normal Weight
Normal Weight	19-25	——
Overweight	27-30	20-40 percent
Obese	31-35	41-100 percent
Seriously Obese	Over 35	>100 percent

Table 4.6
Anatomic Locations of Circumference Measurement Sites

Circumference	Anatomic Site
Abdominal	At the level of the umbilicus
Hips	The largest circumference below the umbilicus
Illiac	Level with the illiac crests
Waist	The narrowest part of the torso.

over their normal weight, and have BMIs between 30.1 and 35. Finally, severely overweight individuals are more than 100 percent above their normal weight, comprise only .5 percent of overweight people and have BMIs greater than 35 (Table 4.5).

Since BMI uses total body weight (i.e., not estimates of fat and lean body mass separately) in the calculation, it does not discriminate between the over-fat and the athletic, more muscled body type. Therefore, body composition assessments should ideally be used in conjunction with BMI.

Anthropometry

Anthropometric assessments of body composition are perhaps the easiest and least expensive methods for assessing body composition. These include circumference and skinfold measures, which are readily used in the field. Anthropometric measures also can be used to estimate body fat and the distribution of body fat (i.e., central vs. peripheral or upper vs. lower body).

Circumference Measures. Circumference measures can easily be used to assess body composition, even with significantly overweight clients. However, to ensure accuracy, the exact anatomical landmarks for taking each circumference measurement must be carefully

utilized (Table 4.6 and Figures 4.2 - 4.5). A thorough review of anthropometric measurement sites and techniques for optimizing accuracy are presented in Lohman et al. (1988).

A cloth or fiberglass (i.e., non-elastic) measurement tape must be used. The tape should be periodically calibrated against a meter stick to ensure it hasn't been stretched. When assessing significantly overweight clients, be sure to use a long enough tape. Pull the tape tight enough to keep it in position without causing an indentation of the skin.

Estimating Body Fat From Circumference Measures. Tran and Weltman (1989) developed a generalized equation for predicting the body density of women from girth measurements. They used the following equation to predict body density (measurements in cm):

Body Density = 1.168297 - (0.002824 x abdomen) + (0.0000122098 x abdomen^2) - (0.000733128 x hips) + (0.000510477 x height) - (0.000216161 x age)

A similar equation was developed to predict body composition in men by Tran et al. (1988). They reported the following equation:

CHAPTER FOUR

BODY
COMPOSITION
ASSESSMENT

$$BF\% = 47.371817 +$$
$$(0.57914807 \times abdomen) +$$
$$(0.25189114 \times hips) +$$
$$(0.21366088 \times iliac) -$$
$$(0.35595404 \times weight)$$

Weltman and colleagues (1988) developed an equation to predict body-fat percentage (BF%) in overweight women (i.e., those with BF% ≤ 40%) using the abdominal circumference measure, height and weight.

$$BF\% = 0.11077 (X_1) -$$
$$0.17666 (X_2) +$$
$$0.14354 (X_3) +$$
$$51.03301$$

X_1= Abdominal girth (cm)
X_2 = height (cm)
X_3 = weight (kg)

Estimating Body-Fat Distribution.
Since upper-body or abdominal obesity is known to increase health risk (Van Itallie, 1988), it is important to assess your client's body-fat distribution. The most widely used technique is the waist-to-hip circumference ratio (WTH), which offers a fast and reliable assessment of fat distribution. The WTH ratio is calculated by dividing the waist measurement by the hip measurement to determine the ratio. Table 4.8 illustrates

Table 4.7
Anatomic Locations of Skinfold Measurement Sites

Skinfold	Anatomic Site
Abdomen	A vertical fold taken 1 inch to the left of the umbilicus
Bicep	A vertical fold taken anteneriorly halfway between the acromian and olecranon processes
Chest	A diagonal fold taken halfway between the armpit and the nipple for men and one-third the distance for women
Subscapular	A diagonal fold taken just below the inferior angle of the scapula
Suprailiac	A diagonal fold taken just above the iliac crest at the midaxillary line
Tricep	A vertical fold taken posteriorly to the bicep skinfold

the relative risk ratings for WTH ratios.

Skinfold Measures. Body-fat percentage can be predicted from a single skinfold site, but is typically derived from a more complex equation using the sum of several skinfolds in combination with other predictors of body-fat distribution. These predictors can include

Figure 4.2
Measuring the abdominal circumference.

Figure 4.3
Measuring the circumference of the hips.

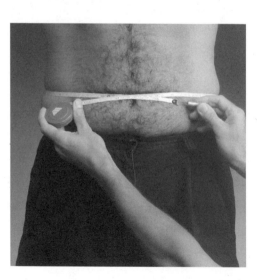

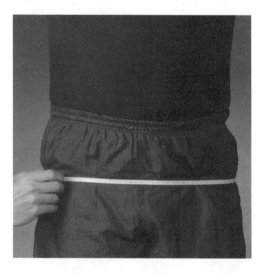

weight, height, age and activity level. The reliability of skinfold measures of body fat is not as high as other methods of estimating body fat since human error tends to be higher with this method. However, test-retest reliability for a skilled anthropometrist can be quite high.

The proper use of skinfold calipers appears deceptively simple. Mastery of the skinfold technique requires formal training and a great deal of practice (Table 4.7, Figures 4.6 - 4.11). For example, Ross and Marfell-Jones (1984) suggest that reasonable skinfold competence can be achieved after triple measurements and spot-checking on 100 or more subjects.

Methodological Issues. Research has proven that different prediction equations can result in highly variable estimates. It has been suggested that many skinfold body-fat prediction models are limited to the volunteers that were used to develop the models. For example, an equation that was derived to predict body fat in male wrestlers is not as accurate in middle-aged men. Thus, skinfold equations will be most accurate when they are gender-, age-, fatness- and fitness- or sport-specific.

The skinfold technique is based upon two assumptions: (a) the thickness of the **subcutaneous** adipose tissue

Table 4.8
Waist-to-Hip Ratios and Associated Level of Health Risks

High Risk	>1.0	> 0.85
Moderately High Risk	0.90-1.0	0.80-0.85
Lower Risk	<0.90	<0.80

Adapted from Van Itallie (1988).

reflects a constant proportion of total body fat, and (b) the site chosen represents the average thickness of adipose tissue throughout the body. Lukaski (1987) noted that neither of these assumptions have been validated experimentally.

It is critical that the anthropometrist obtain the exact anatomical landmark when using the skinfold technique. A good review of the measurement sites and techniques for optimizing accuracy is presented in Lohman et al. (1988).

Obtaining Accurate Skinfold Measures. Have the client relax the underlying musculature as much as possible. When the skinfold site has been determined, use the thumb and index finger to grasp the fold and the underlying fat. Next, "draw up" the fold. It should not be pinched too hard, and the fingers should not compress the fold. The jaws of the calipers should be

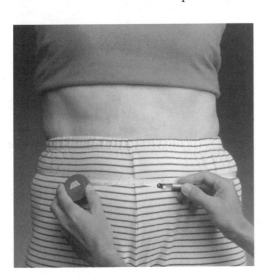

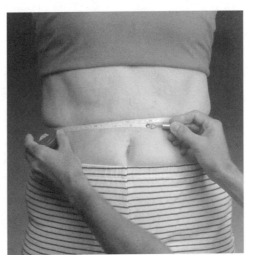

Figure 4.4
Measuring the circumference at the iliac crest.

Figure 4.5
Measuring waist circumference.

Figure 4.6
a. Triceps skinfold
location.

b. Triceps skinfold
measurement.

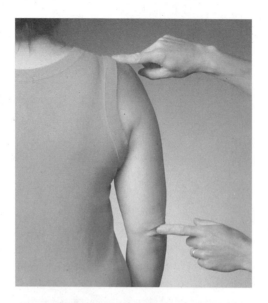

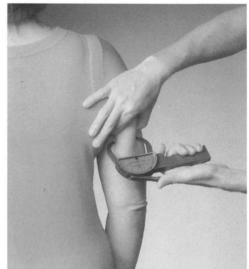

Figure 4.7
Iliac crest skinfold
measurement.

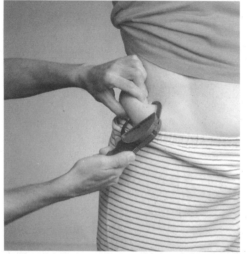

**Sources of Variation Associated
with Skinfold Measurements:**

1. Variability in the way different
   appraisers measure skinfolds
2. Variability in brand of skinfold
   calipers used
3. Variability from different prediction equations
4. Variability in the ratio of subcutaneous to internal fat at different sites on the body

Figure 4.8
a. Thigh skinfold
location — female.

b. Thigh skinfold mea-
surement — female.

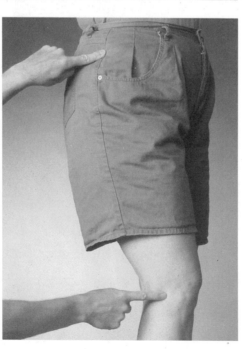

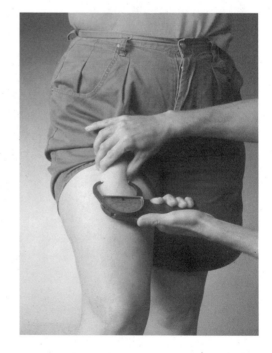

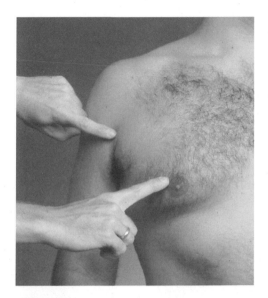

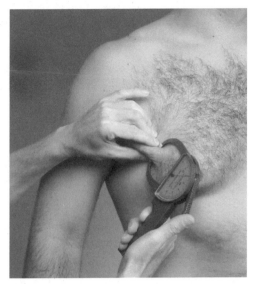

Figure 4.9
a. Chest skinfold location — male.

b. Chest skinfold measurement — male.

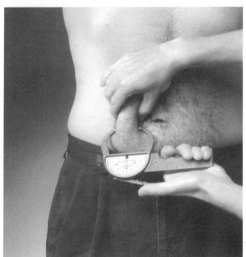

Why Skinfold Measurements are Problematic in Significantly Overweight Individuals

1. The calipers may not open wide enough to measure the entire fold.
2. There is often difficulty determining the amount of tissue to be picked up when forming the fold.
3. There may be difficulty in determining the muscle-to-fat interface.
4. Anatomical landmarks are hard to accurately identify.
5. The compression of fat may affect subsequent measures.
6. Clients may feel discomfort and embarrassment.

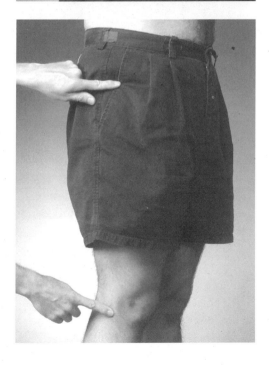

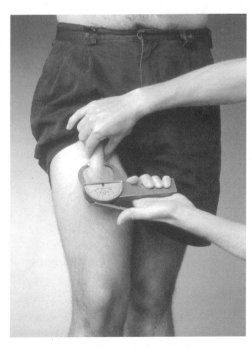

Figure 4.10
Abdominal skinfold measurement — male.

Figure 4.11
a. Thigh skinfold location — male.

b. Thigh skinfold measurement — male.

Table 4.9

Durnin and Womersley Percent Body Fat Estimations for Women

Sum of Skinfolds	Percent Fat	Sum of Skinfolds	Percent Fat	Sum of Skinfolds	Percent Fat	Sum of Skinfolds	Percent Fat
15-16	12	31-33	22	63-66	32	122-130	42
17	13	34-35	23	67-71	33	131-139	43
18	14	36-38	24	72-76	34	140-148	44
19-20	15	39-41	25	77-81	35	149-158	45
21	16	42-44	26	82-87	36	159-168	46
22-23	17	45-47	27	88-93	37	169-180	47
24	18	48-50	28	94-99	38	181-192	48
25-26	19	52-54	29	100-106	39	193-204	49
27-28	20	55-58	30	107-114	40	205-218	50
29-30	21	59-62	31	115-121	41		

Table 4.10

Durnin and Womersley Percent Body Fat Estimations for Men

Sum of Skinfolds	Percent Fat	Sum of Skinfolds	Percent Fat	Sum of Skinfolds	Percent Fat	Sum of Skinfolds	Percent Fat
15-16	5	31-33	15	62-66	25	121-128	35
17	6	34-35	16	67-70	26	129-137	36
18	7	36-38	17	71-75	27	138-146	37
19-20	8	39-40	18	76-81	28	147-156	38
21	9	41-43	19	82-86	29	157-166	39
22-23	10	44-47	20	87-92	30	167-177	40
24	11	48-50	21	93-98	31	178-188	41
25-26	12	51-53	22	99-105	32	189-201	42
27-28	13	54-57	23	106-112	33		
29-30	14	58-61	24	113-120	34		

opened at right angles to the fold. The tips of the calipers should come into contact with the skinfold about 1 centimeter below the point where the skinfold was raised. Maintain pressure on the fold with the fingers and thumb, then release as the calipers take hold. The measurement should be made about four seconds after the caliper settles. Record the thickness of the fold in millimeters. Three measurements should be taken at each measurement site, with the median or middle value used to determine the recorded measurement.

Generalized equations to predict body composition. Body composition can be estimated in men and women using the following Durnin and Womersley (1974) equations.

Here is an example of a male client:

Triceps: 22 mm
Biceps: 18 mm
Subscapular: 26 mm
Suprailliac: 29 mm

Step 1. Calculate the sum of four sites:

22 + 18 + 26 + 29 = 96 mm.

Step 2: Tables 4.9 and 4.10 are provided so you can look-up the estimated body fat percentage from the sum of the four sites used in the Durnin and Womersly formula.

The Jackson and Pollock (1978) and the Jackson, Pollock and Ward (1980) generalized equations are frequently used by anthropometrists to predict body composition. These equations both use age as one of the predictor variables. The equations are as follows:

1. For women (Jackson, Pollock and Ward, 1980):
Body Density = 1.09949921 - 0.0009929 (X1) + 0.0000023 (X2)^2 - 0.0001392 (age in years)

2. For men (Jackson and Pollock, 1978):
Body Density = 1.10938 - 0.0008267 (X2) + 0.0000016 (X2)^2 - 0.0002574 (age in years)

X1 = the sum of the triceps, thigh and suprailliac skinfolds
X2 = the sum of the chest, abdominal and thigh skinfolds
Use Tables 4.11 and 4.12 to determine the estimated body-fat percentage using age and the sum of the three sites used in the Jackson and Pollock and the Jackson, Pollock and Ward formulas.

The Durin and Womersley formula and the Jackson and Pollock formula provide equally accurate results for the middle-age and younger subject. The age coefficient in the Jackson and Pollock equations accounts for the migration of fat from the subcutaneous to the **viscera** in older adults.

Once you have calculated a client's body-fat percentage, use Table 4.13 to determine where they fall within a range of norms. It is generally agreed that a body-fat percentage greater than 25 for men and 32 for women is the cut-off for obesity and is considered to be a health risk. The primary value of estimating body-fat is that it can show change over time. This table gives you some general categories for various body-fat percentages, but all reasonable weight determinations should be based on many factors.

Bio-electric Impedance Analysis

Bio-electric Impedance Analysis (BIA) is a relatively inexpensive, safe and portable method of assessing body composition. Disposable surface electrodes are attached to the hand, wrist, foot and ankle. The analyzer introduces a known current through the **proximal** electrodes that is detected by the **distal** electrodes and offers a measure of resistance. Fat-free tissue is known to be a good conductor of electrical current, whereas adipose tissue is a poor conductor. The result is a significant relationship between both the fat-free tissue and total body water of the individual, and the resistance detected by the analyzer.

BIA Equations. BIA analyzers are often programmed with prediction equations to estimate body composition. These equations vary, but most include variables such as height, weight, sex and age in addition to resistance. Other input variables may include the level of body fatness, phase angle obtained from the analyzer or reactance.

Recent reports have found that generalized BIA equations may not accurately estimate body composition in certain ethnic groups and in significantly under- and overweight individuals. For example, Eckerson and colleagues (1992) found that body weight alone estimated **fat-free mass** (FFM) as accurately as eight different BIA equations in lean males. Thus, the use of the BIA analyzer did not improve the accuracy

Table 4.11

Percent Body Fat Estimations for Women — Jackson and Pollock Formula

Sum of Skinfolds (mm)	Age Groups								
	Under 22	23-27	28-32	33-37	38-42	43-47	48-52	53-57	Over 57
23-25	9.7	9.9	10.2	10.4	10.7	10.9	11.2	11.4	11.7
26-28	11.0	11.2	11.5	11.7	12.0	12.3	12.5	12.7	13.0
29-31	12.3	12.5	12.8	13.0	13.3	13.5	13.8	14.0	14.3
32-34	13.6	13.8	14.0	14.3	14.5	14.8	15.0	15.3	15.5
35-37	14.8	15.0	15.3	15.5	15.8	16.0	16.3	16.5	16.8
38-40	16.0	16.3	16.5	16.7	17.0	17.2	17.5	17.7	18.0
41-43	17.2	17.4	17.7	17.9	18.2	18.4	18.7	18.9	19.2
44-46	18.3	18.6	18.8	19.1	19.3	19.6	19.8	20.1	20.3
47-49	19.5	19.7	20.0	20.2	20.5	20.7	21.0	21.2	21.5
50-52	20.6	20.8	21.1	21.3	21.6	21.8	22.1	22.3	22.6
53-55	21.7	21.9	22.1	22.4	22.6	22.9	23.1	23.4	23.6
56-58	22.7	23.0	23.2	23.4	23.7	23.9	24.2	24.4	24.7
59-61	23.7	24.0	24.2	24.5	24.7	25.0	25.2	25.5	25.7
62-64	24.7	25.0	25.2	25.5	25.7	26.0	26.7	26.4	26.7
65-67	25.7	25.9	26.2	26.4	26.7	26.9	27.2	27.4	27.7
68-70	26.6	26.9	27.1	27.4	27.6	27.9	28.1	28.4	28.6
71-73	27.5	27.8	28.0	28.3	28.5	28.8	29.0	29.3	29.5
74-76	28.4	28.7	28.9	29.2	29.4	29.7	29.9	30.2	30.4
77-79	29.3	29.5	29.8	30.0	30.3	30.5	30.8	31.0	31.3
80-82	30.1	30.4	30.6	30.9	31.1	31.4	31.6	31.9	32.1
83-85	30.9	31.2	31.4	31.7	31.9	32.2	32.4	32.7	32.9
86-88	31.7	32.0	32.2	32.5	32.7	32.9	33.2	33.4	33.7
89-91	32.5	32.7	33.0	33.2	33.5	33.7	33.9	34.2	34.4
92-94	33.2	33.4	33.7	33.9	34.2	34.4	34.7	34.9	35.2
95-97	33.9	34.1	34.4	34.6	34.9	35.1	35.4	35.6	35.9
98-100	34.6	34.8	35.1	35.3	35.5	35.8	36.0	36.3	36.5
101-103	35.3	35.4	35.7	35.9	36.2	36.4	36.7	36.9	37.2
104-106	35.8	36.1	36.3	36.6	36.8	37.1	37.3	37.5	37.8
107-109	36.4	36.7	36.9	37.1	37.4	37.6	37.9	38.1	38.4
110-112	37.0	37.2	37.5	37.7	38.0	38.2	38.5	38.7	38.9
113-115	37.5	37.8	38.0	38.2	38.5	38.7	39.0	39.2	39.5
116-118	38.0	38.3	38.5	38.8	39.0	39.3	39.5	39.7	40.0
119-121	38.5	38.7	39.0	39.2	39.5	39.7	40.0	40.2	40.5
122-124	39.0	39.2	39.4	39.7	39.9	40.2	40.4	40.7	40.9
125-127	39.4	39.6	39.9	40.1	40.4	40.6	40.9	41.1	41.4
128-130	39.8	40.0	40.3	40.5	40.8	41.0	41.3	41.5	41.8

Source: Jackson, A.S. & Pollock, M. L (1985). *Practical Assessment of Body Composition*.
Reprinted with permission of McGraw-Hill.

Table 4.12

Percent Body Fat Estimations for Men — Jackson and Pollock Formula

Sum of Skinfolds (mm)	Age Groups								
	Under 22	23-27	28-32	33-37	38-42	43-47	48-52	53-57	Over 57
8-10	1.3	1.8	2.3	2.9	3.4	3.9	4.5	5.0	5.5
11-13	2.2	2.8	3.3	3.9	4.4	4.9	5.5	6.0	6.5
14-16	3.2	3.8	4.3	4.8	5.4	5.9	6.4	7.0	7.5
17-19	4.2	4.7	5.3	5.8	6.3	6.9	7.4	8.0	8.5
20-22	5.1	5.7	6.2	6.8	7.3	7.9	8.4	8.9	9.5
23-25	6.1	6.6	7.2	7.7	8.3	8.8	9.4	9.9	10.5
26-28	7.0	7.6	8.1	8.7	9.2	9.8	10.3	10.9	11.4
29-31	8.0	8.5	9.1	9.6	10.2	10.7	11.3	11.8	12.4
32-34	8.9	9.4	10.0	10.5	11.1	11.6	12.2	12.8	13.3
35-37	9.8	10.4	10.9	11.5	12.0	12.6	13.1	13.7	14.3
38-40	10.7	11.3	11.8	12.4	12.9	13.5	14.1	14.6	15.2
41-43	11.6	12.2	12.7	13.3	13.8	14.4	15.0	15.5	16.1
44-46	12.5	13.1	13.6	14.2	14.7	15.3	15.9	16.4	17.0
47-49	13.4	13.9	14.5	15.1	15.6	16.2	16.8	17.3	17.9
50-52	14.3	14.8	15.4	15.9	16.5	17.1	17.6	18.2	18.8
53-55	15.1	15.7	16.2	16.8	17.4	17.9	18.5	19.1	19.7
56-58	16.0	16.5	17.1	17.7	18.2	18.8	19.4	20.0	20.5
59-61	16.9	17.4	17.9	18.5	19.1	19.7	20.2	20.8	21.4
62-64	17.6	18.2	18.8	19.4	19.9	20.5	21.1	21.7	22.2
65-67	18.5	19.0	19.6	20.2	20.8	21.3	21.9	22.5	23.1
68-70	19.3	19.9	20.4	21.0	21.6	22.2	22.7	23.3	23.9
71-73	20.1	20.7	21.2	21.8	22.4	23.0	23.6	24.1	24.7
74-76	20.9	21.5	22.0	22.6	23.2	23.8	24.4	25.0	25.5
77-79	21.7	22.2	22.8	23.4	24.0	24.6	25.2	25.8	26.3
80-82	22.4	23.0	23.6	24.2	24.8	25.4	25.9	26.5	27.1
83-85	23.2	23.8	24.4	25.0	25.5	26.1	26.7	27.3	27.9
86-88	24.0	24.5	25.1	25.7	26.3	26.9	27.5	28.1	28.7
89-91	24.7	25.3	25.9	26.5	27.1	27.6	28.2	28.8	29.4
92-94	25.4	26.0	26.6	27.2	27.8	28.4	29.0	29.6	30.2
95-97	26.1	26.7	27.3	27.9	28.5	29.1	29.7	30.3	30.9
98-100	26.9	27.4	28.0	28.6	29.2	29.8	30.4	31.0	31.6
101-103	27.5	28.1	28.7	29.3	29.9	30.5	31.1	31.7	32.3
104-106	28.2	28.8	29.4	30.0	30.6	31.2	31.8	32.4	33.0
107-109	28.9	29.5	30.1	30.7	31.3	31.9	32.5	33.1	33.7
110-112	29.6	30.2	30.8	31.4	32.0	32.6	33.2	33.8	34.4
113-115	30.2	30.8	31.4	32.0	32.6	33.2	33.8	34.5	35.1
116-118	30.9	31.5	32.1	32.7	33.3	33.9	34.5	35.1	35.7
119-121	31.5	32.1	32.7	33.3	33.9	34.5	35.1	35.7	36.4
122-124	32.1	32.7	33.3	33.9	34.5	35.1	35.8	36.4	37.0
125-127	32.7	33.3	33.9	34.5	35.1	35.8	36.4	37.0	37.6

Source: Jackson, A.S. & Pollock, M.L (1985) *Practical Assessment of Body Composition*.
Reprinted with permission of McGraw-Hill.

of estimating FFM from body weight alone. Furthermore, the manufacturer's equations have been found to underestimate body-fat percentage in overweight women (Heyward et al., 1992; Andersen et al., 1994). When using BIA to assess overweight individuals, fat- and gender-specific equations (Segal et al., 1988) have been shown to significantly improve estimates of body composition in this group (Andersen et al., 1994).

The Segal Equation for women with greater than 30 percent fat is as follows:

FFM = 9.4 + 0.000912 (ht²) - 0.0147 (resistance) + 0.299 (wt) - 0.070 (age)

Height in cm
Resistance in ohms
Weight in kg
Age in years

The Segal Equation for men with greater than 20 percent fat is as follows:

FFM = 9.4 + 0.000664 (ht²) - 0.0212 (resistance) + 0.628 (wt) - 0.124 (age)

BIA analyzers produced by different manufacturers may yield different estimates of resistance in healthy student populations (Graves et al., 1989). Differences in resistance as large as 50 ohms have been reported between analyzers used on overweight individuals (Andersen et al., 1994).

Improving BIA Accuracy. Recently, investigators have found that moving the proximal leads from the wrist and ankle to the antecubital (elbow) and popliteal (knee) space may decrease the error of the estimate (Steen et al., 1995; Lukaski et al., 1994). The theory behind changing the electrode placement is that the distal arm and leg offer more than half of the resistance detected by the BIA analyzer. However, the contribution of these limbs to the total body mass is minimal. Regardless,

the proposed proximal lead configuration allows the current to travel through tissue that more closely reflects the total body. New equations are currently being developed with this lead configuration.

Additionally, BIA analyzers have historically used a frequency of 50 kHz. Companies are now developing multiple-frequency impedance analyzers, which may allow a better estimate of both body composition and total body water.

Near Infrared Interactance

Near infrared interactance (NIR) uses the principles of light absorption and reflection to estimate body composition. This technique was developed using very sophisticated and expensive computerized equipment in research and hospital settings. Recently, less expensive NIR equipment has been developed (e.g., Futrex™) for use in field testing, weight-loss centers and health clubs. These low-cost NIR systems gather light-interactance information via an optic probe that is typically placed over the belly of the biceps muscle. The NIR data, height, weight, activity level and frame size are entered into a prediction equation to estimate body composition.

There are several problems with the single-site, less-expensive NIR equipment. First, it is relatively inaccurate and does not predict body composition as well as skinfold measures. Second, the technique uses a generalized prediction equation that does not provide accurate predictions for significantly under- and overweight individuals.

Research and Laboratory Methods

Field estimates of body composition simply divide the body into two components: fat and fat-free mass.

Researchers and healthcare professionals are interested in further compartmentalizing the body. For example, it is common for obesity researchers to examine the changes in fat, fat-free tissue, bone mass and total body water that typically accompany weight loss. Following are some of the most commonly used methods to accurately estimate body composition in clinical and research settings.

Densitometry (Underwater or Hydrostatic Weighing)

Densitometry is one of the oldest techniques for estimating body composition and, for years, has been used as the "gold standard" against which new methods or equations to predict body composition were compared. This procedure divides the body into two compartments: fat and fat-free mass. Underwater body weight and scale-measured weight are used to estimate body density. Individuals are immersed in a heated, water-filled tank while sitting on a chair that is suspended from a scale. While completely submerged, subjects exhale all of the air in the lungs and attempt to remain as still as possible while underwater. (Subjects who have never undergone underwater weighing may require extra time to practice the technique.) A minimum of six attempts should be made, since underwater weight tends to improve as subjects become more comfortable with being underwater without air. The most commonly duplicated reading of underwater weight is used to calculate body density.

Most research laboratories measure residual lung volume during or before underwater weighing. This is important since it allows underwater weight to be corrected for differences in **residual air** (which affect buoyancy). Because water density varies, a correction for water temperature also must be used when

Table 4.13
General Body-fat Percentage Categories

Classification	Women (% fat)	Men (% fat)
Essential Fat	10-12%	2-4%
Athletes	14-20%	6-13%
Fitness	21-24%	14-17%
Acceptable	25-31%	18-25%
Obese	32 and higher	25 and higher

calculating body density. A diver's belt is often secured to the chair or around the overweight person's waist to ensure that the individual does not involuntarily float to the surface during the procedure.

Calculations of body density assume that fat in the body has a density of 0.9007 g/cc and that fat-free mass has a uniform density of 1.100 g/cc. While fat density tends to remain fairly constant, the density of fat-free mass can vary considerably among different populations. Young black males have been found to have a fat-free mass that is denser than 1.100 g/cc, whereas elderly women may have less. The densitometry model assumes that all of the components of the FFM are in constant proportions. For example, bone is thought to make up a constant 17 percent of the FFM. Again, a **post-menopausal** woman with **osteoporosis** would have different bone density than a mature athlete with dense bones.

Once whole-body density has been determined, the fraction of fat and fat-free weight can be estimated. The following equation is commonly used to estimate body fat:

$$\text{Body fat \%} = \left(\frac{4.95}{\text{Body density}} - 4.5 \right) \times 100$$

The weight of fat-free mass can be calculated as follows:

Fat-free mass =
Body weight (kg) -
Fat-weight (kg)

The weight of fat mass can be calculated as follows:

$$\text{Fat Weight (kg)} = \frac{\text{Body Weight (kg) x Percent Fat}}{100}$$

Dual Energy X-ray Absorptiometry (DEXA)

Dual Energy X-ray Absorptiometry (DEXA) has become a popular method for assessing body composition. This is due, in large part, to its relative accuracy. This technique uses a very-low-dose X-ray to separate the body into three compartments: fat, fat-free tissue and bone mineral. Regional measurements of fat (e.g., arms, legs and trunk) also are possible with DEXA. Many body composition experts believe that DEXA will replace densitometry as the standard of measurement.

DEXA systems are costly ($70,000 - $100,000) and in some states, a licensed x-ray technician is required to operate DEXA equipment. A sample report from a DEXA assessment is presented in Figure 4.12.

Total Body Water

Fat-free mass can be estimated by measuring total body water (TBW), since almost all of the body's water is located in fat-free tissue. This method assumes that fat-free tissue has a constant proportion of water (e.g., 73.2 percent). Fat-free mass can be estimated by using the following formula:

$$\text{FFM} = \frac{\text{TBW}}{0.732}$$

So, if you found that a 60 kg woman had 35 liters of body water you could calculate that she had 47.8 kg of FFM. For example:

$$\frac{35 \text{ liters}}{0.732} = 47.8 \text{ kg of FFM}$$

In order to measure TBW, the individual must allow a radioactive tracer to settle proportionately throughout the entire body. An absolute volume of a tracer is either injected or ingested. Once the tracer has settled, TBW can be estimated by measuring the concentration of the tracer in the urine, blood or saliva. Small fluctuations (~2 percent) in total body water will occur during the menstrual cycle.

Imaging Techniques

Fat and fat-free regional tissue mass can be accurately quantified by using imaging techniques. These techniques also can distinguish between visceral and subcutaneous fat. Computed axial tomography (CT) and magnetic resonance imaging (MRI) are the most widely used methods. Both procedures are costly and time consuming, and the CT scans involve exposure to radiation.

Using Body Composition Results to Determine a Reasonable Body Weight

Helping clients determine a goal weight that is realistic and achievable is one the biggest challenges that you may face as a lifestyle and weight management consultant. When working with mildly overweight individuals, determining a reasonable body weight is relatively straightforward. For individuals who have small to moderate amounts of weight to lose (i.e., up to 20 pounds for women and 25 pounds for men) and do not have a long history of weight problems some simple arithmetic calculations based on body composition results are helpful.

Dan, for example, is a 32-year-old executive who works long hours and travels frequently. He has recently gained weight and is seeking advice on how to shed some pounds. During an initial interview, Dan reveals that he played varsity basketball and would like to regain the body he had in college. Your initial assessment established that he is 6'3" tall and weighs 225 pounds — his highest lifetime weight. Bio-electric impedance analysis measures of body composition in men indicates that about 25 percent of Dan's weight is body fat. After determining that 15 percent fat is a reasonable body-fat percentage for Dan, the following calculations can be made:

Note: Remember that you must convert percentages to decimals to manipulate them in these equations. To do this, divide the percent by 100; the quotient will be a decimal number that you can use (i.e., 25 percent divided by 100 equals 0.25).

Current weight = 225 lbs
Fat weight = 225 lbs x 0.25 = 56.25 pounds of fat

Fat-free weight = 225 lbs - 56.25 lbs = 168.75 pounds fat-free tissue

Ideal weight based upon 15% fat =

$$\frac{168.75}{0.85\ [1.00 - .15]} = 198 \text{ pounds}$$

The above example illustrates a reasonable weight for Dan. Remember, he hasn't struggled with his weight for very long, and he has only a moderate amount (less than 25 pounds) of weight to lose.

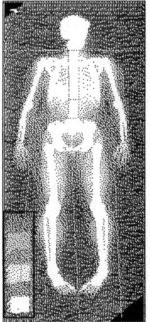

CHILDREN'S HOSPITAL OF PHILADELPHIA

Z10239518   Mon Oct 23 16:39 1995
Name:
Comment: wt loss 2nd scan
I.D.:   wt loss 6   Sex: F
S.S.#:   - -   Ethnic: C
ZIPCode: Height: 163.15 cm
Scan Code: BSZ Weight: 73.50 kg
BirthDate: 12/07/56   Age: 38
Physician: ANDERSEN
Image not for diagnostic use
  ?
 F.S.   68.00%   0(10.00)%
 Head assumes 17.0% brain fat
 LBM 73.2% water

Region	Fat (grams)	Lean+BMC (grams)	% Fat (%)
L Arm	1811.5	1559.6	53.7
R Arm	1707.6	1744.8	49.5
Trunk	11338.2	21147.9	34.9
L Leg	6590.2	7927.6	45.4
R Leg	6888.7	7907.5	46.6
SubTot	28336.3	40287.4	41.3
Head	715.2	3221.9	18.2
TOTAL	29051.5	43509.4	40.0

·Oct 23 17:07 1995 [333 x 152]
Hologic QDR-2000 (S/N 2219)
Enhanced Array Whole Body V5.67A

HOLOGIC

Figure 4.12
A sample report from a DEXA assessment.

Realistic Body Weight for Overweight Clients

Reasonable or realistic weight versus ideal weight is crucial for you to understand when working with overweight clients. Many unfortunate situations have occurred when naive healthcare providers (exercise specialists, weight-loss counselors, dietitians, physicians, nurses, etc.) assigned unrealistically low goal weights for their clients. Individuals who have a lifetime history of obesity (e.g., childhood-onset obesity), a strong family history of obesity, or have medical or other conditions that make weight management more difficult (e.g., use of specific medications) will be unlikely to maintain their "ideal weight" for more than a short period.

Lisa provides a good example. Lisa is 5'4" tall and is 35 years old. She has four children and has been overweight since she was about 2 years old. Both her mother and her father are significantly overweight, as are one sister and a brother. (Another sister exercises and diets strenuously and has maintained a low weight throughout most of her adult life.)

While reviewing Lisa's weight and dieting history, you establish that in college she weighed about 175 pounds. With the birth of each child, she gained more than 60 pounds, and was able to lose only about 35 to 40 pounds afterward. She now weighs 250 pounds. Lisa has dieted down to 150 pounds in the past, but maintained that weight only two weeks before starting to regain.

Underwater weighing determined that Lisa's body-fat percentage was 47 percent. After seeing an article in a popular women's magazine, Lisa seeks your services, stating that she wants to reach her "ideal" weight of 130 pounds with a body-fat percentage of 15 percent to 18 percent fat. She tells you that even at 150 pounds, she still felt "too fat."

Current weight = 250 lbs
Fat weight = 250 lbs x
.47 [47 percent] = 117.5 lbs

Fat-free weight = 250 lbs - 117.5 lbs = 132.5 lbs

Ideal weight based upon 18 % fat =

$$\frac{132.5 \text{ lbs}}{.82 \ [1.00 - .18]} = 161.6 \text{ lbs}$$

A quick glance back at the Metropolitan Life Height-Weight Tables on page 74 reveals that the recommended weight for a medium-framed woman of Lisa's height would be between 124 and 138 pounds. As the above calculations illustrate, this is the present weight of her fat-free mass. In essence, Lisa wants to lose ALL the fat in her body (a physiological impossibility).

These simple calculations illustrate how unrealistic "ideal" weights may be for significantly overweight individuals. There are many reasons why it is unlikely that Lisa could maintain a weight as low as 130 pounds for any significant period of time. For example, as body weight increases beyond 140 percent of ideal weight, a strong probability exists that both her fat cell number and size have increased. The increased number of fat cells will make it very difficult for her to maintain a traditional "ideal" weight.

Setting Weight-loss Goals with Overweight Clients

Our society covets lean, athletic, beautiful bodies. Many clients begin a weight-loss program with a specific "goal" weight in mind. It is important to determine how this goal weight was selected and whether it is realistic.

Caution must be used in assigning an "ideal" or "goal" weight. As a lifestyle and weight management consultant you should help people set a primary goal of reducing their body weight by 10 percent. After this primary goal has been met, it is easier to identify the next reasonable and achievable goal, taking into account how the individual fared with lifestyle changes made so far. Wadden and Foster (1992) have suggested that the overweight adult's initial goal weight should be no lower than the client's lowest weight achieved since the age of 21 that they successfully maintained for one year.

For Lisa, a long-term goal may be to reduce her body weight to 175 pounds since that was her lowest weight since age 21. A weight loss of this magnitude is frequently associated with significantly improved health status, such as positive changes in **cholesterol**, blood pressure, **lipid profiles**, etc. (Andersen et al., 1995). Helping Lisa achieve and maintain a weight of 175 pounds would be an important step to improving her health and fitness. Though her stated goal is to lose 120 pounds, it is important to help her realize that the loss of 75 pounds is no small task and indeed worthwhile.

Helping clients understand the importance of losing and keeping off any amount of excess weight is the greatest challenge. Clients often more readily accept goal weights that are unrealistic, though socially desirable, than those that are realistic and achievable. It is often discouraging for clients to hear that modest weight-loss goals (e.g., 10 percent of present weight) may be the most realistic. However, it is important for you to establish realistic and attainable goals from the outset.

Body Composition and the Drive for Excessive Leanness: A Caution

It is well known that excess body fat impedes performance in athletes. This can be more of an issue in sports such as wrestling, light rowing, gymnastics and dancing. Yet few sports have escaped the notion that there is an optimal body weight that will maximize both performance and the aesthetic appeal.

Unfortunately, the drive for excessive leanness is not limited to athletes. A glance at both male and female models on popular magazine covers reveals extremely lean and muscled bodies. You must exercise extreme caution when offering advice to people of seemingly normal weight who are driven to become more "lean and cut." Crash dieting, fluid restriction and excessive exercise can all lead to significant health problems, and may signal the presence of a formal eating disorder.

Your role as a lifestyle and weight management consultant is not to uncover or develop the "dream body" hidden within every client. Rather, your background and training should promote discussion about the merits of sensible, healthy eating, in conjunction with moderate, safe exercise. It should be stressed that if you suspect that a client is developing or may have an eating disorder, the client must be referred to an appropriate mental healthcare professional who specializes in the treatment of these potentially life-threatening psychiatric disorders. It is beyond your professional scope to help or treat such individuals (see Chapter 4).

Summary

An accurate body composition estimation can offer valuable information to both you and your client and can become the cornerstone of a successful weight-management program. By understanding the limitations and strengths of assessing body composition, you can help your clients set realistic, attainable goals that result in both weight loss and, ultimately, long-term weight management.

References

Andersen, R., Wadden, T., Bartlett, S. & Weinstock, R. (1995).The effects of weight loss and exercise on changing blood lipid and lipoprotein profiles in obese women. *American Journal of Clinical Nutrition, 62*, 350-357

Andersen, R., Miles, D., Wadden, T., Kendrick, Z., Bartlett, S. & Buckenmeyer, P. (1994). Accuracy of Bioelectric Impedance Analyzers for Body Composition Assessment in Obese Women. *Medicine and Science in Sports and Exercise, 26*, Supplement 417.

Andersen, R., Brownell K. & Haskell W. (1992). *Health and Fitness Leaders Guide: Administering a Weight Management Program.* Dallas: American Health Publishing.

Durnin, J. & Womersley, J. (1974). Body fat assessed from total body density and its estimation form skinfold thicknesses: Measurements on 481 men and women aged 16 to 72 years. *British Journal of Nutrition, 32*, 77-97.

Eckerson, J., Housh, T. & Johnson, G. (1992). Validity of bioelectric impedance equations for estimating fat-free weight in lean males. *Medicine and Science in Sports and Exercise, 24*, 1298-1302.

Graves, J., Pollock, M., Colvin, A., Van Loan, M. & Lohman, T. (1989). Comparison of different bioelectric impedance analyzers in the prediction of body composition. *American Journal of Human Biology, 1*, 603-611.

Heyward, V., Cook, K., Hicks, V., et al. (1992). Predictive accuracy of three field methods for estimating relative body fatness of non-obese and obese women. *International Journal of Sports Nutrition, 2*, 75-86.

Jackson, A. & Pollock, M. (1978). Generalized equations for predicting body density in men. *British Journal of Nutrition, 40*, 497-504.

Jackson, A., Pollock, M. & Ward, A. (1980). Generalized equations for predicting body density in women. *Medicine Science in Sports and Exercise, 12*, 175-182.

Lohman, T., Roche, A. & Martorell, R. (eds). (1988). *Anthropometric Standardization Reference Manual.* Champaign: Human Kinetics.

Martin, A. & Drinkwater, D. (1991). Variability in the measures of body fat: Assumptions or technique? *Sports Medicine, 91,11*, 277-288.

Metropolitan Life Insurance Company. (1983). Height -Weight Tables. New York.

Ross, W. & Marfell-Jones, M. (1982). Kinanthropometry. In MacDougal J.D., Wenger H.A., Green H.J. (eds). *The physiological testing of the elite athlete.* Canadian Association of Sport Sciences.

Segal, K., Van Loan, M., Fitzgerald, P., et al. (1988). Lean body mass estimation by bioelectric impedance analysis: A four site cross validation study. *American Journal of Clinical Nutrition, 47*, 7-14.

Tran, Z. & Weltman, A. (1989). Generalized equation for predicting body density of women from girth measurements. *Medicine Science in Sports and Exercise, 21*, 101-104.

Tran, Z., Weltman, A. & Seip, R. (1988). Predicting body composition of men from girth measurements. *Human Biology, 88, 60*, 167-176.

Wadden T. & Foster G. (1992). Behavioral Assessment and Treatment of Markedly Obese Patients. In Wadden T. & VanItallie, T. *Treatment of the seriously obese patient.* (Eds): New York: Guilford Press.

Weltman, A., Levine, A., Seip R. & Tran Z. (1988). Accurate assessment of body composition in obese females. *American Journal of Clinical Nutrition, 48*, 1179-1183.

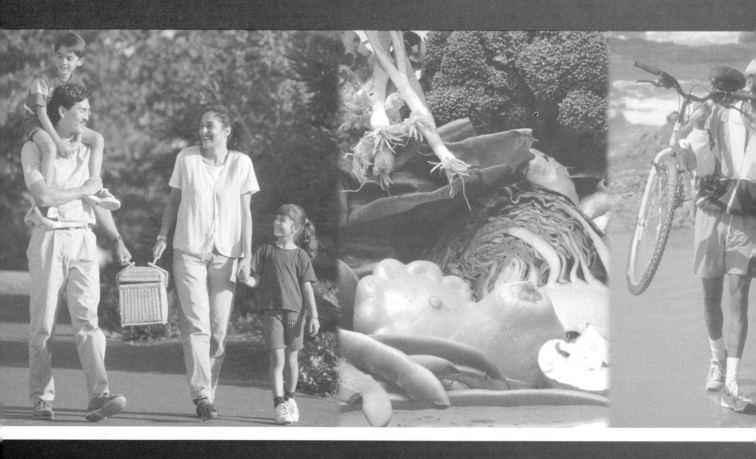

CHAPTER FIVE

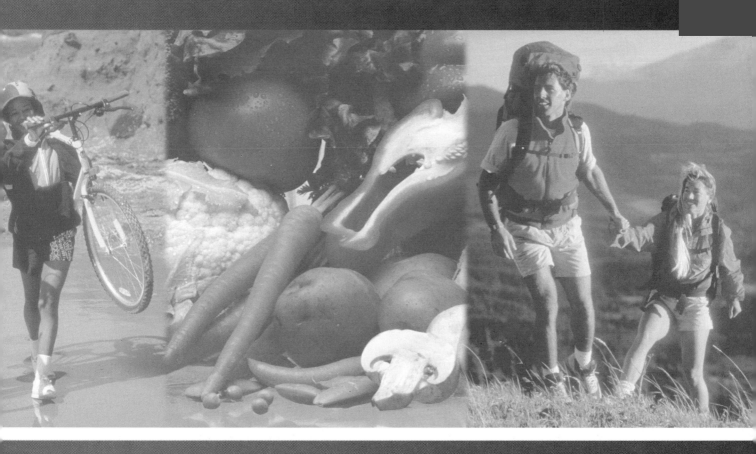

PHYSIOLOGY OF *Obesity*

Ross E. Andersen

Ross E. Andersen, Ph.D., is an assistant professor of medicine at Johns Hopkins University, and focuses on the treatment of obesity. His research areas include the changes in resting metabolism, body composition and fitness that accompany weight-loss and exercise programs. His work is supported by the National Institutes of Health, and his articles have appeared in Redbook *and* Reader's Digest *as well as other publications.*

Introduction

Obesity or overweight is a major cause of health risks such as hypertension, hyperlipidemia, osteoarthritis and coronary artery disease. It also places a significant burden on the healthcare system. In the United States alone, the estimated cost of illnesses associated with obesity are in excess of $39 billion a year. These findings are paralleled by another alarming statistic — the increased prevalence of over-weight American adults. In fact, the incidence of obesity has more than doubled during the past century, regardless of the fact that Americans now consume 3 per-cent to 10 percent fewer calories than they did at the turn of the century (Wadden & Brownell, 1992). Despite our nation's intense preoccupation with weight and dieting, the percent-age of overweight individuals increased from 25 percent to 33 percent between the 1976/1980 and the 1988/1991 National

Health and Nutrition Examination Surveys (NHANES). During this period, the average body mass index (BMI) (kg/M²) increased from 25.3 to 26.3, while the mean body weight was 3.6 kg heavier. Current estimates place the overall prevalence of overweight (defined as a BMI greater than 27.8 for men and 27.3 for women) at 31 percent of men and 33 percent of women.

Prevalence of Overweight Among Races

For all race and ethnic groups combined, the prevalence of overweight is similar for men and women. However, in Mexican American and African American subgroups, a significantly greater proportion of women than men are classified as overweight. Figure 5.1 shows that 36 percent of Mexican American males are overweight. Similarly, 32 percent of Caucasian men and 31 percent of African American men also are classified as being overweight. Among women, however, the prevalence ranged from 33 percent of Caucasian women, to 47 percent of Mexican American women and 49 percent of African American women. Scientists have found that overweight leads to similar health problems in all populations. However, recent reports suggest that diabetes in association with overweight may be more common among minority than among Caucasian populations.

You should understand that the concept of "desirable" or "normal" weight will vary across ethnic groups. In many cases, weight management programs designed to treat Caucasian populations do not work for other ethnic groups. A recent survey of African American women (Kumanyika, 1993) found that they are more likely than Caucasian women to feel that their weight is not under their control. Comparisons of

dieting attempts by African American and Caucasian women revealed that they are equally frequent among both groups. However, the attempts by African American women have been reported to be less drastic. Eating disorders and preoccupation with dieting also are less common among African American women.

There is a greater tolerance of overweight among minority populations. For example, many of the African American women that we have treated in research trials and in our clinic are satisfied with modest weight losses that leave them lighter but still overweight. This attitude is perhaps healthier than the constant drive for the "perfect" body that seems to exist in the Caucasian community.

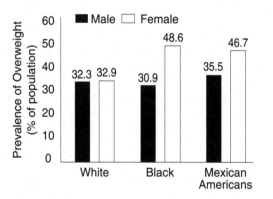

Figure 5.1
Prevalence of overweight in the U.S.

The Genetic Link

Most of us know someone who constantly seems to be eating high-fat food and candy yet still remains thin. Conversely, some individuals seem destined to be overweight. For years, it was thought that the sole reason people became overweight was because they simply ate too much food. But we have come to realize that a complex interaction of factors, such as genetics and environmental, social and racial influences, determine whether or not people can manage their weight.

Dr. Albert Stunkard at the University of Pennsylvania has provided convincing evidence of the strong genetic link to obesity. Stunkard examined 540 Danish adoptees who were reared apart from their biological parents. He found a strong association between the weight class of the adoptee and the body mass index (BMI) of their biological parents, but not between the adoptee and their adoptive parents. In another study of

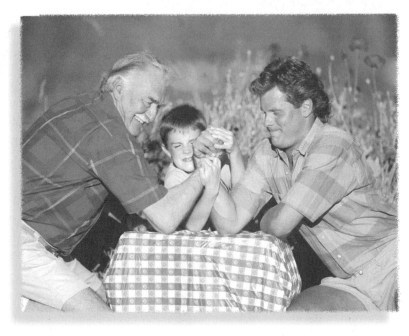

It is important to realize that genetics play a central role in the development of obesity.

1,974 identical and 2,097 fraternal twins, Stunkard found that the identical twins were twice as likely to have similar body weights compared to fraternal twins, and he estimated that as much as 80 percent of the variance in BMI in the twins could be accounted for by genetic factors.

Claude Bouchard at Laval University in Quebec, Canada, gave a group of overweight twins a fixed diet based on their total daily energy expenditure. He found that the pairs of identical twins lost almost identical amounts of weight, whereas there was tremendous variability in the amount of weight lost between pairs of fraternal twins (Bouchard et al., 1990). Again, these data point to the

strong genetic links to obesity. The mechanisms through which genetics may effect weight gain include reduced dietary-induced **thermogenesis**, lower resting metabolic rate, decreased thyroid functioning, decreased **lipoprotein lipase** activity, lower basal body temperatures and decreased amounts of more metabolically active **brown fat**.

While it is impossible to determine exactly how much genetics contributes to an individual's weight problem, it is important for you to realize that genetics play a central role in both the development of obesity and the rate at which people lose weight.

Health Risks of Obesity

Obesity is associated with several health problems (Table 5.1). As the severity of obesity increases, so do medical complications, especially cardiovascular disease, stroke, gallbladder disease, diabetes, respiratory disease and arthritis.

Cardiovascular Disease

Coronary artery disease, angina, myocardial infarction and sudden death are more common in obese individuals. This may be partially explained by higher-fat diets and sedentary living.

High blood pressure has also been associated with weight gain. For every 10 kg increase in body weight, there will be a 3 mmHg rise in **systolic** and a 2 mmHg rise in **diastolic blood pressure** (Pi-Sunyer, 1995). Furthermore, the longer an individual is obese, the greater their likelihood of developing **hypertension.** Persons with abdominal obesity (e.g., apple-shaped individuals) also are more likely to develop hypertension than those with gynoid obesity (e.g., pear-shaped). Research indicates that weight reduction is one of the most effective ways to reduce and, ultimately, control elevated blood pressure.

Stroke

The risk of stroke increases exponentially as body weight increases and is higher in obese people as compared to those who are not obese.

Dyslipidemia obesity results in the elevation of total cholesterol, **LDL cholesterol** and triglycerides. Low **HDL cholesterol** is commonly reported in overweight persons as well. An elevated LDL to HDL ratio has been related to both arteriosclerosis and coronary artery disease, both of which can lead to a stroke. Serum **lipid** levels are related to most measures of body composition including body-fat percentage, **BMI** and **waist-to-hip ratio**. Caloric excess also is thought to be partially responsible for both **hyperlipidemia** and hypertriglyceridemia. Decreased production of the enzyme lipoprotein lipase also may result in elevated lipid and lipoprotein levels.

Weight loss and a low-fat diet have been found to dramatically improve lipid profiles (Andersen et al., 1995). HDL cholesterol may actually be depressed while a person is actively losing weight. This reduction is not thought to indicate an increased risk of atherosclerosis, since the HDL cholesterol will typically increase above pre-dieting levels once dieting stops and the individual's weight stabilizes.

Diabetes

There is a strong relationship between the presence of type II diabetes mellitus (adult onset) and obesity. In fact, almost 80 percent of type II diabetics are obese. Young, overweight adults are nearly four times more likely to develop diabetes as compared to age-matched, normal-weight persons. Insulin production is much greater in the obese individual. However, as body fat increases, insulin does not act effectively on the cells to reduce blood glucose levels. There are fewer active insulin

---

Table 5.1
Medical Problems Associated with Obesity

1. Increased risk of coronary artery disease (CAD)
2. Hypertension
3. Elevated total cholesterol, LDL cholesterol and triglycerides
4. Lower HDL cholesterol
5. Stroke
6. Type II diabetes
7. Gout
8. Cancer - Common in women:
         breast, endometrial,
         ovarian and cervical
   Common in men:
         colon, rectal and prostate
9. Sleep apnea
10. Arthritis
11. Gallbladder disease
12. Potential social and psychological consequences
13. Diaphoresis (excessive sweating)
14. Fatigue
15. Orthopnea (need to sit up to breathe)
16. Digestive distress
17. Menstrual abnormalities
18. Infertility

---

receptor sites and a reduced insulin sensitivity. This combination results in an overproduction of insulin in an effort to control blood glucose levels. Furthermore, the sedentary lifestyle commonly associated with obesity can lead to decreased capillary blood flow and promote insulin resistance.

The complex interactions between obesity, insulin resistance and blood sugar remain unclear. However, weight loss appears to improve glucose tolerance, decrease insulin resistance and reduce **hyperglycemia**.

Gallbladder Disease

Bile in the gallbladder can become super-saturated with cholesterol, and bile salts are decreased relative to the cholesterol concentration. Weight gain decreases the motility of the gallbladder, resulting in less efficient emptying. The net effect is an increased risk of gallstone formation in the obese individual. And overweight women tend to have a higher incidence of gallstones than overweight men. Dieting, particularly low-fat dieting, has been found to increase the formation of gallstones in some individuals, but unless an

Overweight individuals with diabetes who lose 10 percent to 20 percent of their body weight through a combination of diet and regular exercise often can reduce or discontinue the use of diabetic medications.

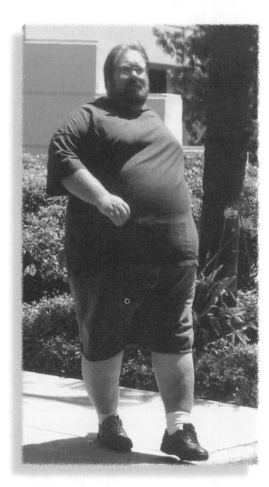

ultrasound is obtained prior to beginning a diet, it cannot be known whether the gallstones were a pre-existing condition.

Respiratory Disease

Respiratory function in the obese person is frequently impaired. Increased fat in the chest decreases the mechanical efficiency of the respiratory system, and excess fat in the viscera may compromise the efficient motion of both the diaphragm and the rib cage. Total lung capacity and **forced vital capacities** tend to be lower than average in the obese person, whereas **residual lung volumes** may be greater. Fatty tissue may obstruct or occlude the large airways, leading to **sleep apnea**.

Arthritis

Stress on the weight-bearing joints increases as weight increases and often leads to arthritis. Knee, hip and low-back problems are frequently reported by obese persons. Excessive wear on the cartilage of the knees and hip can lead to the degeneration of these joints, particularly as the severity and duration of obesity increases.

Health-related quality of life is dramatically effected as mobility and simple daily tasks are much more difficult for the obese person (Table 5.2).

The 10-Percent Solution

Weight loss has been found to improve a number of the medical problems associated with obesity. Clients may feel that the only way to resolve these medical conditions is to reduce their weight to their "ideal" range, which in many cases is not reasonable or realistic. Fortunately, recent clinical evidence suggests that even modest weight loss can eliminate many obesity-related disorders.

Caloric restriction and exercise have been found to improve the body's ability to use insulin and to normalize blood glucose levels. Overweight individuals who lose and maintain weight losses of 10 percent to 20 percent often can reduce or discontinue the use of diabetic medications.

Modest weight reductions also have been found to improve blood pressure. One study reported that a long-term,

5 percent reduction in body weight was enough to significantly reduce blood pressure and allow participants to discontinue the use of antihypertensive medication. Dieting and lifestyle changes that are typically associated with healthier eating, such as low sodium and reduced fat consumption also help to reduce blood pressure.

Weight reductions of 5 percent to 10 percent often result in large reductions in serum cholesterol and triglycerides. It was recently reported that body-weight losses of 11 percent resulted in triglyceride and cholesterol reductions of 23 percent and 16 percent, respectively (Andersen et al., 1995). Interestingly, greater reductions were seen in persons whose pre-dieting levels were considered high. Hence, individuals whose lipid levels put them at the greatest risk, benefited the most from weight loss.

Modest weight losses also can reduce back pain and **osteoarthritis**, especially in the knees, and finally, a 5 percent to 10 percent weight reduction has been shown to significantly improve mood, self-esteem, **self-efficacy** and body image.

Unsafe Approaches to Weight Loss

Your obese clients may have tried any number of approaches to weight loss that may not have been safe or effective. It is important that you are aware of these methods and how they do or do not work.

Fad Diets

It seems that every year brings along a new "quick and easy approach" to weight loss. If you follow the best-sellers list at your local book store, you will probably notice that there is at least one diet book on the list at any given time.

Table 5.2

The Effects of Obesity on Health-related Quality of Life

---

1. Increased shortness of breath

2. Decreased mobility and range of movement

3. Diminished capacity for exercise and activity

4. Increased ankle swelling

5. Lower level of physical self-efficacy (i.e., one's perception of their ability to exercise)

6. Decreased agility and balance

It is important for you to stay on top of the trends in the popular press, since your clients will no doubt have many questions about the pros and cons of the latest diets. Some of these diets make the authors very wealthy, but, unfortunately, may put the public at risk. New diets often limit or emphasize the consumption of certain foods, using half-truths to describe their importance for weight control. For example, the Scarsdale Diet is a low-calorie, high-protein diet that can promote dramatic weight losses, primarily due to the increased water loss that accompanies this type of diet. Weight is quickly regained when the consumption and storage of carbohydrates resumes. The Fit-For-Life diet promotes the consumption of certain raw foods at special times of the day. You should be aware of the nutrient composition of the diets that your clients may be consuming. One of the greatest hazards of fad diets is that they may be nutritionally inadequate. An optimal diet program should produce results without inducing additional health risks.

Most diets and weight-loss programs work by either reducing caloric consumption, increasing energy output or a combination of the two. Be leery of new diets that claim to include "magic" fat-burning foods or unique combinations of vitamin or mineral supplements to speed weight loss. Perhaps the best way to judge a popular diet is to examine how effective it is at helping the dieter keep weight off after they have lost it. In general, a sound weight-loss program should include each of the following components:

✔ decreased fat consumption
✔ reduced caloric consumption (through portion control)
✔ high carbohydrate and fiber content in the diet
✔ adequate nutrition
✔ palatable food choices
✔ a more active lifestyle
✔ change of behaviors that lead to becoming overweight
✔ establishment of lasting eating patterns

A single approach to weight loss will not work for all people. An optimal program takes into account an individual's needs, risks and dieting history. Some individuals require a great deal of support and attention to lose weight while others do not. Individuals who appear to be self-motivated and concerned with cost may benefit from a sensible, self-directed diet.

Calories Per Day

When developing a nutrition program for your client, keep in mind that as the level of caloric restriction increases, so do the health risks. The Michigan Health Council (1990) suggests that calories per day should not be less than 1,000 kcal/d at Level I; 800 kcal/d at Level II; and 600 kcal/d at Level III. The weight-loss food plan should provide the participant with between 0.8 and 1.5 grams of protein per kilogram of desirable body weight. Fewer than

30 percent of the calories should come from fat. Daily fluid intake should consist of at least 24 ounces. The program should offer choices that provide 100 percent of the client's **Recommended Dietary Allowances (RDA)**. Avoid mega-doses (i.e., those significantly exceeding 100 percent of RDA) of vitamins or minerals. Make the food plan practical with easily obtainable foods, and focus on the development of safe and healthy eating patterns.

The American Heart Association recently established a Scientific Statement on Guidelines for Weight Management Programs in Healthy Adults (1994), which may help you develop programs for your clients. It suggests that "The nutritional recommendations for each participant's treatment should include a personal food plan that takes into account current eating habits, lifestyle, ethnicity and culture, energy needs, any diet prescription related to medical treatment and potential nutrient-drug interactions." Caloric intake should be adjusted to allow for a safe rate of weight loss, which they deem to be an average of 1 pound per week, and that women should not consume less than 1,200 kcal/d and men should not eat less than 1,500 kcal/d. It also advises that less than 30 percent of energy consumed should come from fat, 15 percent from protein and at least 55 percent from carbohydrates.

Fasting

Fasting for extended periods of time is clearly not a healthy way to lose weight. While fasting can lead to large weight losses in severely overweight persons, as much as 50 percent of the weight lost comes from lean mass — an undesirable outcome. Fasting also has been reported to cause severe degenerative changes in the heart muscle. Studies examining long-term weight maintenance following a fast are disappointing, since the weight lost during a fast is typically quickly regained. Starvation or fasting diets are no longer considered a safe or acceptable method of weight loss in the medical community.

Diet Pills

"Diet pills" were popular for the short-term treatment of obesity in the 1960s. These pills, which were usually amphetamines, acted as appetite suppressants. Amphetamines are now seldom used for the treatment of obesity, since they have a high potential for abuse and, ultimately, drug dependence. Drugs that work specifically on the hypothalamus to decrease hunger and increase satiety, however, have been the topic of much interest to both the scientific community and lay persons. The combination of the drugs Phentermine and Fenfluramine (trade names are Ionomin and Pondimin) has recently been successful in helping overweight people maintain lower weights. This drug combination appears to help individuals lose and keep off approximately 10 percent of their body weight for as long as the drugs are taken. Weight regain is rapid once the drugs are discontinued, though it is lost again when the drugs are reintroduced. Since obesity is considered by most experts to be a "chronic disease," it has prompted many to suggest that the long-term use of these drugs is an appropriate treatment. Research on the effectiveness of these drugs, combined with all of the components of an effective weight-loss and relapse-prevention program, will be the focus of several studies in the near future.

Very-low-calorie Diets

Very-low-calorie diets (VLCDs) have been used by the medical community as a last resort for seriously obese persons. They are inappropriate for prepubertal adolescents, pregnant or lactating women, the elderly or those with psychiatric illness. The VLCD approach typically involves the consumption of several liquid meals throughout the day, which together contain less than 800 kcal/d. These meals typically contain high-quality protein to attenuate the loss of lean tissue, and 100 percent of the RDA of essential vitamins and minerals. It is important to emphasize that VLCDs can only be used when the dieter is under the care and supervision of a physician. The caloric content of these meals usually ranges between 420 and 800 kcal/d. Interestingly, participants who carefully follow a VLCD report significant decreases in hunger and interest in food after one or two weeks. The long-term follow-up evaluations following VLCDs reflect disappointing maintenance results, but combining the VLCD with a behavior

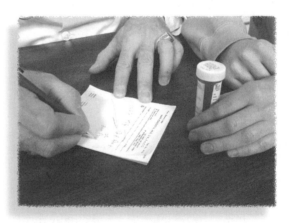

While some people benefit from the use of diet pills, the lost weight generally returns once use of the drugs is discontinued.

modification and a weight-maintenance program has been found to improve the long-term prognosis of persons on these diets.

You should be on the lookout for clients who may be using over-the-counter, commercially available liquid shakes as a VLCD (i.e., consuming shakes only, without a solid meal). It should be stressed that persons who are following a VLCD need continual medical supervision that is beyond the scope of care that you can provide.

In a recent study, a modified VLCD was used with very promising results (Wadden et al., 1995). Participants had a combination of liquid meals for breakfast and lunch and a low-fat prepackaged entree with a garden salad for dinner. Subjects' average caloric consumption was about 950 kcal/d. It was interesting that the weight losses in the study were similar to those of a standard VLCD (22 pounds in eight weeks and 31.5 pounds by week 17). Thus, it appears that aggressively controlled portions result in large weight losses similar to those achieved on a VLCD, and a lower loss of lean tissue than that reported in traditional VLCDs.

Based on these findings, Wadden (1995) has suggested the following recommendations concerning the use of modified VLCDs:

1. The use of VLCDs, as commonly defined, should be discontinued with most patients in favor of low-calorie diets that provide at least 800 kcal/d (and ample protein) but retain the form of the VLCD (i.e., portion- and calorie-controlled servings).

2. All significantly obese individuals seeking treatment using a modified VLCD should have a thorough medical examination. If found to be in good health, the individual's schedule of medical monitoring can be reduced.

3. Preliminary findings indicate that it may be beneficial to add a daily meal of conventional food to liquid-diet regimens. The inclusion of this meal is likely to reduce patients' anxiety and the incidence of problem eating during the refeeding period.

4. Low-calorie formula diets should only be used in a program of lifestyle modification designed to increase physical activity, reduce consumption of dietary fat and improve coping skills. Moreover, these diets should only be used with patients who have failed to reduce their weight using more con-

servative interventions. With either approach, both you and your client must be prepared to devote as much effort to the maintenance of weight loss as to its induction.

Exercise and Weight Management

The treatment of obesity requires consuming less energy than is expended, and usually focuses on either the consumption of fewer calories, increasing caloric expenditure or, ideally, a combination of the two. The prevalence of overweight has increased steadily over the past century, and has paralleled our moves from an agrarian to an industrial and, finally, to an information society. Consequently, it appears that reduced physical activity is partly responsible for the weight gain seen in most modern societies; overweight people tend to be less active.

There is abundant evidence to suggest that exercise, without diet and lifestyle modifications, is an ineffective way to lose substantial amounts of weight. In 1983, Wilmore reviewed 55 studies that tried to do just that, and reported an average loss of only 1.6 percent fat. Most exercise-alone studies result in average weight losses of about six pounds over the course of the program. A few studies that used very intense and lengthy exercise protocols reported losses of 12 to 25 pounds. However, the volume of activity used in these investigations would not be practical for most overweight individuals.

While it is true that exercise alone may not be an effective way for obese people to lose a great deal of weight, it may offer a good long-term solution for the individual who wants to lose a relatively small amount of weight, and it can result in positive cosmetic and body composition changes. Exercise-alone programs have been found to modestly increase fat-free mass and decrease body-fat percentage, while weight on the scale remains unchanged.

Diet Plus Aerobic Exercise

In some studies, adding aerobic exercise to a weight-loss program has been found to increase the rate of weight loss, while others have not found differences compared to a diet-alone protocol. The level of caloric restriction of the diet may help to explain why these differences exist. When calorie restriction is moderate, adding aerobic exercise may enhance weight loss. However, with severe calorie restriction, exercise does not appear to increase the rate of weight loss. This may partly be explained by the fact that the body is making an effort to preserve itself while under the severe stress of a low-calorie diet. Interestingly, Foster et al. (1992) found no differences in weight loss in subjects who consumed either a 420, 660 or 800 kcal/d liquid diet, but the type of weight lost may be different in those persons who add exercise to their diet regimen. The diet-plus-aerobic exerciser may lose less of their total weight from the fat-free mass.

The Influence of Exercise on Resting Metabolism

To understand the role that exercise plays in metabolism, it is important to understand each of the components that make up total daily energy expenditure. These include resting metabolic rate (RMR), the thermic effect of feeding (TEF) and the thermic effect of physical activity (TEA) (Figure 5.2).

RMR can be defined as the energy required to sustain bodily functions and maintain body temperature at rest. RMR represents the largest portion of the total daily energy expenditure (typically 60 percent to 75 percent). The thyroid hormones largely regulate

and control RMR. It is usually measured first thing in the morning on a metabolic cart, a device used to measure oxygen consumption, after a 12-hour fast and at least a 24-hour rest from exercise.

TEF can be described as the metabolic cost of ingesting, digesting and storing food. This constitutes approximately 10 percent of the total daily energy expenditure. TEA can be explained as the additional energy expended above RMR and the TEF, due to physical activity. It is the most variable of the energy expenditure components. In sedentary individuals it represents approximately 15 percent of

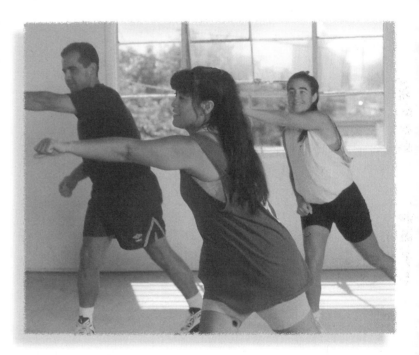

daily expenditure, while in active individuals this number may be as high as 35 percent.

One of the key benefits of aerobic exercise is the increased calories that are burned beyond resting levels. For example, a beginning exerciser may expend calories at a rate that would be 10 times above their resting level, while a trained athlete can exercise at 15 to 20 times their resting level. This is encouraging for weight management clients as their RMR does not plunge

Aerobic exercise, when combined with moderate caloric restriction, may enhance weight loss by elevating the metabolism both during and after the exercise session.

back to resting levels after a bout of aerobic exercise. In fact, resting metabolism has been found to be significantly higher the day after an intense bout of exercise than it is the morning after several days of rest. Figure 5.3 shows a hypothetical plot of energy consumption before, during and after a bout of exercise. Once the workout begins, the resting metabolism rises quickly to meet the increased energy demands of the exercise. The body then settles into a

Figure 5.2
The three major components of daily energy expenditure: RMR, resting metabolic rate; TEF, thermic effect of feeding; and TEA, thermic effect of activity. (Adapted from Poehlman, 1989.)

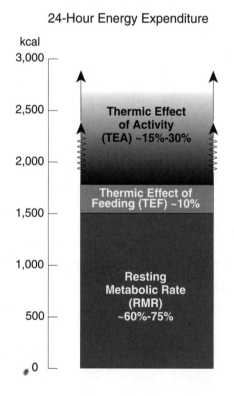

24-Hour Energy Expenditure

steady state, burning calories at a rate far greater than the resting level. Note how the metabolism remains significantly elevated for 10 to 15 minutes after the bout of exercise and then gradually returns to baseline. However, if you look closely at the graph, you will note that the resting oxygen consumption is still slightly higher than the baseline resting levels, even two hours after the bout of exercise is completed (Gillette et. al., 1994).

Cross-sectional studies show that

athletes demonstrate a higher RMR than sedentary individuals, and training studies suggest that sedentary individuals who are not restricting calories can increase their RMR by beginning a regular exercise program. There may, however, be a threshold of exercise intensity necessary to derive this increase in RMR, since low-intensity exercise has not been found to produce the same effect. This is partially due to the fact that there is a metabolic cost associated with replenishing fuels expended (i.e., glycogen) and repairing tissues damaged during vigorous exercise. Furthermore, Poehlman (1989) suggests that the energy requirements of "active metabolic tissue" may be altered with high levels of aerobic training.

The effects of weight loss on each of the components of total energy expenditure has been the focus of many studies. Obese individuals tend to have higher RMR values compared to non-obese persons, when they are matched for age and height. This is due to their greater overall abundance of metabolically active tissue. However, when obese people are matched per unit of body weight, they tend to have lower RMR measures. This is partially explained by the fact that they have proportionally less metabolically active lean tissue.

Exercise, Dieting and RMR

Little can be done to increase RMR while fat-free mass (FFM) remains constant, since RMR is directly related to the amount of FFM a person has. Thus, a drop in FFM will usually result in a drop in RMR. A recent meta-analysis found that roughly 24 percent to 28 percent of weight lost will come from the FFM in non-exercising dieters, while only 11 percent to 13 percent of weight loss will come from the FFM in persons who simultaneously exercise and diet (Ballor and Poehlman, 1994). Hence, exercise appears to attenuate, but not totally prevent, the loss of lean mass.

In a recent study conducted at the University of Pennsylvania, 128 obese women were randomly assigned to either a 1) diet only; 2) diet-plus-aerobic exercise; 3) diet-plus-resistance training; or 4) diet-plus-aerobic and resistance training regimen (Wadden et al., 1996). All subjects received the same 950 kcal/d diet, while the exercising subjects trained three days per week. It was hypothesized that exercise would spare the loss of lean tissue, which also would prevent the typical drop in RMR. Interestingly, there were no differences in weight loss across the four conditions at weeks eight, 24 or 48. There also were no significant differences at any time in body composition. Subjects who exercised aerobically had smaller reductions in RMR at week 24 than those who received resistance training, but there were no other metabolic differences at any time. Thus, researchers were not able to attenuate the loss of lean tissue with exercise, and exercise did not prevent the drop in RMR which is typically seen in dieters (Wadden et al., 1996).

Resistance training has been found to significantly increase both RMR and FFM in sedentary elderly persons who are not restricting calories. Future studies are needed to examine the role that moderate calorie restriction has on both RMR and body composition.

Resistance Training

Resistance training has recently become a popular and important component of exercise programs for healthy adults (Campbell et al., 1994). In fact, the American College of Sports Medicine (ACSM) now suggests that adults include two resistance training sessions in their exercise routines each week. Weight training was initially added to weight-loss programs in an effort to

reduce or prevent the loss of FFM during caloric restriction, which in theory would attenuate the drop in RMR typically seen with weight loss. The results of studies in this area are equivocal and require interpretation.

One of the first studies was done by Ballor and colleagues (1988) when he reduced calories by 1,000 kcal/d and assigned subjects to treatment by either 1) diet only; 2) diet-plus-resistance training; or 3) resistance training only. They found no differences in weight loss between the diet-only and diet-plus-resistance training group after eight

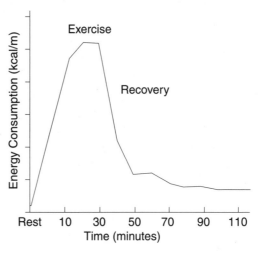

weeks (4.47 vs. 3.89 kg). However, the diet-only group lost 0.9 kg of FFM while the diet-plus-resistance training group gained 0.4 kg. The resistance-training-only group lost a small amount of fat and gained more lean mass than the diet-plus-resistance training group. Thus, it appears that resistance training plus modest calorie restriction for short periods of time may result in an increase or sparing of lean mass. Unfortunately, these investigators did not measure RMR before and after weight loss.

Several studies have examined the potential muscle-sparing effects of resistance training on subjects who followed more restrictive diets (i.e., less

Figure 5.3
Energy consumption before, during and after a bout of aerobic exercise.

than 1,000 kcal/d). Well-designed studies have consistently demonstrated no differences in weight loss or body composition between diet-only and diet-plus- resistance training groups. The mechanism by which resistance training would spare or attenuate the loss of skeletal muscle is complex. Contractile proteins synthesize and **hypertrophy** in response to the stress of resistance training. Bodybuilders and athletes know that in order to increase lean mass, they must combine the consumption of sub-stantial amounts of food with high-quality training. In the case of the dieter, it appears that if the metabolic needs of the body are not being met, the contractile proteins will not synthesize or hypertrophy. Several studies have reported that diet-plus-resistance training results in significant strength increases, despite the fact that muscle mass had been lost. This would suggest that improved neural responses may be partially responsible for the strength increases seen in dieting adults.

The Critical Role of Exercise in Weight Management

Current research on the role of exercise in weight control often yields conflicting results. While exercise alone appears largely ineffective in producing a significant weight loss, combined with moderate caloric restriction, regular exercise may enhance weight loss. If the calories are restricted too severely, however, exercise appears to have a negligible effect on weight loss. More research is needed to identify optimal levels of caloric restriction and exercise required to produce the desired metabolic changes.

Still, exercise should play a central role in most weight-loss programs for several reasons:

✔ Exercise is a key determinant for long-term success at weight management. Studies have shown that individuals who have lost weight are much less likely to regain it if they are exercising (Blair, 1993; Kayman et al., 1990; Pavlou et al., 1989).

✔ Physical activity can potentially mitigate the negative health consequences of overweight. Exercise can reduce hypertension, improve lipid profiles and lower overall mortality and morbidity risks (IOM, 1995).

✔ Regular exercise may increase resting energy expenditure and fat oxidation (IOM, 1995), and contribute to a negative energy balance while helping preserve lean body tissue.

✔ Exercise positively influences mood and enhances psychological well-being (IOM, 1995).

Tailoring exercise interventions to meet the unique physical and psychosocial needs of overweight individuals may help them become more physically active. For instance, a strong focus on increasing daily physical activity may help an otherwise busy person to become more active. Lifestyle exercise also may increase feelings of exercise self-efficacy (the belief that one is able to exercise competently). As self-efficacy increases, individuals are more likely to adopt and maintain a traditional exercise program.

Because physical activity plays a central role in the regulation of body weight, one of your primary goals as a lifestyle and weight management consultant is to help your clients adopt and maintain a more active lifestyle.

Donnelly et al. (1993) recently reported that diet-plus-resistance training resulted in total body loss of FFM. However, muscle biopsies taken before and after training reported that both the fast-twitch and slow-twitch muscle fibers increased significantly with the diet and resistance training combination. Research is needed to determine optimal interactions of the level of caloric restriction and volume of resistance training that results in the desired sparing of lean tissue.

The Thermic Effect of Food

The thermic effect of food can be measured by giving a person a meal consisting of a known **macronutrient** and caloric content. Typically, it will be a simple liquid supplement. After consuming this meal, the individual's oxygen consumption is monitored on a metabolic cart for several hours while resting. Energy expended above resting values is assumed to be the thermic effect of food. As mentioned earlier, there is a metabolic cost to ingesting, digesting and storing food. Research has shown that obese individuals may have a more efficient thermic response to a meal compared to a normal-weight person. Reports have suggested that TEF differences between obese and normal-weight persons is approximately 30 kcal/d. These differences are not great, but over time they may result in energy surpluses and, therefore, extra weight.

Researchers also have compared the effect of exercise on TEF in lean and obese persons. It has been demonstrated that exercise will double the thermic effect of food in lean persons and has little or no effect on obese women. The differential thermic responses to a meal with exercise may partially explain the difficulties that obese and formerly obese individuals have in managing their weight (Poehlman, 1989).

The Thermic Effect of Activity

The metabolic picture, so far, may appear gloomy for your overweight clients. It is true that sometimes a "sluggish" RMR and a decreased TEF will contribute to the development and persistence of obesity. These two components of total energy expenditure are not under your control or your client's. The last component of total energy expenditure is the energy cost of activity, and is the one component that we can influence. Differences in RMR and TEF may be offset through increased activity via a safe and sensible exercise prescription. Figure 5.4 demonstrates the typical metabolic responses that

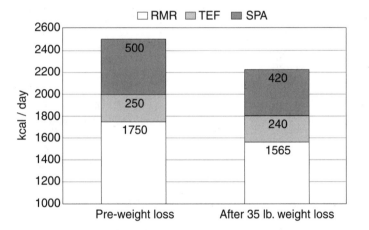

may accompany weight loss in a sedentary individual. Note that RMR, TEF and the metabolic cost of spontaneous daily activity (SPA) all decrease when body weight is reduced.

Exercise or increased lifestyle activity may help to undo some of the metabolic changes that take place with weight loss. For example, the 30 kcal/d difference in TEF could be countered by simply encouraging clients to take the stairs instead of the elevator. The 185 kcal/d drop in RMR described in Figure 5.4 could be equalized in clients who deliberately get off the bus one stop earlier before and after work and walk the rest of the way. They can also take a series of three-minute walks throughout the day.

Figure 5.4

The effects of weight loss on daily energy expenditure.

Of course, more intense, programmed exercise could provide a metabolic advantage through: 1) expending calories at a greater rate; 2) possibly increasing RMR once participants are weight stable; and 3) increasing **post-exercise oxygen consumption**. Figure 5.5 demonstrates the hypothetical metabolic changes that would take place if the same individual described in Figure 5.4 took part in a 16-week aerobic class once her weight was stable. We can see that her RMR is increased significantly, her TEF is up slightly and the metabolic cost of spontaneous activity does not change, but the 228 kcal/d are expended with voluntary physical activity. This exercising individual is now expending almost 2,600 kcal/d, whereas she was only expending 2,500 kcal/d before she began her weight-loss program.

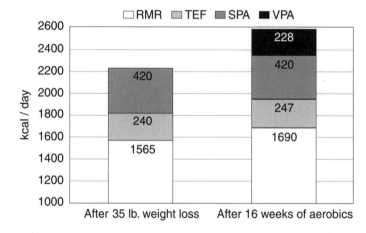

Figure 5.5
The metabolic changes that might occur if the individual described in Figure 5.4 took part in a 16-week aerobic class once her weight was stable.

Research on underfeeding has revealed that when humans are underfed or starved they become less active in an effort to conserve energy and regulate their energy balance. Time/motion studies, which examine spontaneous physical activity throughout the day, have revealed that obese people tend to move less to conserve energy. People who move and fidget more will expend more calories each day than their sedentary counterparts. Investigators have found that the daily energy cost of physical activity could be increased by

17 percent to 29 percent depending on the position that subjects assumed (i.e., laying, sitting or standing). Thus, teaching clients to focus on activity, and deliberately increasing energy expenditure and becoming more spontaneously active (even in the posture they assume) can ultimately help them learn to manage their weight more effectively (Andersen, 1995).

Theories that Address the Causes of Obesity

For years, scientists have been trying to understand what causes obesity. Several theories have attracted the attention of both the popular press and obesity researchers. It is important that you understand the basis of these theories so that you can discuss them with clients who have been confused by the media.

Weight Cycling

Since the mid-1980s, **weight cycling** has received much attention from both researchers and the popular press. The weight-cycling theory was developed as researchers noticed that many individuals reported increased difficulty losing weight with each subsequent attempt at weight loss. People who frequently went on and off diets became known as "yo-yo" dieters. Brownell (1986) reported from a study of rats that with each attempt at dieting, there is a slower rate of weight loss and a faster rate of weight regain. It also has been shown that wrestlers who were "weight cyclers" had lower RMRs than their weight-stable counterparts. At the time, researchers speculated that the metabolic efficiency that was being reported in the weight cyclers was due to the fact that the yo-yo dieters were losing approximately 25 percent of their weight as fat-free mass (which is metabolically active tissue) that was not being resynthesized when weight was regained.

Recent work has disproved some of the elements of the original theory, despite the fact that the body does seem to make some adaptation to protect its energy stores. Scientists have shown that approximately 25 percent of weight lost from dieting without exercise will come from the fat-free tissue. However, when weight is regained, approximately 25 percent of the increased weight will again be lean tissue. This may be explained by the fact that the obese individual requires extra muscle mass for support and movement.

A recent joint consensus statement released by the National Task Force on the Prevention and Treatment of Obesity and the National Institutes of Health (1994) concluded that weight cycling did not lead to long-term metabolic damage. However, they did note that several observational and cross-sectional studies have shown a relationship between variation in body weight and increased morbidity and mortality. In a recent review by Wing et al. (1992), it was concluded that most recent studies show no adverse effects of weight cycling on body composition, metabolism, body fat distribution or future attempts at weight loss. However, the evidence on the ill effects of weight cycling is not sufficiently compelling to override the health benefits of moderate weight loss in significantly obese persons. They also suggested that obese persons should not allow their concerns of the hazards of weight cycling to deter them from efforts to control their weight.

Set-point Theory

The **set-point theory** of weight loss and regain attempts to explain the resistance that humans and animals demonstrate toward weight gain and loss. If animals or humans are overfed or underfed, they will either gain or lose weight accordingly. It is typical, however, for the individual or animal to quickly return to their normal weight once regular eating resumes. Proponents of the set-point theory argue that the body has an internal control mechanism to regulate body weight, which is probably located in the brain's hypothalamus. This mechanism is thought

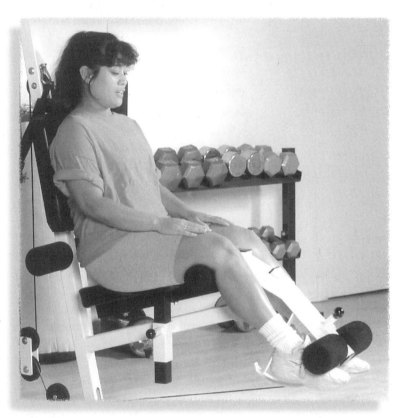

to drive the body to maintain a certain body weight. When body weight is reduced below a given "set-point," the body makes a series of internal adjustments to resist weight change and conserve fat stores. For example, we discussed the well-documented drop in RMR that accompanies weight loss in the preceding section. Researchers have found that many overweight people decrease levels of spontaneous physical activity once they are at a lower weight.

Can the set point be altered? It appears that long-term overfeeding can

By increasing lean body mass, resistance training can help counteract the drop in resting metabolic rate that often accompanies weight loss.

move the set-point upward to allow for a greater body weight. Smoking cessation may increase the set-point as well, since nicotine suppresses feelings of hunger. Aging also appears to change the set-point, since weight gain is common from young adulthood into middle age, and weight loss is common in the elderly. As mentioned previously, pharmacological treatment of the seriously obese individual may help to adjust the set-point to a lower weight.

Development of Fat Cells

Studies of adipose cellularity have examined the cellular characteristics in both obese and non-obese populations. They have determined that excess calories can be stored as fat by: 1) depositing more fat in existing cells (hypertrophy); 2) by forming new cells (hyperplasia); or 3) a combination of hypertrophy and hyperplasia. Fat biopsy studies have revealed that the fat content within a fat cell is approximately 35 percent greater in the obese compared to the non-obese, and that the total number of fat cells in an obese person is as much as three times greater than in a normal-weight person (Katch and McArdle, 1988). Figure 5.6 demonstrates that an obese individual may have 75 billion fat cells in their body, whereas the non-obese person will average 27 billion.

It appears that weight loss in the obese individual results in decreased fat cell diameter, but not in a decreased number of fat cells. One of the reasons that formerly obese persons have such a difficult time maintaining large weight losses is that the size of their reduced fat cells is somehow linked to the appetite center in the brain.

Conversely, overfeeding studies have examined the role of excessive caloric intake on the size and number of fat cells. When normal weight individuals are deliberately overfed it seems that the size of the fat cells increases as body fat stores increase. Moderate weight gain (i.e., less than 25 pounds) through deliberate overeating does not appear to increase the number of fat cells. Hyperplasia occurs when massive overfeeding continues and the fat cells reach maximal size. Avoiding hyperplasia is critical from a weight management perspective, since it makes both weight reduction and weight management increasingly more difficult.

Body-fat Distribution

Body fat is stored in different regions of the body, and the pattern of its distribution can actually alter the health risks of obesity. For example, central or android-type obesity is associated with an increased risk of coronary artery disease, and all-cause mortality, whereas, weight gain in the thighs and hips (peripheral or gynoid obesity) does not have the same magnitude of increased risk. The preferential fat storage in the body may be partly explained by the activity of the enzyme lipoprotein lipase (LPL) which is produced in the adipocyte and is responsible for transporting fat into the adipocyte for storage. LPL activity in women is higher in hip and thigh regions and tends to be elevated in the abdominal region in men. The lower body fat patterning in women seems to be related to reproductive function since the expansion of the abdomen is reserved for fetal growth and the lower body-fat stores serve as an energy reserve for pregnancy and lactation.

The **waist-to-hip ratio (WTH)** can be used to help you assess the degree of risk associated with fat patterning in your clients. The WTH can be measured with a non-stretchable measuring tape at the waist (smallest circumference below the rib cage) and the largest circumference around the buttocks. A WTH above 1.0 in men and 0.80 in women has been associated with a

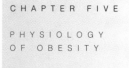

higher risk to health than weight gain alone. Chapter 4 explains WTH in greater detail.

Influence of Exercise on Fat Cells

Several animal studies have examined the role that intense exercise plays on fat weight, fat cell size and fat cell number. In young, growing rats, exercise has been reported to slow the rate of fat gain, fat cell size and fat cell number. At maturity, animals who have exercised through their youth will have lower weights, less total fat and smaller and fewer fat cells. Thus, it appears that exercise may attenuate the rate of proliferation of fat cells in young animals. This is an important point, since entering adulthood with a reduced number

cise, since there appears to be no way to reduce the number of adipocytes once they have proliferated.

Spot Reduction

If you have worked with overweight individuals or the general public, you have no doubt had clients ask you "Could you give me an exercise to help me firm up my tummy?" Women frequently ask for help with toning and shaping their thighs, buttocks and arms, while men may request help with melting away their beer belly. This is called **spot reduction**. The theory behind spot reduction is that contracting muscles will preferentially and selectively reduce locally stored fat in the area where the exercise was performed.

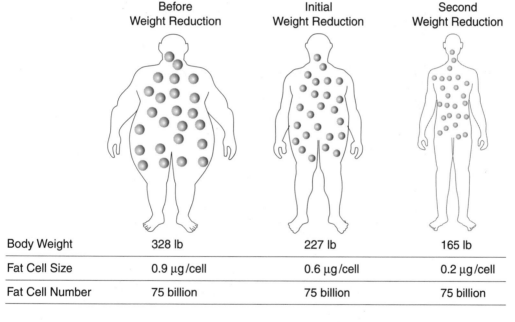

	Before Weight Reduction	Initial Weight Reduction	Second Weight Reduction
Body Weight	328 lb	227 lb	165 lb
Fat Cell Size	0.9 µg/cell	0.6 µg/cell	0.2 µg/cell
Fat Cell Number	75 billion	75 billion	75 billion

Figure 5.6
Changes in adipose cellularity wth weight reduction in obese subjects (Data from Hirsch, J. 1971. Adipose cellularity in relation to human obesity. *Advances in Internal Medicine,* 17. Edited by G.H. Stollerman, Chicago, Year Book).

of fat cells will help to reduce the likelihood of becoming an overweight adult (Katch and McArdle, 1988).

Exercise in adult animals has also been found to significantly reduce the total body weight, fat weight and size of the fat cells. The number of adipocytes, however, does not appear to be altered by vigorous exercise. Again this speaks to the need for early prevention of obesity through sensible eating and exer-

The promise of spot reduction is very attractive from both an aesthetic and business perspective, as evidenced by the plethora of commercial products available. We can watch 30-minute infomercials that flog specially designed abdominal toning equipment that guarantees "wash-board" abdominal muscles by simply following their program. There are literally hundreds of exercise videos designed to tone and shape "problem areas." In fact, many health clubs have added very popular "ab, butt and thigh" toning classes to their exercise class lineup. Each of these special devices and exercise routines claim that exercising the muscles beneath fat storage areas will help mobilize and get rid of stubborn fat in that area.

Unfortunately, the research literature in this area does not support this theory. One classic study examined the muscle and fat mass in the right and left arms of high-caliber tennis players before the two-handed backhand became so popular. At that time, the

Figure 5.7
A comparison of the exercise habits of weight maintainers, relapsers and individuals who have never been obese. (Kayman et al, 1990.)

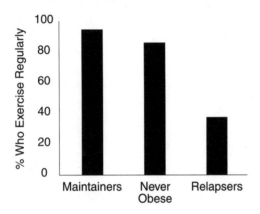

diameter and muscle mass of the dominant playing arm in professional tennis players was much greater than the non-dominant playing arm. If spot-reduction truly worked, we would expect to see less fat storage in the dominant playing arm. However, no differences were found between the sum of multiple skinfold measures of either forearm. Thus, sustained exercise in the playing arm did not result in reduced fat storage over the exercised muscle (Gwinup et al., 1971).

Katch and colleagues (1984) examined the effects of a vigorous sit-up exercise program on adipose cell size and adiposity. They had subjects perform more than 5,000 sit-ups over a period of 28 days. Skinfold thickness, body composition and circumference

measures were taken before and after the exercise program. They also took fat biopsies from the abdominal, buttocks and subscapular regions to assess the number and size of the cells in each area at baseline and after the vigorous training program. The extensive sit-up routine resulted in no changes in skinfold thickness, body composition or circumferences. Interestingly, the fat biopsy data did not find any selective differences in the preferential use or reduction in fat cell size or number in the abdominal region compared to the subscapular or buttocks regions.

Weight Maintenance

One of the biggest challenges facing both dieters and the professionals who treat them is the maintenance of weight loss. Unfortunately, after a successful weight-loss program, most dieters relapse into the old eating, behavioral and lifestyle habits that led them to be overweight in the past. There are a number of strategies that you can try with your clients to help them maintain their weight loss.

Continued Contact

Research has shown that continued contact with weight management professionals following a weight-reduction program is a strong predictor of weight maintenance. Group or individual bi-weekly meetings for a year after weight loss may help to keep your client focused. The continued contact can help reinforce the need for continuing the important dietary and lifestyle changes that are required to maintain weight loss.

Weight-Maintenance Strategies

Successful weight maintainers have developed skills to help them anticipate and cope with situations that put them at risk for relapsing into old behaviors.

If an individual lacks the skills to handle high-risk situations, such as holiday eating, a sense of hopelessness can set in.

Successful maintainers also tend to watch their weight more closely and notice small weight gains. When people are losing weight, weigh-ins can be discouraging since the scale does not always give the desired feedback, but frequent weight checks after weight loss can help prevent weight gain in the weight-stable maintainer.

Exercise

Exercise adherence is commonly cited as the strongest predictor of long-term success in weight management. In a recent study, weight maintainers, relapsers (weight regainers) and individuals who had never been obese were compared (Kayman et al., 1990). One of the most striking findings of this study was that most maintainers (90 percent) and women who never had a weight problem (82 percent) reported exercising regularly (at least three times per week). In contrast, only 34 percent of relapsers reported regular exercise (Figure 5.7), and those who did trained less frequently and at lower intensities than the weight maintainers.

Pavlou and colleagues (1989) also examined the role that exercise played in helping a group of slightly overweight police officers both lose and manage their weight. The subjects were randomly assigned to one of four diet conditions and to either an exercise (90 minutes of supervised exercise, three times per week) or non-exercise condition. After eight weeks of dieting, there were no differences between the diet-alone and diet-plus-exercise subjects. However, 18 months after treatment, the non-exercisers had regained all of their weight, whereas the exercisers had maintained their weight loss. This stresses the need for adding an exercise or activity component to the weight-maintenance phase of any weight-management program.

Summary

Obesity is a common and serious health problem. The risks of obesity can be dramatically reduced with a safe, sensible weight-management program that focuses on permanent change. Exercise can help overweight clients lose weight, improve health, possibly spare the loss of lean body mass as the weight is lost, and ultimately manage their weight. Finally, you will have to design treatment plans that integrate the client's genetic, psychological and physiological factors into the program.

References

American College of Sports Medicine. (1993). Position stand: physical activity, physical fitness and hypertension. *Medicine & Science in Sports and Exercise,* 10, i-x.

American Heart Association. (1994). Scientific statement on guidelines for weight management program in healthy adults. *Heart Disease and Stroke,* 3, 221-228.

Andersen, R. (1995). Is exercise/activity necessary for weight loss and weight management? *Medicine, Exercise, Nutrition and Health,* 4, 57-59.

Andersen, R., Brownell, K. & Haskell, W. (1992). *The Health and Fitness Leaders Guide: Administering a Weight Management Program.* Dallas: American Health Publishing.

Andersen, R., Wadden, T., Bartlett, S., Vogt R. & Weinstock, R. (1995). Relation of weight loss to changes in serum lipids and lipoproteins in obese women. *American Journal of Clinical Nutrition,* 62, 350-357.

Ballor, D., Katch, V.L., Becque, M. & Marks, C. (1988). Resistance weight training during caloric restriction enhances lean body weight maintenance. *American Journal of Clinical Nutrition,* 47, 19-25.

Ballor, D. & Poehlman, E. (1994). Exercise training enhances fat-free mass preservation during diet induced weight loss: a meta-analytic finding. *International Journal of Obesity,* 18, 35-40.

Blackburn, G. (1995). Effects of weight loss on weight-related risk factors. In: K.D.Brownell & C.G. Fairburn (Eds). *Eating Disorders and Obesity: A Comprehensive Handbook.* New York: Guilford Press.

Blackburn, G. & Rosofsky, W. (1992). Making the connection between weight loss, dieting and health: The l0-percent solution. *Weight Control Digest,* 2, 1-10.

Bouchard, C., Tremblay, A., Depres, J., Nadeau, A., Lupien, P., Theriault, G., Moojani, S., Pinault, S. & Fournier, G. (1990). The response to long term overfeeding in identical twins. *New England Journal of Medicine,* 322, 1477-1482.

Brownell, K. (1995). Matching individuals to treatments. In: K.D. Brownell & C. Fairburn (Eds). *Eating Disorders and Obesity: A Comprehensive Handbook.* New York: Guilford Press.

Brownell, K., Greenwood, M., Stellar, E. & Shrager, E. (1986). The effects of repeated cycles of weight loss and regain in rats. *Physiology and Behavior,* 38, 459-464.

Brownell, K. & Wadden, T. (1992). Etiology and treatment of obesity: Understanding a serious, prevalent and refractory disorder. *Journal of Clinical and Consulting Psychology,* 60, 505-517.

Campbell, W., Crim, M., Young, V. & Evans W. (1994). Increased energy requirements and changes in body composition with resistance training in older adults. *American Journal of Clinical Nutrition,* 60, 167-175.

Donnelly, J., Sharp, T., Houmard, J., et al. (1993). Muscle Hypertrophy with large scale weight loss and resistance training. *American Journal of Clinical Nutrition,* 58, 561-565.

Dwyer, J. (1995). Popular Diets. In: K.D. Brownell & C.G. Fairburn (Eds). *Eating Disorders and Obesity: A Comprehensive Handbook.* New York: Guilford Press.

Foster, G., Wadden, T., Peterson, F., Letizia, K., Bartlett, S. & Conill, A. (1992). A controlled comparison of three very low-calorie-diets: Effects on weight, body composition, and symptoms. *American Journal of Clinical Nutrition,* 55, 811-817.

Gillette, C., Bullough, R. & Melby, C. (1994). Post Exercise energy expenditure in reponse to acute aerobic or resistive exercise. *International Journal of Sports and Nutrition,* 4,3, 47-50.

Katch, F. & McArdle, W. (1988). *Nutrition, Weight Control, and Exercise.* Philadelphia: Lea and Febiger.

Katch, F., Clarkson, P., Kroll, W., McBride, T. & Wilcox, A. (1984). Preferential effects of abdominal exercise training on regional adipose cell size. *Research Quarterly in Exercise and Sports,* 55, 242-247.

Kayman, S., Bruvold, W. & Stem, J. (1990). Maintenance and relapse after weight loss in women: behavioral aspects. *American Journal of Clinical Nutrition,* 52, 800-807.

Kuczmarski, R., Flegal, K., Campbell, S. & Johnson, C. (1994) Increasing prevalence of overweight among US adults: The National Health and Nutrition Examination Surveys, 1960 to 1991. *Journal of the American Medical Association,* 272, 205-211.

Kumanyika, S., Wilson, J. & Guilford-Davenport, M. (1993). Weight-related attitudes and behaviors of black women. *Journal of the American Dietetic Association,* 93, 416-422.

Michigan Health Council. (1990). Toward safe weight loss: Recommendations for adult weight loss programs in Michigan. East Lansing Michigan.

Pi-Sunyer, F. (1995). Medical complications of obesity. In: K.D. Brownell & C.G. Fairburn (Eds). *Eating Disorders and Obesity: A Comprehensive Handbook.* New York: Guilford Press.

Poehlman, E. (1989). Exercise and its influence on resting metabolism in man. *Medicine and Science in Sports and Exercise,* 21, 515-525.

Stunkard, A., Sorensen, T., Hanis, C., Teasdale, T., Chakraborty, R., Schull, W. & Schulsinger, F. (1986). An adoption study of human obesity. *New England Journal of Medicine,* 314, 193-198.

Stunkard, A., Foch, T. & Hrubec, Z. (1986). A twin study of human obesity. *Journal of American Medical Association,* 256, 51-54.

Wadden, T. (1995). Very-Low-Calorie Diets: Appraisal and recommendations. In: K.D. Brownell & C.G. Fairburn (Eds). *Eating Disorders and Obesity: A Comprehensive Handbook.* New York: Guilford Press.

Wadden, T., Vogt, R., Andersen, R., et al. (1996). Exercise in the Treatment of Obesity: Effects of Four Interventions on Body Composition, Resting Energy Expenditure, Appetite, and Mood. *Journal of Clinical and Consulting Psychology.*

Wilmore, J. (1983). Body Composition in Sport and Exercise: Directions for future research. *Medicine and Science in Sports and Exercise,* 15, 21-31.

Wing, R. (1993). Weight cycling: the public concern and the scientific data. *Obesity Research,* 1, 390-391.

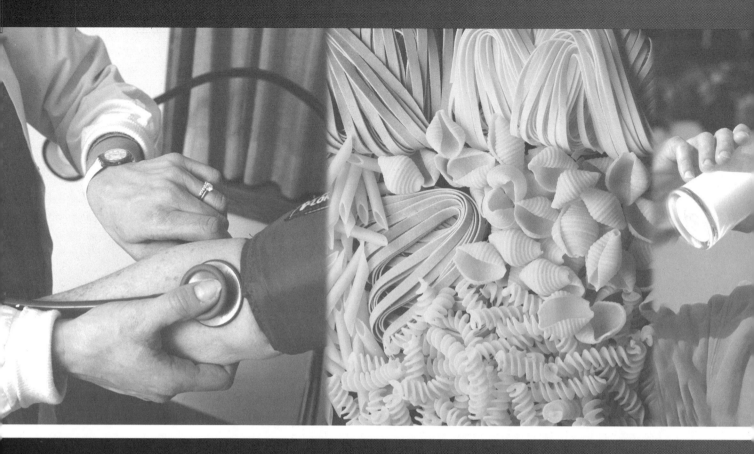

CHAPTER SIX

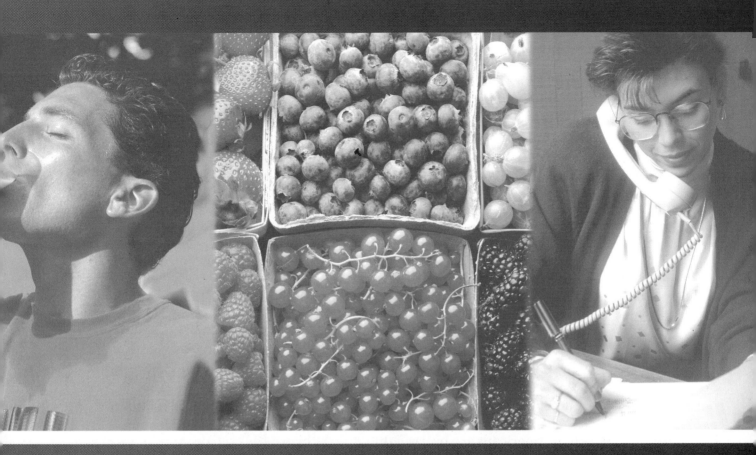

SCREENING, ASSESSMENT AND Referral

Susan J. Bartlett

Susan J. Bartlett, Ph.D., is a post-doctoral fellow at the Johns Hopkins School of Medicine, and associate director of clinical psychology with the Johns Hopkins Weight Management Center in Baltimore, Md. Dr. Bartlett also served as a member of the ACE Lifestyle & Weight Management Consultant Certification Examination Committee.

Ross E. Andersen

Ross E. Andersen, Ph.D., F.A.C.S.M, is an assistant professor of medicine at Johns Hopkins University, and focuses on the treatment of obesity. His research areas include the changes in resting metabolism, body composition and fitness that accompany weight-loss and exercise programs. His work is now supported by the National Institutes of Health, and his articles have appeared in Redbook and Reader's Digest as well as other publications.

Lawrence J. Cheskin

Lawrence J. Cheskin, M.D., F.A.C.P., is director of the Johns Hopkins Weight Management Center in Baltimore, Md. He is an associate professor of medicine at the Johns Hopkins University School of Medicine and holds a joint appointment in International Health (Human Nutrition) at the Johns Hopkins School of Hygiene and Public Health.

Introduction

Obesity is a serious threat to one's health and well-being. Medical risks associated with overweight include diabetes, hypercholesterolemia, gall bladder disease, hypertension, some forms of cancer and cardiovascular disease (see Chapter 5). It is estimated that more than 34 million Americans are overweight (31 percent of men and 35 percent of women), and the prevalence is increasing (Kuczmarski et al., 1994). The economic, medical and psychological costs to our society are staggering.

A record number of individuals are now attempting to control their weight. Recent surveys indicate that up to 45 percent of women and 25 percent of men report that they are currently trying to lose weight (Williamson et al., 1992). However, dieting and weight-loss practices are not without important health and economic consequences (see Chapter 4). The pervasiveness of dieting in our culture has led to a multi-billion dollar weight-loss industry and sparked congressional investigations into the activities and efficacy of many commercial programs.

Lifestyle and weight management consultants (LWMCs) offer a unique service combining information from nutritional, behavioral and exercise sciences to help clients manage their weight. The hallmark of ACE-certified consultants is their ability to work safely and effectively in promoting lifestyle change for a wide variety of individuals. However, not all clients who seek your services can and should be treated by you. The purpose of this chapter is to: 1) assist in screening for potential contraindications to weight loss treatment; 2) provide a framework for the assessment of potential clients; and 3) identify appropriate referral sources.

The Importance of a Thorough Screening and Assessment

There are many factors that influence whether an individual will become overweight. Identifying underlying contributors to a client's weight problem is important because it will influence the type of treatment you recommend for them. For example, Joe is the chief counsel in a large firm of attorneys. His work frequently takes him on the road for several weeks at a time. Trials are often preceded by weeks of long work days and are followed by a couple of weeks of relaxation. Though once a highly fit, athletic individual, Joe has gained about 50 pounds over the past 10 years. You surmise that Joe's "fast food" lifestyle and lack of regular exercise are major contributors to his weight difficulties.

On the other hand, consider Sam.

Sam is the chief operating officer of a major manufacturing plant. Recently separated from his wife, he is finding it increasingly difficult to return to an empty apartment each evening and has begun to work longer hours each day without breaking for lunch or dinner. Once home, however, he finds himself consumed with thoughts of eating and

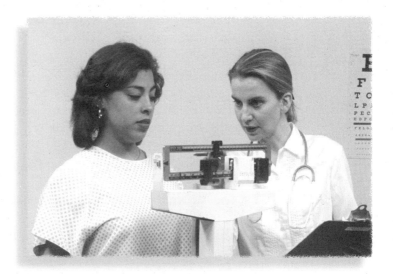

binges nearly every night on food and alcohol. As a result, he has gained nearly 50 pounds in six to nine months. He confides to you that he feels his eating is increasingly out of control and that he feels powerless to stop.

Both Joe and Sam need to lose similar amounts of weight. The excess 50 pounds they are carrying confers a significant health risk, and weight gain is likely to continue unless specific changes are made. Joe's lifestyle choices are clearly affecting his weight. More appropriate food choices and behavioral strategies to reduce his calorie and fat consumption, in combination with a regular program of physical activity, will be the cornerstone of his weight-management program. However, Sam's weight difficulties appear more complex. His weight problem results from more than careless eating patterns or a **sedentary** lifestyle (though these may be

You and your client must decide how to best measure their progress. For some, this may mean weekly weigh-ins, while others may prefer to have their measurements taken on a monthly basis. Regardless of what method is chosen, it must be performed consistently in order to give the client both encouragement and incentive to stick to their new lifestyle.

important factors for later weight maintenance). You may suspect Sam has an underlying depressive disorder that is complicated by both his current stressors (the separation) and excessive eating and drinking patterns. Depression, current major stressors and uncontrolled bingeing are potential contraindications for weight loss and may require the assistance of a mental health professional before weight loss is attempted. To best meet the needs of the overweight client, it is important to match each client's needs with the appropriate level of care. The next section presents an overview of the various types of **obesity** programs currently available.

Types of Programs

Many clients you work with will require no direct involvement of healthcare professionals. However, to work with some clients appropriately, you may need to seek support from healthcare providers such as physicians, mental health specialists (e.g., psychologists, psychiatrists, psychiatric nurses and psychiatric social workers), dietitians and exercise physiologists. To understand when and whom to involve in your client's care, you must understand the spectrum of services available for treating overweight. The various approaches to obesity treatment can be broadly broken down into three categories: 1) self-help programs, 2) non-clinical programs and 3) clinical approaches (Institute of Medicine, 1995). While clients with no special medical or psychological problems can be treated appropriately in any of these three categories, those with problems may be best served by more intensive clinical programs that employ only licensed professionals.

Self-help programs are widely used and vary in format. Examples may include the use of meal-replacement shakes or frozen entrees, participation in support or self-help groups (e.g., Overeaters Anonymous, church-based groups), popular diet books, manuals, magazine articles or increased exercise. The safety, effectiveness and quality of such approaches varies greatly. In general, among self-help programs, one approach is recommended for everyone with little or no individualization.

Non-clinical programs are typically more structured and tailored than self-help programs. Most non-clinical programs are commercial-based franchises. The parent company provides the structure, materials and, in some cases, the food for clients to utilize. Consultants are then employed to present the program to participants. The training of such consultants varies widely and in some cases counselors are simply program graduates with some additional training provided by the company. Consultants may or may not be supervised by experienced weight-loss professionals. While some attempt may be made to individualize treatment, most programs allow only minimal deviation from a well-defined plan.

In clinical programs, treatment is provided largely by licensed professionals such as psychologists, registered dietitians and physicians. The clinician may work alone and refer to allied health professionals as needed, or, more typically, be part of a multidisciplinary team. Clinical programs may be commercially based (e.g., Optifast, Medifast) or affiliated with a hospital or university. They are characterized by a thorough medical and psychological assessment and are best suited to treat complicated or recalcitrant cases of obesity. Treatment may be highly individualized to meet the unique medical and psychological needs of the participants.

Standards of Care for Weight-Management Programs

New "diets" that promise fast, easy, large weight losses have been a part of our culture for decades. The next time you are standing in line at the supermarket, conduct an informal survey of the top women's magazines; most will feature at least one article about diet and weight loss on the cover. New weight-loss books can frequently be found among the top 10 best-sellers. As a result, the weight-loss industry has grown tremendously, and with this growth has come the need to oversee both the safety and efficacy of the increasing number of approaches. Recently, several regulatory bodies have developed guidelines to regulate the practices and advertising claims of weight-loss providers.

The Department of Consumer Affairs (DCA) of New York City was the first to document deceptive practices of many rapid-weight-loss centers. These ranged from working with inappropriate candidates (i.e., underweight individuals) and offering false and misleading statements to outright quackery (Winner, 1991). The result was the first "Truth-in-Dieting" regulation which mandated specific requirements for all centers promoting rapid weight loss (e.g., more than 1½ to 2 pounds per week, or the loss of more than 1 percent of body weight per week after the second week of participation). Specifically, such centers were required to post a "Weight-Loss Consumers Bill of Rights" (Table 6.1) and provide all consumers with a wallet-size card outlining them. In addition, programs were required to disclose all costs and the recommended length of treatment.

At about the same time, the Michigan Department of Public Health developed its own set of guidelines for weight-loss programs (Drewnowski,

Table 6.1

The Weight-loss Consumers' Bill of Rights

1. WARNING: Rapid weight loss may cause serious health problems. (Rapid weight loss is weight loss of more than 1½ to 2 pounds per week, or weight loss of more than 1 percent of body weight per week after the second week of participation in a weight-loss program.)

2. Only permanent lifestyle changes—such as making healthful food choices and increasing physical activity—promote long-term weight loss.

3. Consult your personal physician before starting any weight-loss program.

4. Qualifications of this provider's staff are available upon request.

5. You have a right to
   ✔ ask questions about the potential health risks of this program, its nutritional content, and its psychological support and educational components;

   ✔ know the price of treatment, including the price of extra products, services, supplements and laboratory tests; and

   ✔ know the program duration that is being recommended for you.

Source: New York Department of Consumer Affairs (1992).

1990). The Michigan guidelines applied to all non-clinical and clinical programs and were even more detailed than those developed in New York City. The Michigan Guidelines made several key recommendations:

1. That all clients be screened to verify that they have no medical or psychological conditions that could make weight loss inappropriate. Depending on the client, such screening would range from a simple health checklist to a complete physical exam.

2. That clients be classified not only by excess body weight, but also by overall health risks to ensure that the individual would receive the appropriate

Table 6.2

Criteria for Evaluating Weight-management Programs

Criterion	Program	Person
1. The match between program and consumer	Who is appropriate for this program?	Should I be in this program given my goals and characteristics?
2. The soundness and safety of the program	Is my program based on sound biological and behavioral principles, and is it safe for its intended participants?	Is the program safe for me?
3. Outcomes of the program	What is the evidence of success of my program?	Are the benefits I am likely to achieve from the program worth the effort and cost?

Source: Institute of Medicine. (1995). *Weighing the Options: Criteria for Evaluating Weight-management Programs.* Washington: National Academy Press.

level of care. Level I was intended for low-risk clients, Level II for the moderate-risk client who required medical monitoring, and Level III was reserved for the seriously obese or high-risk individual.

3. That care should be provided by appropriately trained individuals. The qualifications of weight-loss staff should be commensurate with the level of health risk of the client. Thus, programs that accepted clients with high health risks required highly trained healthcare professionals.

Specific recommendations were made concerning daily caloric intake, dietary composition, use of appetite suppressant drugs and the inclusion of exercise. An emphasis also was placed on individualizing the programs and including a maintenance phase to promote long-term weight management.

At a national level, the Food and Nutrition Board of the Institute of Medicine (IOM), National Academy of Sciences, commissioned a committee to develop criteria for evaluating the effectiveness of weight-loss approaches in both preventing and treating obesity.

World-renowned researchers in nutrition, psychology, medicine and exercise science participated on the committee. The book summarizing their results, *Weighing the Options: Criteria for Evaluating Weight-Management Programs* (IOM, 1995), set forth three primary criteria, as shown in Table 6.2.

Criterion 1 of the IOM recommendations — the match between program and consumer — addresses the importance of matching individuals to appropriate treatment strategies. Treatment for weight disorders can be seen as ranging on a continuum from the least invasive and costly to strategies requiring intensive, expensive professional care. To better match individual needs and treatment options, Dr. George Blackburn, a leading obesity researcher, developed a **stepped-care model** (IOM, 1995). Stepped-care models are widely used in medicine and are based on the premise that treatment can be cumulative or incremental.

As shown in Figure 6.1, Step one utilizes a low-fat diet, physical activity and lifestyle change to promote a healthy and reasonable weight loss of up to

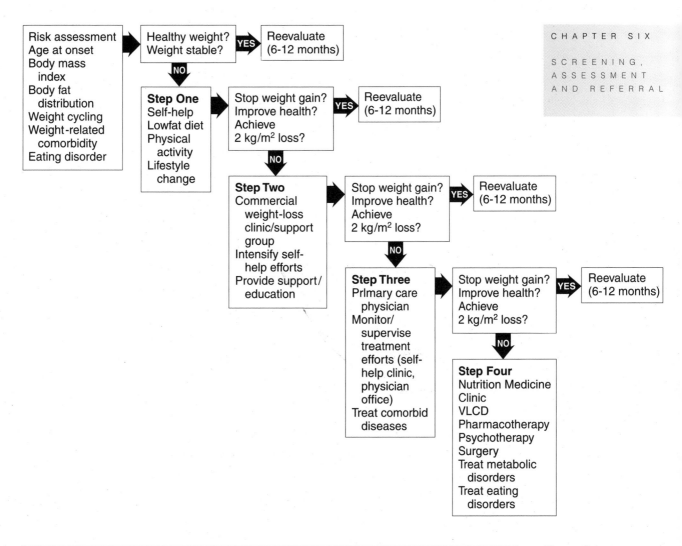

Source: Institute of Medicine. (1995). *Weighing the Options: Criteria for Evaluating Weight-management Programs.* Washington: National Academy Press.

Figure 6.1
Stepped levels of care for obesity treatment.

10 pounds. Step two involves a more detailed assessment of health risks and screening by the client's primary care physician, and utilizes more intensive efforts to help clients change their lifestyles while promoting a larger weight loss. When individuals have comorbid disease or are at high risk of weight-related diseases, more intensive monitoring of the individual is required, as shown in Step three. The client's primary care physician may also participate more actively in the weight-management program through supervision and monitoring. Step four provides the most intensive and aggressive interventions

for weight loss including the use of **very-low-calorie diets**, medication, psychotherapy and even surgery as indicated. Step four incorporates all of the goals of Steps one through three, while maximizing the loss of excess body fat and enhancing metabolic fitness.

Where does the work that you do fit within the stepped model? It is possible that you may work with clients through all four steps, depending on the setting, the level of professional support available to you and your education. However, as a lifestyle and weight management consultant, you are ideally suited to promote lifestyle change in Steps one, two and three through education, support and structure. Also, as health-care becomes increasingly oriented toward the prevention of illness, you can potentially assume a primary role in working with individuals at Step one who are at risk for becoming over-weight and later developing obesity-related illnesses, but are currently free of such problems.

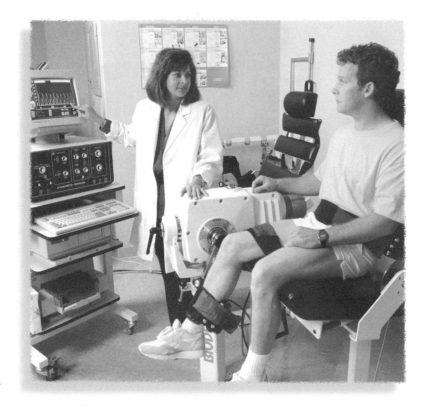

Some clients may require testing that is beyond your capabilities. In these cases, refer them to an appropriate professional for clearance, and always follow their recommendations when developing your client's program.

Criterion 2 of the IOM recommendations — the soundness and safety of the program — proposes **standards of care** or minimum expectations of a credible weight-loss approach. Specifically, the following four areas are identified:

✔ assessment of physical health and psychological status (including assessment of a client's knowledge and attitudes related to weight, and a periodic reassessment to determine if they are still committed to losing weight and learning the facts and skills necessary to succeed)

✔ attention to diet
✔ attention to physical activity
✔ ensuring program safety

The IOM offers two additional recommendations supporting the importance of small weight losses to reduce health risks and placing an emphasis on long-term maintenance of weight losses:

"We recommend that ... the goal of obesity treatment should be refocused from weight loss alone, which is often aimed at appearance, to weight management, achieving the best weight possible in the context of overall health. [Weight-loss programs] should be judged more by their effects on the overall health of participants than by their effects on weight alone" (IOM, 1995, p. 5).

How can you ensure the soundness and safety of your program for potential clients? A thorough assessment of physical and psychological health (which may or may not involve the client's personal physician) is an important beginning. Attention to dietary intake and physical activity to safely promote either an appropriate energy deficit (for weight loss) or **energy balance** (for weight maintenance) also is required. The IOM recommends that reassessment of diet and activity patterns be conducted at the beginning and end of the weight-loss phase of treatment, and every six months during the maintenance phase.

You must also be aware of both the known and hypothetical risks associated with dieting. In general, the more restrictive the diet, the greater the associated risks. For example, the risk of gall-bladder disease is greatest with very-low-calorie diets and rapid weight loss. Caloric intake of fewer than 1,200 kcal/day may not meet nutritional guidelines and should not be promoted. Diets of 800 kcal/day must only be used under a physician's supervision (IOM, 1995).

Criterion 3 of the IOM recommendations — outcomes of the program — focuses on four components of a successful program: 1) long-term weight loss; 2) improvement in obesity-related risk factors; 3) improved health practices (e.g., increased physical activity, improved eating habits); and 4) monitoring of adverse effects that might result from the program (IOM, 1995). To successfully monitor outcome, it is critical that the initial and subsequent client assessments are thorough and well documented.

In the interest of consumer protection, the IOM suggests that all details of a weight-loss program be disclosed. This includes rate of weight loss, outline of treatment plan, cost estimates, professional credentials of program staff and the risks associated with treatment. Claims that weight losses will be maintained over time should be backed up with scientifically valid documentation, not "satisfied client" claims.

Screening Issues

Many factors must be considered when assessing the suitability of a potential client, including medical and psychological status, motivation, readiness to change and timing. For instance, think back to the example of Joe and Sam. Even though Joe (the lawyer) appears to be a good candidate for your services, if the timing is inappropriate (e.g., if he is just beginning a lengthy trial), he is much less likely to succeed. Certain factors may clearly signal that a potential client is not well suited to your services. (For a more thorough review of the LWMC **scope of practice**, see State Regulation of Healthcare — Permitted and Unpermitted Activities and Legal and Professional Duties and Responsibilities in Chapter

11.) All clients who undertake weight management should be both screened and assessed.

Screening is the initial process by which you separate individuals who may be appropriate for your services from those who clearly are not. Assessment is the process of determining the significance or importance of various factors that contribute to, or complicate, your client's weight-management needs. A thorough screening and assessment process protects both you and the consumer by ensuring that the needs of a potential client can be met by the services you can legitimately and ethically provide.

Is this Client Appropriate for this Setting?

Brownell and Wadden (1992) suggest that the degree of overweight, the type of treatment or program, and client characteristics all are factors that should be used to match individuals with treatment protocols. One of your foremost responsibilities is to determine the appropriateness of a potential client for your program. Though lifestyle and weight management consultants may be found in all types of settings, the greatest responsibility will lay with the consultant who is essentially practicing without the formal support of any health professional. Examples of this would include the consultant who works independently or provides services in a health club or commercial franchise setting.

Assessment Issues

An assessment of medical and psychological status, diet and activity level is strongly advised for all clients. The scope and depth of the assessment will vary with the program setting and level of care provided. This section will

Figure 6.2
Sample health
history checklist.

Health History Checklist

Place an X next to any of the following conditions that you have now or have ever had:

_____ High blood pressure
_____ Heart disease
_____ Chest pain
_____ Shortness of breath
_____ Irregular heart beat
_____ Dizziness or fainting spells
_____ Stroke
_____ Severe headaches
_____ Seizures or convulsions
_____ Numbness or tingling
_____ Fainting
_____ Indigestion
_____ Liver disease (hepatitis)
_____ Gallbladder disease
_____ Diabetes
_____ Hypoglycemia
_____ Thyroid disease
_____ High cholesterol level
_____ High triglyceride level
_____ Anemia
_____ Arthritis
_____ Gout
_____ Pain/swelling in joints
_____ Kidney disease
_____ Chronic cough
_____ Asthma
_____ Swelling of feet/ankles
_____ Difficulty breathing
_____ Allergies
_____ Depression
_____ Anxiety
_____ Use of laxatives or water pills
_____ Psychological difficulties
_____ Alcoholism/substance abuse
_____ Other (please explain)

_____
_____
_____

present information on the basic or minimum evaluation of physical and psychological health, readiness to exercise, fitness parameters and motivation or readiness to change (see Chapter 9).

Assessing Physical Health

Since weight-management practices can potentially help or harm the health of your clients (IOM, 1995), some type of physical and psychological health assessment is required for all individuals with whom you work. Physical health can only be assessed by a physician. Physicians, physician assistants and nurse practitioners are best able to review health history and conduct a physical exam to detect obesity-related illnesses.

Criteria for Medical Clearance. Though it is recommended that all clients receive their physician's clearance before beginning a weight-loss program, it is especially important for individuals with the following conditions (see Chapter 10):

✔ hypertension
✔ elevated **cholesterol** or **triglyceride** levels
✔ **diabetes**
✔ significant emotional problems
✔ **BMI** greater than 27
✔ insulin-dependent diabetes
✔ chronic kidney failure
✔ cardiovascular disease, including **angina**, **arrhythmias** and congestive heart failure
✔ liver disease
✔ pregnancy — present or planned
✔ hyperthyroidism or hypothyroidism
✔ substance abuse

The Basic Health Screen. For apparently healthy clients who report no significant current or past medical problems, it may be sufficient to obtain the following health data:

✔ height and weight
✔ **body mass index**
✔ **waist-to-hip ratio**
✔ blood pressure and resting heart rate
✔ current medications
✔ chronic illnesses
✔ medical history
✔ family health history
✔ health-related habits (e.g., cigarette, alcohol and recreation drugs)

Height and weight can be compared against the 1983 Metropolitan Life Insurance table of suggested weights for adults. (See Chapter 4 for the Metropolitan Life Insurance table and information on the calculation and interpretation of body mass index and the waist-to-hip ratio.) A simple health history checklist, which includes current medications, illnesses and a family health history such as the one shown in Figure 6.2, can be included as part of your client application forms. Having clients complete such forms and obtain physician clearance prior to their first meeting with you can save time during the initial consultation. Be sure to review all of this information with the client to ensure nothing has been omitted. This also provides an excellent opportunity to identify and record risk factors that the client may or may not be aware of having.

Measuring Blood Pressure and Resting Heart Rate. Two additional components of physical health that you can effectively screen are resting blood pressure and resting heart rate. Blood pressure reflects the force of the heartbeat and the resistance of the arteries to the pumping action of the heart. It should be measured using a medical grade sphygmomanometer after a client has been seated with both feet flat on the floor for two full minutes. The cuff should be smoothly and firmly wrapped around the arm with its lower margin

Table 6.3

Classification of Blood Pressure for Adults

Systolic Reading*	Diastolic Reading*	Category
<130	<85	Normal
130-139	85-89	High normal
140-159	90-99	Mild hypertension
160-179	100-109	Moderate hypertension
180-209	110-119	Severe hypertension

*In mmHg

Source: Fifth Report of the Joint Committee on Detection, Evaluation, and Treatment of High Blood Pressure (JNCV) (1993). *Archives of Internal Medicine*, 153:154-183.

about one inch above the antecubital space. (Use an appropriate-sized cuff as very obese clients may have falsely elevated blood pressure readings with small, standard-sized cuffs.) The arm should be comfortably supported on either an arm chair or by you at an angle of 10 to 45 degrees. Rapidly inflate the cuff to 20 to 30 mmHg above the radial palpatory pressure (i.e., until 20 to 30 mmHg above the point when the pulse can no longer be felt at the wrist). Place the stethoscope over the brachial artery using a minimal amount of pressure so as not to distort the artery. The stethoscope should not touch the cuff or its tubing. Release the pressure at a rate of about 2 mmHg per second, listening for sounds. The **systolic pressure** is determined by the first perception of sound. The **diastolic pressure** is determined when the sounds cease to be heard or when they become muffled. A duplicate measurement should be made using the other arm. Normative values for blood pressure readings are presented in Table 6.3.

Resting heart rate also is considered to be a crude indicator of physical health and cardiovascular fitness. The average resting heart rate is 72 beats per minute (bpm) with a range of 60 to

Table 6.4
Common Psychotropic Medications

Drug Name	Trade Names(s)	Major Use
alprazolam	Xanax	Anti-anxiety
amitriptyline	Elavil	Antidepressant
amoxapine	Asendin	Antidepressant
bupropion	Wellbutrin	Antidepressant
buspirone	Buspar	Anti-anxiety
carba-mazepine	Tegretol	Mood stabilizer, Anticonvulsant
chlordiaz-epoxide	Librium	Anti-anxiety
clomipramine	Anafranil	Antidepressant
clonazepam	Klonopin	Anti-anxiety
clonidine	Catapres	Anti-anxiety
desipramine	Norpramin, Pertofrane	Antidepressant
dex-fenfluramine	Redux	Anti-appetite
diazepam	Valium	Anti-anxiety
doxepin	Sinequan, Adapin	Antidepressant
fenfluramine	Pondimin	Anti-appetite
fluvoxamine	Luvox	Antidepressant
fluoxetine	Prozac	Antidepressant
haloperidol	Haldol	Antipsychotic
imipramine	Tofranil	Antidepressant
lithium	Eskalith, Lithonate, Lithobid	Mood stabilizer
lorazepam	Ativan	Anti-anxiety
nefazodone	Serzone	Antidepressant
nortriptyline	Pamelor, Aventyl	Antidepressant
oxazepam	Serax	Anti-anxiety
paroxetine	Paxil	Antidepressant
phenelzine	Nardil	Antidepressant (MAOI)
phentermine	Fasting Lonamin	Anti-appetite
sertraline	Zoloft	Antidepressant
triazolam	Halcion	Anti-anxiety, Hypnotic
valproate	Dapakene, Depakote	Mood stabilizer

Note: This list is not intended to be exhaustive. Always consult with the client's physician (with the client's written permission) if you have any questions regarding medication use.

100 bpm. Generally, the more fit an individual is, the lower their resting heart rate. (However, it is important to recognize that certain medications such as **beta blockers** may slow both resting and non-resting heart rates.) The client should be quietly seated for two full minutes with both feet flat on the floor. Either place a stethoscope firmly to the left of the sternum or feel for the pulse at the thumb side of the wrist. Determine the heart rate using a 15-second count. Multiply this count by four to calculate the resting pulse (in bpm). In the event that the resting heart rate is above 100 bpm, wait another five minutes and take the pulse again. If it is still above 100 bpm, refer the client to their physician before any aerobic or muscular endurance fitness tests are performed.

Determining a Reasonable Weight. For many significantly overweight individuals, weight that is lost is often regained. For example, in one controlled study, individuals who lost large amounts of weight regained about two-thirds of it within one year and almost all of it within five years (Wadden et al., 1989). In response to such disappointing outcomes, many weight-management programs have shifted from the premise of having all clients achieve an ideal weight to helping most achieve and maintain a reasonable weight.

Obesity experts have suggested a weight loss of 10 percent of body weight as an initial goal (IOM, 1995). Once this has been achieved, it may be appropriate to set an interval goal of losing an additional 5 percent of body weight, with re-evaluation after each successive interval (Foster, 1995). Alternately, Brownell and Wadden (1992) have suggested a realistic weight should not be less than the client's lowest weight achieved since the age of 21 that was successfully maintained for one year.

While in many cases modest losses will not bring clients to their ideal weight, such losses may nevertheless confer important health benefits and may be more likely to be sustained over time. (For more on reasonable weights see *Weight Loss Goals for Overweight Clients* in Chapter 4 and *Reviewing Client Expectations* in Chapter 3.)

Assessing Psychological Health

The psychological health of all potential clients should be assessed prior to beginning a weight-loss program. This is especially important since several psychiatric disorders such as eating disorders, anxiety disorders and clinical depression can initially appear to be weight-related difficulties. In reality, though food is involved in the expression of symptoms (e.g., by under- or overeating), eating disorders are classified as mental disorders that can be potentially life-threatening and require specialized interventions by skilled mental-health professionals.

Obtaining a psychological history is an important first step. Ask all clients whether they are currently in therapy or have previously received counseling. Keep a record of all counseling experiences including the therapist's name, dates of treatment and reasons for seeking therapy. If your client is currently receiving counseling, it is advisable to contact the therapist (after obtaining the client's written permission) and mutually determine whether weight loss is appropriate at this time. Review the list of medications your client is presently taking. Certain **psychotropic medications** such as antidepressants, anti-anxiety or mood stabilizers all signal the presence of psychological conditions (Table 6.4), and many psychotropic medications may facilitate or hamper weight loss significantly.

Specific training in psychology, psychiatry, medicine or social work is required to adequately evaluate psychological symptoms. However, by exploring psychological status with potential clients you can obtain some indication of the person's likelihood of succeeding at weight loss and determine whether a more comprehensive psychological evaluation is indicated. Several psychological conditions, such as clinical depression and eating disorders (i.e., **anorexia nervosa**, **bulimia nervosa** and **binge eating disorder**), are clear contraindications for weight loss (see *Eating Disorders* in Chapter 3).

Depression. Depression is a psychological disorder in which the person experiences pervasive feelings of sadness, hopelessness, helplessness and worthlessness. Signs of depression include sleep disturbance (e.g., hypersomnia or **insomnia**), eating difficulties (overeating or lack of interest in eating), excessive guilt and tearfulness or crying spells. Individuals who are depressed also may have difficulty concentrating, remembering or thinking clearly (American Psychiatric Association, APA, 1994).

Depression is increasingly associated, in part, with a chemical imbalance in the brain. Effective treatments for depression include psychotherapy alone or in combination with medication and exercise. Weight loss is never an appropriate treatment for depression and, in fact, most obesity specialists believe it is a contraindication for weight-loss treatment (IOM, 1995). Although some persons who are both overweight and depressed believe that the former causes the latter, this is a dangerous oversimplification. It is important to be able to identify signs of a clinical depression and refer the individual for further evaluation by a mental health specialist.

Eating Disorders. Anorexia nervosa is characterized by the refusal to

Table 6.5
**Screening Questions
to Detect Binge Eating**

1. Are there times during the day when you could not have stopped eating, even if you had wanted to?

2. Do you ever find yourself eating unusually large amounts of food in a short period of time?

3. Do you ever feel extremely guilty or depressed afterward?

4. Do you ever feel even more determined to diet or to eat healthier after the eating episodes?

Source: Bruce & Wilfley, 1996.

Table 6.6
**Major Symptoms and Signs Suggestive
of Cardiopulmonary Disease**

1. Pain, discomfort (or other anginal equivalent) in the chest, neck, jaw, arms, or other areas that might be ischemic in nature

2. Shortness of breath at rest or with mild exertion

3. Dizziness or syncope (fainting spells)

4. Orthopnea (shortness of breath when lying flat—often report sleeping on more than one pillow) or paroxysmal nocturnal dyspnea (labored breathing)

5. Ankle edema (swelling)

6. Palpitations or tachycardia (racing heart)

7. Intermittent pain which occurs with walking (claudication)

8. Known heart murmur

9. Unusual fatigue or shortness of breath with usual activities

These symptoms must be interpreted in the clinical context in which they appear, since they are not all specific for cardiopulmonary or metabolic disease.

Source: American College of Sports Medicine, 1995.

maintain a minimally healthy body weight (i.e., at least 85 percent of ideal body weight), a morbid fear of gaining weight, **amenorrhea** and disturbances in the way in which weight and shape are experienced or evaluated by the individual (APA, 1994). Bulimia nervosa is characterized by recurrent episodes of binge eating in which the individual experiences a loss of control over eating followed by compensatory behaviors aimed at avoiding weight gain (e.g., vomiting, laxative or **diuretic** abuse, fasting or excessive exercise) (APA, 1994). As with anorexia nervosa, self-evaluation is unduly influenced by weight and shape. Individuals with bulimia nervosa are often normal weight or slightly overweight. In binge eating disorder (BED, which is classified as Eating Disorder Not Otherwise Specified), the individual also experiences episodes of bingeing coupled with a sense of loss of control over eating, however there is no active attempt at compensating for the binges (APA, 1994). Individuals with binge eating disorder tend to be overweight. In clinical settings, 25 percent to 33 percent of individuals seeking weight-loss treatment suffer from BED (Spitzer et al., 1993). Table 6.5 presents screening questions to help detect binge eating disorder.

It is important to identify eating disorders in potential clients because these individuals are more likely to suffer from other psychological disorders as well (Bruce & Wilfley, 1996). Weight loss or maintenance of an abnormally low body weight is never appropriate for an individual with anorexia nervosa. This is important to remember when working with athletes such as body builders, gymnasts, dancers and runners where a low body weight is

Table 6.7

Coronary Artery Disease Risk Factors*

Positive Risk Factors	Defining Criteria
1. Age	Men >45 years; women >55 or premature menopause without estrogen replacement therapy
2. Family history	Myocardial infarction or sudden death before 55 years of age in father or other male first-degree relative, or before 65 years of age in mother or other female first-degree relative
3. Current cigarette smoking	——
4. Hypertension	Blood pressure >140/90 mmHg, confirmed by measurements on at least 2 separate occasions, or on antihypertensive medication
5. Hypercholesterolemia	Total serum cholesterol >200 mg/dL (if lipoprotein profile is unavailable) or HDL <35 mg/dL
6. Diabetes mellitus	Persons with insulin-dependent diabetes mellitus (IDDM) who are >30 years of age, or have had IDDM for >15 years, and persons with noninsulin-dependent diabetes mellitus (NIDDM) who are >35 years of age should be classified as patients with disease
7. Sedentary lifestyle/ physical inactivity	Persons comprising the least active 25% of the population, as defined by the combination of sedentary jobs involving sitting for a large part of the day and no regular exercise or active recreational pursuits

Negative Risk Factor	Comments
1. High serum HDL cholesterol	>60 mg/dL (1.6 mmol/L)

Notes: (1) It is common to sum risk factors in making clinical judgments. If HDL is high, subtract one risk factor from the sum of positive risk factors, since high HDL decreases CAD risk; (2) Obesity is not listed as an independent positive risk factor because its effects are exerted through other risk factors (e.g., hypertension, hyperlipidemia, diabetes). Obesity should be considered as an independent target for intervention.

Source: American College of Sports Medicine, 1995.
*Adapted in part from *Journal of the American Medical Association* 269:3015-3023, 1993.

coveted. Weight loss is only appropriate in individuals with bulimia when it is accompanied by psychotherapy (or after a successful course of therapy). Recovery from binge eating disorder also appears to require psychotherapy specifically aimed at reducing binge eating (Bruce & Wilfley, 1996). Currently, it is unclear whether dieting complicates or facilitates recovery from binge eating disorder. If you suspect a poten-

tial client may suffer from BED, it is important to consider referral to an eating disorders specialist as a primary step before you attempt to work with the individual. Psychotherapy may increase the client's ability to lose weight and maximize the likelihood of successful maintenance of a lower body weight.

Assessing Exercise Readiness

The American College of Sports

Table 6.8

ACSM Recommendations for Medical Examination and Pre-exercise Testing

A. Medical examination and clinical exercise test recommended prior to:

	Apparently Healthy		Increased Risk[1]		Known Disease[2]
	Younger[3]	Older	No Symptoms	Symptoms	
Moderate exercise[4]	No[5]	No	No	Yes	Yes
Vigorous exercise[6]	No	Yes[7]	Yes	Yes	Yes

B. Physician supervision recommended during exercise test:

	Apparently Healthy		Increased Risk[1]		Known Disease[2]
	Younger[3]	Older	No Symptoms	Symptoms	
Submaximal testing	No[5]	No	No	Yes	Yes
Maximal testing	No	Yes[7]	Yes	Yes	Yes

1 Persons with two or more risk factors (Table 6.7), or one or more signs or symptoms of cardiopulmonary disease (Table 6.6)

2 Persons with known cardiac, pulmonary or metabolic disease

3 Younger implies < 40 years for men; < 50 years for women

4 Moderate exercise as defined by an intensity of 40% to 60% VO_2 max; if intensity is uncertain, moderate exercise may alternately be defined as an intensity well within the individual's current capacity, one which can be comfortably sustained for a prolonged period of time, that is 60 minutes, which has a gradual initiation and progression, and is generally noncompetitive.

5 A "No" response means that an item is deemed "not necessary." The "No" response does not mean that the item should not be done.

6 Vigorous exercise is defined by an exercise intensity of 60% VO_2 max; if intensity is uncertain, moderate exercise may alternately be defined as exercise intense enough to represent a substantial cardiorespiratory challenge, or if it results in fatigue within 20 minutes.

7 A "Yes" response means that an item is recommended. For physician supervision, this suggests that a physician is in close proximity and readily available should there be an emergent need.

ACSM recommendations for (A) medical examination and exercise testing prior to participation and (B) physician supervision of exercise tests.

Source: American College of Sports Medicine, 1995.

Medicine (ACSM) has recently established recommendations concerning the need for a medical examination and exercise testing prior to participation in an exercise program (ACSM, 1995). Historically, many sedentary adults have been sent for a complete physical exam and stress test before beginning an exercise program. Unfortunately, the cost of such assessments, along with the fear they instilled (by conveying the erroneous message that all exercise is dangerous), may have prevented many adults from adopting a more active lifestyle. Thus, it is important for you to clearly understand who does and does not require a thorough medical screening before beginning an exercise program.

The ACSM classifies adults into three levels of risk: 1) apparently healthy, 2) increased risk and 3) those with known disease. Apparently healthy adults are those individuals who have no apparent signs or symptoms of cardiopulmonary disease (Table 6.6) and no more than one major coronary risk factor (Table 6.7). Apparently healthy women under 50, and men under 40 years of age, may begin an unrestricted exercise program without a physician's approval. These people do not require physician supervision for maximal treadmill testing.

Individuals over these age cut-offs

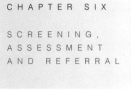

who are apparently healthy also can begin a moderate-intensity exercise program without a physician's approval. The ACSM defines moderate-intensity exercise as 40 percent to 60 percent of **VO₂ max**. Moderate intensity can also be defined as exercise well within the individual's current exercise capacity that can comfortably be sustained for extended periods of time (i.e., 60 minutes) and is non-competitive.

Apparently healthy women over 50 and men over 40 years of age should seek medical approval if they wish to exercise vigorously. The ACSM defines vigorous exercise as being above 60 percent of VO₂ max. If actual exercise intensity is uncertain, vigorous exercise can be defined as an intensity that challenges the aerobic system, or one which results in fatigue after 20 minutes of participation (Table 6.8). Physician supervision is required for maximal exercise testing in apparently healthy older adults, but is not necessary for submaximal assessments.

Individuals with increased risk have one or more signs or symptoms of possible cardiopulmonary or metabolic disease (Table 6.6) and/or two or more major coronary risk factors (Table 6.7). Individuals who are at increased risk but have no symptoms may begin a moderate-intensity exercise program without physician approval; however, these persons require a medical exam and an exercise test before exercising vigorously. Persons with any symptoms should seek physician approval before beginning either a moderate or vigorous exercise program. Physician supervision is required for maximal exercise testing in adults with increased risk.

Individuals with known cardiopulmonary or metabolic disease should consult a physician prior to beginning an exercise program. Physician supervision also is required for both maximal

and submaximal exercise testing in persons with known disease.

Clinical Exercise Testing vs. an Aerobic Fitness Evaluation. Two types of testing are usually used to evaluate readiness to exercise — clinical exercise testing (or stress tests) and aerobic fitness evaluations. Clinical exercise testing is more sophisticated and is typically used to diagnose or rule out cardiopulmonary problems. In addition, persons

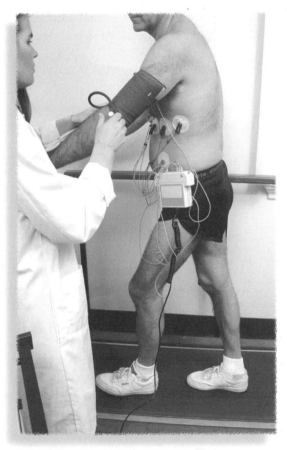

Clinical exercise testing is more sophisticated and is typically used to diagnose or rule out cardiopulmonary problems.

with known disease often undergo clinical exercise testing to determine levels of **ischemia** and establish whether an increase in physical activity is safe. Maximal-capacity clinical exercise tests are typically administered in settings such as human performance laboratories or hospitals by highly trained personnel. Blood pressure, heart rate (via electrocardiogram), **rating of perceived exertion (RPE)** and expired gases are monitored continuously throughout a clinical exercise test.

Contrary to clinical exercise testing, aerobic fitness evaluations are not used to diagnose disease or establish whether or not exercise is safe. Some aerobic fitness evaluations can be readily administered by you, and will provide important information on baseline fitness levels that can be used to help establish an appropriate, safe exercise prescription. Furthermore, knowledge of baseline oxygen capacity (VO_2 max) can help both you and the client in setting realistic, attainable goals.

Traditionally an individual's VO_2 max has been used as the marker of aerobic fitness. The most accurate assessment of VO_2 max is obtained by measuring the volume of expired gases during a maximal-effort, progressive exercise test. However, maximal aerobic testing has three notable drawbacks: it requires highly trained personnel, is time consuming, and poses a higher risk to a sedentary client since most exercise-related complications occur as exercise intensity approaches maximum.

As a result, submaximal exercise tests were developed. VO_2 max can be estimated by knowing the oxygen cost of a given workload. Submaximal exercise testing assumes that there is a linear relationship between work and heart rate or VO_2. By plotting two or more workloads on a graph, you can interpolate and predict what a maximal effort would be based on a predicted maximal heart rate.

A simple way to evaluate whether fitness has improved is by examining repeated measures of the submaximal heart-rate response to a given workload. Thus, if the heart-rate response to a fixed workload decreases after training, it is likely that physical fitness has improved.

For safety, it is recommended that you use only submaximal assessments when determining aerobic fitness in sedentary adults. It also is beyond the scope of practice for you to monitor an ECG for arrhythmias during a fitness evaluation. An ECG should be used to monitor heart rate only. Interpretation of the ECG traces can only be conducted by a physician or a specially trained exercise professional.

Assessing Fitness

Experts have had a difficult time agreeing on a definition of physical fitness over the years. However, most exercise scientists agree that four components are involved in physical fitness: 1) aerobic fitness; 2) muscle and joint flexibility; 3) muscle strength and endurance; and 4) body composition. For a detailed description on methods of assessing body composition, see Chapter 4.

A fitness assessment provides the opportunity to analyze each of these components and is used for any or all of the following:

1. To assess current fitness levels in relation to age and sex
2. To aid in the development of exercise prescriptions
3. To identify areas of health and injury risk, and the need for possible referral to the appropriate healthcare professional
4. To establish realistic, attainable goals and provide motivation
5. To educate the client about physical fitness
6. To evaluate the success of the fitness program through follow-up assessments

Many clients may request that a fitness evaluation be part of their work with you. Some may feel frightened or embarrassed to undergo such an assessment, while others may be overwhelmed and discouraged by the potentially negative feedback provided by baseline

Exercise History and Attitude Questionnaire

Name _____ Date _____

General Instructions: Please fill out this form as completely as possible. If you have any questions, DO NOT GUESS; ask your consultant for assistance.

1. Please rate your exercise level on a scale of 1 to 5 (5 indicating very strenuous) for each age range through your present age:

   15-20 _____   21-30 _____   31-40 _____   41+ _____

2. Were you a high school and/or college athlete?
   ☐ Yes   ☐ No
   If yes, please specify. _____

3. Do you have any negative feelings toward, or have you had any bad experiences with, physical activity programs?
   ☐ Yes   ☐ No
   If yes, please explain. _____

4. Do you have any negative feelings toward, or have you had any bad experiences with, fitness testing and evaluation?
   ☐ Yes   ☐ No
   If yes, please explain. _____

5. Rate yourself on a scale of 1 to 5 (1 indicating the lowest value, and 5 the highest). Circle the number that applies the most.

   Characterize your present athletic ability:
       1   2   3   4   5

   When you exercise, how important is competition?
       1   2   3   4   5

   Characterize your present cardiovascular capacity:
       1   2   3   4   5

   Characterize your present muscular capacity:
       1   2   3   4   5

   Characterize your present flexibility capacity:
       1   2   3   4   5

6. Do you start exercise programs but then find yourself unable to stick with them?
   ☐ Yes   ☐ No

7. How much are you willing to devote to an exercise program?
   _____ minutes/day   _____ days/week

8. Are you currently involved in regular endurance (cardiovascular) exercise?
   ☐ Yes   ☐ No
   If yes, specify the type of exercise(s) _____
   _____ minutes/day   _____ days/week

Figure 6.3
Sample exercise history and attitude questionnaire.

CHAPTER SIX
SCREENING, ASSESSMENT AND REFERRAL

Figure 6.3 continued

Rate your perception of the exertion of your exercise program (circle the number):

1) Light   2) Fairly light   3) Somewhat hard   4) Hard

9. How long have you been exercising regularly?

_____ months   _____ years

10. What other exercise, sport or recreational activities have you participated in?

In the past 6 months? _____

In the past 5 years? _____

11. Can you exercise during your work day?

☐ Yes   ☐ No

12. Would an exercise program interfere with your job?

☐ Yes   ☐ No

13. Would an exercise program beneflt your job?

☐ Yes   ☐ No

14. What types of exercise interest you?

_____ Walking   _____ Jogging   _____ Swimming

_____ Cycling   _____ Dance exercise   _____ Strength training

_____ Stationary biking _____ Rowing   _____ Racquetball

_____ Tennis   _____ Other aerobic   _____ Stretching

15. Rank your goals in undertaking exercise:
What do you want exercise to do for you?

Use the following scale to rate each goal separately.

Not at all important				Somewhat important			Extremely important		
1	2	3	4	5	6	7	8	9	10

a. Improve cardiovascular fltness   _____

b. Body-fat weight loss   _____

c. Reshape or tone my body   _____

d. Improve performance for a speciflc sport   _____

e. Improve moods and ability to cope with stress   _____

f. Improve flexibility   _____

g. Increase strength   _____

h. Increase energy level   _____

i. Feel better   _____

j. Enjoyment   _____

k. Other   _____

16. By how much would you like to change your current weight?

(+) _____ lbs   (-) _____ lbs

Table 6.9

Norms for Three-minute Step Test (Men)

Fitness Category	Age (years)					
	18-25	26-35	36-45	46-55	56-65	65+
Excellent	< 79	< 81	< 83	< 87	< 86	< 88
Good	79-89	81-89	83-96	87-97	86-97	88-96
Above average	90-99	90-99	97-103	98-105	98-103	97-103
Average	100-105	100-107	104-112	106-116	104-112	104-113
Below average	06-116	108-117	113-119	117-122	113-120	114-120
Poor	117-128	118-128	120-130	123-132	121-129	121-130
Very poor	> 128	> 128	> 130	> 132	> 129	> 130

Source: Adapted from Golding, et al. (1986). *The Y's way to physical fitness* (3rd ed.), p. 613. Reprinted with permission of the YMCA of the USA.

Table 6.10

Norms for Three-minute Step Test (Women)

Fitness Category	Age (years)					
	18-25	26-35	36-45	46-55	56-65	65+
Excellent	< 85	< 88	< 90	< 94	< 95	< 90
Good	85-98	88 - 99	90-102	94-104	95 - 104	90 - 102
Above average	99-108	100-111	103-110	105-115	105-112	103- 115
Average	109-117	112-119	111-118	116-120	113-118	116-122
Below average	118-126	120-126	119-128	121 -126	119-128	123- 128
Poor	127-140	127-138	129-140	127-135	129-139	129-134
Very poor	> 140	> 138	> 140	> 135	> 139	> 134

Source: Adapted from Golding, et al. (1986). *The Y's way to physical fitness* (3rd ed.), p. 114. Reprinted with permission of the YMCA of the USA.

testing results. It is important to respect a client's sensitivity to, and interest in, a thorough fitness assessment. However, the minimum evaluation that you should take new clients through is an assessment of cardiovascular risk factors, resting heart rate and resting blood pressure to assess readiness for aerobic exercise. Also explore the client's activity history, attitudes toward exercise and stated fitness goals. A sample *Exercise History and Attitude Questionnaire* is shown in Figure 6.3.

Assessing Aerobic Fitness. Two submaximal tests that are easily administered and readily interpreted are recommended for assessing aerobic fitness: the YMCA Step Test and the Rockport Walking Test. Though both require little or no equipment, they are not as accurate as cycle ergometer or treadmill tests. Also, little comparative data is available. (For more information on administering cycle ergometry and treadmill assessments see the *ACE Personal Trainer Manual.*)

Table 6.11

Estimated Maximal Oxygen Uptake (mL$_2$/Kg·bw/min) for Men and Women, 20-69 Years Old

Heart Rate					Minute/Mile						
	10	11	12	13	14	15	16	17	18	19	20
Men (20-29)											
120	65.0	61.7	58.4	55.2	51.9	48.6	45.4	42.1	38.9	35.6	32.3
130	63.4	60.1	56.9	53.6	50.3	47.1	43.8	40.6	37.3	34.0	30.8
140	61.8	58.6	55.3	52.0	48.8	45.5	42.2	39.0	35.7	32.5	29.2
150	60.3	57.0	53.7	50.5	47.2	43.9	40.7	37.4	34.2	30.9	27.6
160	58.7	55.4	52.2	48.9	45.6	42.4	39.1	35.9	32.6	29.3	26.1
170	57.1	53.9	50.6	47.3	44.1	40.8	37.6	34.3	31.0	27.8	24.5
180	55.6	52.3	49.0	45.8	42.5	39.3	36.0	32.7	29.5	26.2	22.9
190	54.0	50.7	47.5	44.2	41.0	37.7	34.4	31.2	27.9	24.6	21.4
200	52.4	49.2	45.9	42.7	39.4	36.1	32.9	29.6	26.3	23.1	19.8
Women (20-29)											
120	62.1	58.9	55.6	52.3	49.1	45.8	42.5	39.3	36.0	32.7	29.5
130	60.6	57.3	54.0	50.8	47.5	44.2	41.0	32.7	34.4	31.2	27.9
140	59.0	55.7	52.5	49.2	45.9	42.7	39.4	36.1	32.9	29.6	26.3
150	57.4	54.2	50.9	47.6	44.4	41.1	37.8	34.6	31.3	28.0	24.8
160	55.9	52.6	49.3	46.1	42.8	39.5	36.3	33.0	29.7	26.5	23.2
170	54.3	51.0	47.8	44.5	41.2	38.0	34.7	31.4	28.2	24.9	21.6
180	52.7	49.5	46.2	42.9	39.7	36.4	33.1	29.9	26.6	23.3	20.1
190	51.2	47.9	44.6	41.4	38.1	34.8	31.6	28.3	25.0	21.8	18.5
200	49.6	46.3	43.1	39.8	36.5	33.3	30.0	26.7	23.5	20.2	16.9
Men (30-39)											
120	61.1	57.8	54.6	51.3	48.0	44.8	41.5	38.2	35.0	31.7	28.4
130	59.5	56.3	53.0	49.7	46.5	43.2	39.9	36.7	33.4	30.1	26.9
140	58.0	54.7	51.4	48.2	44.9	41.6	38.4	35.1	31.8	28.6	25.3
150	56.4	53.1	49.9	46.6	43.3	40.1	36.8	33.5	30.3	27.0	23.8
160	54.8	51.6	48.3	45.0	41.8	38.5	35.2	32.0	28.7	25.5	22.2
170	53.3	50.0	46.7	43.5	40.2	36.9	33.7	30.4	27.1	23.9	20.6
180	51.7	48.4	45.2	41.9	38.6	35.4	32.1	28.8	25.6	22.3	19.1
190	50.1	46.9	43.6	40.3	37.1	33.8	30.5	27.3	24.0	20.8	17.5
Women (30-39)											
120	58.2	55.0	51.7	48.4	45.2	41.9	38.7	35.4	32.1	28.9	25.6
130	56.7	53.4	50.1	46.9	43.6	40.4	37.1	33.8	30.6	27.3	24.0
140	55.1	51.8	48.6	45.3	42.1	38.8	35.5	32.3	29.0	25.7	22.5
150	53.5	50.3	47.0	43.8	40.5	37.2	34.0	30.7	27.4	2¢.2	20.9
160	52.0	48.7	45.4	42.2	38.9	35.7	32.4	29.1	25.9	22.6	19.3
170	50.4	47.1	43.9	40.6	37.4	34.1	30.8	27.6	24.3	21.0	17.8
180	48.8	45.6	42.3	39.1	35.8	32.5	29.3	26.0	22.7	19.5	16.2
190	47.3	44.0	40.8	37.5	34.2	31.0	27.7	24.4	21.2	17.9	14.6

Heart Rate	Men (40 - 49)										
120	57.2	54.0	50.7	47.4	44.2	40.9	37.6	34.4	31.1	27.8	24.6
130	55.7	52.4	49.1	45.9	42.6	39.3	36.1	32.8	29.5	26.3	23.0
140	54.1	50.8	47.6	44.3	41.0	37.8	34.5	31.2	28.0	24.7	21.4
150	52.5	49.3	46.0	42.7	39.5	36.2	32.9	29.7	26.4	23.1	19.9
160	51.0	47.7	44.4	41.2	37.9	34.6	31.4	28.1	24.8	21.6	18.3
170	49.4	46.1	42.9	39.6	36.3	33.1	29.8	26.5	23.3	20.0	16.7
180	47.8	44.6	41.3	38.0	34.8	31.5	28.2	25.0	21.7	18.4	15.2

Heart Rate	Women (40 - 49)										
120	54.4	51.1	47.8	44.6	41.3	38.0	34.8	31.5	28.2	25.0	21.7
130	52.8	49.5	46.3	43.0	39.7	36.5	33.2	29.9	26.7	23.4	20.1
140	51.2	48.0	44.7	41.4	38.2	34.9	31.6	28.4	25.1	21.8	18.6
150	49.7	46.4	43.1	39.9	36.6	33.3	30.1	26.8	23.5	20.3	17.0
160	48.1	44.8	41.6	38.3	35.0	31.8	28.5	25.2	22.0	18.7	15.5
170	46.5	43.3	40.0	36.7	33.5	30.2	26.9	23.7	20.4	17.2	13.9
180	45.0	41.7	38.4	35.2	31.9	28.6	25.4	22.1	18.9	15.6	12.3

Heart Rate	Men (50 - 59)										
120	53.3	50.0	46.8	43.5	40.3	37.0	33.7	30.5	27.2	23.9	20.7
130	51.7	48.5	45.2	42.0	38.7	35.4	32.2	28.9	25.6	22.4	19.1
140	50.2	46.9	43.7	40.4	37.1	33.9	30.6	27.3	24.1	20.8	17.5
150	48.6	45.4	42.1	38.8	35.6	32.3	29.0	25.8	22.5	19.2	16.0
160	47.1	43.8	40.5	37.3	34.0	30.7	27.5	24.2	20.9	17.7	14.4
170	45.5	42.2	39.0	35.7	32.4	29.2	25.9	22.6	19.4	16.1	12.8

Heart Rate	Women (50 - 59)										
120	50.5	47.2	43.9	40.7	37.4	34.1	30.9	27.6	24.3	21.1	17.8
130	48.9	45.6	42.4	39.1	35.8	32.6	29.3	26.0	22.8	19.5	16.2
140	47.3	44.1	40.8	37.5	34.3	31.0	27.7	24.5	21.2	17.9	14.7
150	45.8	42.5	39.2	36.0	32.7	29.4	26.2	22.9	19.6	16.4	13.1
160	44.2	40.9	37.7	34.4	31.1	27.9	24.6	21.3	18.1	14.8	11.5
170	42.6	39.4	36.1	32.8	29.6	26.3	23.0	19.8	16.5	13.2	10.0

Heart Rate	Men (60-69)										
120	49.4	46.2	42.9	39.6	36.4	33.1	29.8	26.6	23.3	20.0	16.8
130	47.9	44.6	41.3	38.1	34.8	31.5	28.3	25.0	21.7	18.5	15.2
140	46.3	43.0	39.8	36.5	33.2	30.0	26.7	23.4	20.2	16.9	13.6
150	44.7	41.5	38.2	34.9	31.7	28.4	25.1	21.9	18.6	15.3	12.1
160	43.2	39.9	36.6	33.4	30.1	26.8	23.6	20.3	17.0	13.8	10.5

Heart Rate	Women (60-69)										
120	46.6	43.3	40.0	36.8	33.5	30.2	27.0	23.7	20.5	17.2	13.9
130	45.0	41.7	38.5	35.2	31.9	28.7	25.4	22.2	18.9	15.6	12.4
140	43.4	40.2	36.9	33.6	30.4	27.1	23.8	20.6	17.3	14.1	10.8
150	41.9	38.6	35.3	32.1	28.8	25.5	22.3	19.0	15.8	12.5	9.2
160	40.3	37.0	33.8	30.5	27.2	24.0	20.7	17.5	14.2	10.9	7.7

Note: Calculations assume 170 lb for men and 125 lb for women. For each 15 lb beyond these values, subtract 1 ml. Adapted from Kline et al. (1987).

Source: Howley, E.T. & Franks B.D. (1992). *Health Fitness Instructor's Handbook*. (2nd ed.) Champaign: Human Kinetics.

The YMCA's Three-minute Step Test was developed by Dr. Fred Kasch of San Diego for mass testing of participants. The procedure involves the delivery of a measured aerobic stimulus controlled by stepping to a standardized cadence. The following equipment is needed to administer the test:

✔ 12-inch-high step/bench
✔ a metronome for accurate pacing (96 bpm)
✔ a timer for timing the three-minute test and the one-minute recovery
✔ test forms to record data

The YMCA Step Test is an easily administered and readily interpreted submaximal test used to assess aerobic fitness.

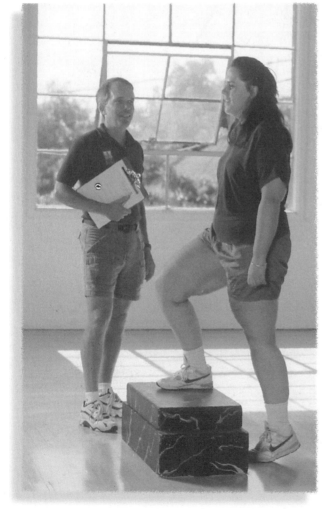

Before administering the test, you should demonstrate the stepping procedure for the client. With the

metronome set to 96 bpm (24 stepping cycles per minute), start stepping to a four-beat cycle — up, up, down, down. It does not matter which foot begins the cycle, although both feet must contact the top of the bench on the up portion, and both feet must contact the floor during the down portion. The lead foot may change during the test. Give the client a short practice session in which to step in place without the bench or, if necessary, with the bench, with adequate recovery afterward.

To begin the test itself, have the client face the bench, and then remind them that they will be stepping for three minutes and that they will be seated immediately afterward for a one-minute pulse count. Have the client step in place in time with the metronome. Start the timing of the three minutes when the client begins stepping on the bench. Check stepping rhythm throughout the test, announcing when one minute, two minutes, and two minutes and 40 seconds have elapsed. To further assist the client, you may want to provide additional verbal cues by clapping your hands or saying "up, up, down, down" in cadence with the metronome. At the end of the three-minute stepping period, immediately begin counting the heart rate of the seated subject for one minute. The one-minute post-exercise heart rate is used to score the test and can be compared to the norms in Tables 6.9 or 6.10, and previous test results if appropriate.

The Rockport Fitness Walking Test involves a timed 1-mile walk and run on a smooth and level surface (preferably a quarter-mile running track). The only other equipment necessary is a timing device and a form for recording results. An advantage of this test over the lab tests, which measure parameters (e.g., estimated VO_2 workload or heart rate), is that it evaluates performance, which gives a good indication of how well an individual will perform during aerobic activity. Limitations of the test lie in the fact that pacing ability and body-fat weight may adversely affect performance. The test is based on data for 170-pound men and 125-pound women. (If the client weighs substantially more, cardio-vascular fitness will be slightly overesti-mated.) Since the test requires that the mile be walked as fast as possible, lack of motivation or pacing difficulty may result in an underestimation of cardio-vascular fitness.

The test should begin with a warm-up consisting of walking and light stretch-ing. After the warm-up, explain to the client that this test requires a near-maximal effort, but for safety reasons they should not walk to exhaustion and should stop at any time if necessary. Elapsed times should be announced with every lap. Immediately upon com-pletion of the mile, take a 10-second exercise pulse. This 10-second value and its corresponding per-minute pulse (the 10-second pulse times six) should be recorded along with the time it took to complete the mile walk. After test completion, have the client walk for at least five minutes to cool down.

In addition to completion time and immediate post-exercise heart rate, a maximal perceived exertion also can be recorded to provide an indication of effort and for comparison to subse-quent tests. Completion time and min-ute pulse rate are used to score the test using the proper chart for age and sex (Table 6.11).

Assessing Muscle and Joint Flex-ibility. **Flexibility** is a measure of the range of movement about a joint or group of joints, and is often the most neglected component of physical fit-ness. It also is the component that responds fastest to a training program.

Table 6.12

Flexibility Rating Scale for Trunk Flexion (cm)

Classification	Males	Females
Excellent	≥45	≥47
Good	36-44	37-46
Minimum	25-35	27-36
Below minimum	15-24	17-26
Poor	≤14	≤16

Source: Fitness Canada. CSTF Operations Manual.

Table 6.13

Isometric Combined Rating Scale for Hand Grip Strength (lbs)

Classification	Men	Women
Excellent	260+	160+
Good	210-259	130-159
Minimum	185-209	95-129
Below Minimum	<185	<95

Source: Fitness Canada. CSTF Operations Manual.

The trunk forward flexion (sit and reach) test is the most commonly used index of overall flexibility and has well-established norms available for compar-ison. A low-intensity warm-up should precede any tests of flexibility. Ask your client to perform some slow, static stretches before attempting a test of the range of movement. Ideally, flexibility assessments should follow an aerobic assessment when the muscles are fully warmed up.

A Wells and Dillon flexometer is typically used to perform the sit-and-reach test. Have your client sit on the floor with their feet together and placed flat against a bench turned on its side. The ruler arm is attached at the 25-centimeter mark with the zero centimeter mark closest to the client. Keeping their knees fully extended,

Figure 6.4
Sit-and-reach
flexibility test.

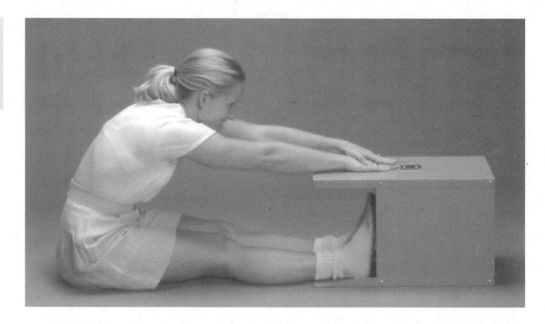

arms evenly stretched and palms facing down, the client should reach forward (without bouncing or jerking) along the ruler with the fingertips extended as far as possible. Advise them that lowering their head will maximize the distance reached. The position should be held for two seconds. Repeat the test twice. Do not allow bouncing movements, and do not attempt to hold the client's legs or knees down. Record the maximal distance reached to the nearest 0.5 centimeter. Persons with low back pain or other orthopedic ailments should avoid this assessment.

The sit-and-reach test, which has well-established norms for comparison, can also be administered with a meterstick and tape (Table 6.12). Place the meterstick on the floor and put a piece of tape at least 12 inches long at a right angle to the stick between the legs with the zero mark toward the body. The feet should be approximately 12 inches apart and the heels aligned with the tape at the 15-inch mark on the yardstick (Figure 6.4). Have the client place one hand on top of the other, with their tips of the fingers aligned, exhale and slowly lean forward by dropping the head toward or between the arms.

The fingers should be kept in contact with the yardstick and their knees kept straight.

Assessing Muscle Strength and Endurance. Two components of muscular fitness testing are muscular strength and muscular endurance. Adequate muscular strength and endurance are necessary for both optimal health and to enhance quality of life.

Muscle strength is measured by the amount of force that can be produced by a single maximal effort. Strength has historically been assessed using maximal lifts such as the bench press or leg squat in the weight room. This type of assessment would not be practical or safe for you to use with overweight, sedentary adults. A better alternative is the handgrip dynamometer, which measures grip strength.

The dynamometer should be adjusted to the most comfortable setting for the client's hand. The second joint of the fingers should fit snugly under the handle and take the weight of the instrument (Figure 6.5). The dynamometer should be firmly gripped and squeezed vigorously, exerting a maximal force. During the test, neither the dynamometer nor the hand should be

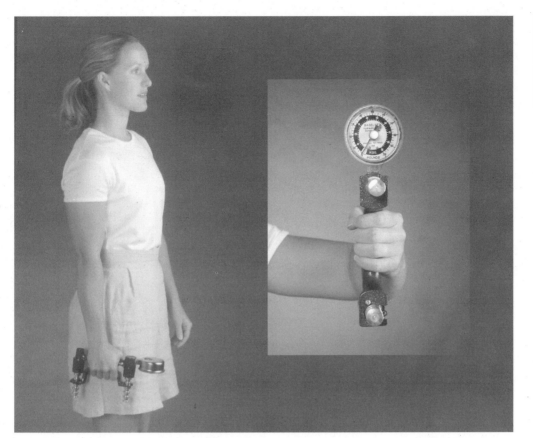

Figure 6.5
Proper hand and finger positioning for handgrip dynamometer.

allowed to touch the body or any other surface. Measure both hands alternately, testing each hand twice. Add the best score from each hand together and record as a single score. The rating scale for the combined grip scores is shown in Table 6.13.

Readiness to Change

A key factor to assess with clients is whether this is an appropriate time in their life to make a serious attempt at losing weight. Readiness to change is a complex phenomenon that encompasses an individual's motivation to lose weight, their commitment to restructuring their life and their current life circumstances. Success is more likely when a client's readiness to change is high (Brownell, 1994). Ideally, potential clients have carefully thought through these issues prior to meeting with you. Realistically, however, many factors will lead people to seek your help, including the need to please others (e.g., spouse, physician) or to find a quick fix for major problems in their life.

Readiness to change can be assessed in several ways. The simplest way is to have clients carefully evaluate what benefits may be obtained through weight loss against what sacrifices may need to be made. Two psychologists, Dr. James Prochaska and Dr. Carlo DiClemente, have developed a sophisticated model in which they identify discrete **stages of change**. (For a more detailed discussion, see *Stages of Change* in Chapter 3.) The Stages of Change model suggests that a complicated period of psychological preparation precedes true readiness to commit to lifestyle change. Thus, even though clients may not appear fully committed to losing weight, for many, motivation increases early on as they enjoy some success and witness the benefits of lifestyle change (see Chapter 1).

Figure 6.6
Sample weight loss
readiness quiz.

Weight Loss Readiness Quiz

Are you ready to lose weight? Your attitude about weight loss affects your ability to succeed. Take this Readiness Quiz to learn if you need to make any attitude adjustments before you begin. Mark each item true or false. Be honest! It's important that these answers reflect the way you really are, not how you would like to be. A method for interpreting your readiness for weight loss follows:

1. ____ I have thought a lot about my eating habits and physical activities to pinpoint what I need to change.

2. ____ I have accepted the idea that I need to make permanent, not temporary, changes in my eating and activities to be successful.

3. ____ I will only feel successful if I lose a lot of weight.

4. ____ I accept the idea that it's best if I lose weight slowly.

5. ____ I'm thinking of losing weight now because I really want to, not because someone else thinks I should.

6. ____ I think losing weight will solve other problems in my life.

7. ____ I am willing and able to increase my regular physical activity.

8. ____ I can lose weight successfully if I have no "slip-ups."

9. ____ I am ready to commit some time and effort each week to organizing and planning my food and activity programs.

10. ____ Once I lose some initial weight, I usually lose the motivation to keep going until I reach my goal.

11. ____ I want to start a weight loss program, even though my life is unusually stressful right now.

Scoring the Weight Loss Readiness Quiz.

To score the quiz, look at your answers next to items 1, 2, 4, 5, 7 and 9. Score "1" if you answered "true" and "0" if you answered "false."

For items 3, 6, 8, 10 and 11, score "0" for each true answer and "1" for each false answer.

To get your total score add the scores of all questions.

No one score indicates for sure whether you are ready or not to start losing weight. However, the higher your total score, the more characteristics you have that contribute to success. As a rough guide, consider the following recommendations:

1. If you scored 8 or higher, you probably have good reasons for wanting to lose weight now and a good understanding of the steps needed to succeed. Still, you might want to learn more about the areas where you scored a "0" (see "Interpretation of Quiz Items" below).

2. If you scored 5 to 7, you may need to reevaluate your reasons for losing weight and the methods you would use to do so. To get a start, read the advice given below for those quiz items where you received a score of "0".

3. If you scored 4 or less, now may not be the right time for you to lose weight. While you might be successful in losing weight initially, your answers suggest that you are unlikely to sustain sufficient effort to lose all the weight you want or to keep off the weight that you do lose. You need to reconsider your weight loss motivations and methods and perhaps learn more about the pros and cons of different approaches to reducing. To do so, read the advice below for those quiz items where you marked "0".

Interpretation of Quiz Items.

Your answers to the quiz can clue you in to potential stumbling blocks to your weight loss success. Any item score of "0" indicates a misconception about weight loss, or a potential problem area. While no

Figure 6.6 continued

individual item score of "0" is important enough to scuttle your weight-loss plans, we suggest that you consider the meaning of those items so you can best prepare yourself for the challenges ahead.

1. It has been said that you can't change what you don't understand. You might benefit from keeping records for a week to help pinpoint when, what, why and how much you eat. This tool also is useful in identifying obstacles to regular physical activity.

2. Making drastic or highly restrictive changes in your eating habits may allow you to lose weight in the short-run, but be too hard to live with permanently. Similarly, your program of regular physical activity should be one you can sustain. Both your food plan and activity program should be healthful and enjoyable.

3. Most people have fantasies of reaching a weight considerably lower than they can realistically maintain. Rethink your meaning of "success." A successful, realistic weight loss is one that can be comfortably maintained through sensible eating and regular activity. Take your body type into consideration. Then set smaller, achievable goals. Your first goal may be to lose a small amount of weight while you learn eating habits and activity patterns to help you maintain it.

4. If you equate success with fast weight loss, you will have problems maintaining your weight. This "quick fix" attitude can backfire when you face the challenges of weight maintenance. It's best — and healthiest — to lose weight slowly, while learning the strategies that allow you to keep the weight off permanently.

5. The desire for and commitment to weight loss must come from you. People who lose and maintain weight successfully take responsibility for their own desires and decide the best way to achieve them. Once this step is taken, friends and family are an important source of support, not motivation.

6. While being overweight may contribute to a number of social problems, it is rarely the single cause. Anticipating that all your problems will be solved through weight loss is unrealistic and may set you up for disappointment. Instead, realize that successful weight loss will make you feel more self-confident and empowered, and that the skills you develop to deal with your weight can be applied to other areas of your life.

7. Studies have shown that people who develop the habit of regular, moderate physical activity are most successful at maintaining their weight. Exercise does not have to be strenuous to be effective for weight control. Any moderate, physical activity that you enjoy and will do regularly counts. Just get moving!

8. While most people don't expect perfection of themselves in everyday life, many feel they must stick to a weight loss program perfectly. This is unrealistic. Rather than expecting it and viewing lapses as catastrophes, recognize them as valuable opportunities to identify problem triggers and develop strategies for the future.

9. Successful weight loss is not possible without taking the time to think about yourself, assess your problem areas, and develop strategies to deal with them. Success takes time. You must commit to planning and organizing your weight loss.

10. Do not ignore your concerns about "going the distance" because they may indicate a potential problem. Think about past efforts and why they failed. Pinpoint any reasons, and work on developing motivational strategies to get you over these hurdles. Take your effort one day at a time; a plateau of weight maintenance within an ongoing weight-loss program is perfectly OK.

11. Weight loss itself is a source of stress, so if you are already under stress, it may be difficult to successfully implement a weight-loss program at this time. Try to resolve other stress sources in your life before you begin a weight-loss effort.

Source: National Center for Nutrition and Dietetics of The American Dietetic Association.

Table 6.14

Inappropriate Candidates Who Must be Referred to Healthcare Specialists

Inappropriate Candidates	Potential Referral Sources
Pregnant and lactating women	Primary healthcare provider (obstetrician, family practitioner, nurse practitioner, midwife), dietitian
Underweight or anorexic individuals	Primary healthcare provider, mental health specialist, dietitian
Children	Primary healthcare provider, dietitian, mental health specialist, clinical weight-loss program specializing in children
Bulimia, eating disorders, and other psychological/ psychiatric disorders	Mental health specialist, specialized eating disorders program
Significant cardiovascular, renal or medical problems; diabetes	Healthcare provider, dietitian, clinical weight-loss program

The American Dietetics Association has developed a Weight Loss Readiness Quiz that addresses attitudes toward weight loss (Figure 6.6).

It is important to recognize that for most, change is never easy. In his book, *Weight Loss Through Persistence,* psychologist Dr. Daniel Kirschenbaum reviews some startling statistics surrounding our difficulty in making lifestyle changes — even when one's life may depend on it! For example, when medications are prescribed by physicians for their patients, approximately 33 percent are never even filled. Parents fail to ensure that their children complete a directed course of medications 50 percent of the time. Seventy percent of those with high blood pressure do not follow their physician's advice. And statistics demonstrate that 65 percent of Americans fail to use seat belts properly. Thus, it is very important to carefully review with clients the natural tendency within all of us to resist change. Kirschenbaum argues that a strong commitment to persistence is needed to make change possible. Discuss candidly with your clients their previous attempts at changing their lifestyle to ensure that their readiness is not merely a reflection of superficial enthusiasm or the naive wish that their lifestyle could be different.

Making Appropriate Referrals

Some individuals are clearly inappropriate candidates for weight loss and should always be referred to a proper healthcare specialist for clearance before beginning a weight-loss program. Table 6.14 presents a list of such individuals and potential referral sources. Table 6.15 presents a brief description of healthcare specialties.

Case Examples

The following are three examples of individuals who may seek your help with a weight-loss program. Try to determine the critical issues to be addressed in each assessment.

Janet. Janet is 35 years old, married with no children and works as a secretary for a cardiologist. She is 5'8" and weighs 260 pounds. She is coming to see you at the insistence of her employer who says he is worried about her health. She says she is in good health at the present time, but reports taking medication to control her blood pressure and chronic heartburn. During the assessment, she tells you that she has been on "every diet known to man" and does well for the first three to four months, then returns to her old eating habits and regains all the weight and then some. She has exercised on occasion to facilitate weight loss, but has never stayed with any program of activity for more than a few weeks. She confides during the interview that she is very unhappy about her weight as her husband makes constant reference to it. To avoid his criticism, she eats very little in front of him, then sneaks out to fast food restaurants or convenience stores to get "what I really want to eat" (e.g., ice cream, fried foods, candy bars). She has gained 20 pounds in the past six months. When you ask about her perceptions of eating, she tells you, "Of course I'm out of control. If I was in control, would I eat this way?" She denies that she is depressed but is tearful at times during your meeting.

Approach to Assessing Janet. You need to find out more information about a number of things. You'll want to explore her motivation very carefully; is she coming to you out of desperation, or to appease her employer or husband? If pleasing others is a major factor, you'll need to carefully explore with her the burden of attempting lifestyle change at this time and mutually determine if she is really ready to undertake this challenge. Also, there are some red flags that her eating may be especially problematic. You'll want to assess the presence of potential binge eating very carefully. Ask her to review several days of eating with you, noting everything she ate and the times and

places she associates with eating. Explore the secretive eating. Is she doing this out of shame and embarrassment, or to avoid criticism? Is she unhappy about her eating? Does she really "lose" control when she is eating, or does she simply eat on impulse (i.e., without thinking about what she is eating and why). Talk about the tearfulness. Does this happen frequently when she thinks about herself, her weight and her eating? You will need to have a good understanding of each of these issues before you can comfortably assume she is an appropriate client for you to work with.

Billy. Billy is a 25-year-old lean construction worker who would like advice on how to optimize his training program and weight for competitions. He has been weight lifting for about a year in his basement and is satisfied with his progress. (His maximal bench press is 255 pounds and he can squat 375 pounds.) Billy feels that his strength improvements have plateaued over the past two months and would like your advice on how to get past this to prepare for an upcoming show. He would also like a spotter when he is lifting heavier weights since he sometimes feels dizzy during or immediately after his heavy lifts.

Approach to Assessing Billy. Billy's youth and active lifestyle may be somewhat deceptive. According to Table 6.6, Billy's dizziness is a major symptom of cardiopulmonary disease. Thus, in spite of his age and apparent fitness, according to the ACSM recommendations (Table 6.8), persons with any major symptoms of disease must undergo both a medical exam and exercise testing before beginning an exercise program under your supervision. It will be important not to scare Billy, but you will have to let him know that he must consult with his physician about the dizziness he is experiencing during exercise. You can tell him that this is not a normal response to exercise and that you want to be cautious and certain that he can safely train for the upcoming event.

After obtaining Billy's written permission, contact his physician before proceeding further. Outline your concerns, including the intensity of Billy's program, his current response to exercise and his stated goals. You will need to have documentation from his physician that it is safe for Billy to proceed with exercise and that his current training regimen is medically appropriate at this time.

Mary. Mary is a 52-year-old single lawyer who has come to you for help with improving her health and losing weight. Her blood pressure is 138/88 and her body fat is 37 percent of her total weight. She has never been physically active in the past and feels that she is quite uncoordinated. Furthermore, she is wary about exercising since her 62-year-old uncle died suddenly while shoveling snow last winter.

Approach to Assessing Mary. It is safe for you to begin working with Mary since she is under 55 years of age and her sedentary lifestyle is her only major risk factor. (Her uncle is 62 and not a first-degree relative.) Her blood pressure is high to normal and she is carrying excess body fat. However, these do not qualify as risk factors that would prevent her from beginning a moderate exercise program without her physician's clearance. You could have Mary perform an aerobic fitness test (e.g., the YMCA Step Test or the Rockport Walking Test) to establish her baseline fitness levels and determine an appropriate starting point for exercise. When administering a submaximal aerobic fitness test, monitor heart rate closly to ensure that the activity remains "moderate" as defined in Table 6.8.

Since Mary does not feel that she is a competent exerciser, it will be important for her to begin exercising gradually with activities that require little athletic skill. Walking outdoors and stationary cycling are good modes of activity to train the aerobic system. Stair-climbing machines, rowing ergometers, aerobic step classes and cross-country ski machines can be introduced as physical fitness and self-confidence improve. Resistance training on machines also is an excellent way for persons with no history of programmed exercise to train the musculoskeletal system since it requires little skill and offers results quickly.

Establishing a Referral Network

For lifestyle and weight management consultants who work relatively independently, it is very important to establish a network of allied healthcare professionals to whom you can refer clients. You also have an ethical responsibility to ensure that the professionals you refer your clients to are appropriately qualified to treat the problem. For example, if you identify uncontrolled hypertension in a client, the appropriate referral is to a healthcare provider such as a physician or nurse practitioner.

It is always best to refer your clients to professionals you personally know and trust. A referral for dietary counseling to "Sarah Jones, a registered dietitian who specializes in weight management and has worked with several previous clients" is always preferable to a referral to "the dietary department" at the local hospital. When establishing your referral sources, speak with the professional directly. You'll want to determine whether their views on the importance of lifestyle change compliment yours. Garner their assistance in supporting the changes your client is attempting to make. For example, a brief comment by a physician during an

Table 6.15

Allied Healthcare Professionals

Primary Health

✔ Primary healthcare providers are comprised of physicians, physician assistants and nurse practitioners. They are licensed by state boards of professional standards to provide medical care. Physicians hold a doctoral degree, M.D. or D.O., and receive the most extensive training. Physician's assistants (P.A.s) usually receive four years of training after high school and may treat patients only under the supervision of a licensed physician. They may not prescribe medications. Nurse practitioners (N.O.s) are registered nurses who have at least two years of additional training. In many states, N.O.s may be licensed to practice medicine in a limited fashion independently of a physician and may prescribe certain types of medications.

Mental Health

✔ Psychologists have completed doctoral level training in clinical or counseling psychology and have passed both a national and state exam certifying their competence. Only psychologists who are licensed to practice psychology may legally use the title "psychologist." In some states, master's level practitioners who have completed additional training and supervision in addition to the other requirements have been "grandfathered" and are able to use the title licensed psychologist. Ethical standards of practice are set forth by the American Psychological Association. The State Board of Psychology for each state maintains a listing of all licensed psychologists along with their areas of expertise.

✔ Psychiatrists are physicians who have completed a residency in psychiatry. Board certified psychiatrists have met additional requirements set forth by the American Board of Psychiatry and Neurology. Some psychiatrists also have received additional specialized training in the treatment of eating disorders.

✔ Social workers have completed bachelor, master's or doctoral level training in social work at an accredited college or university and have passed a licensure examination. The State Board of Social Work Examiners maintains a list of licensed social workers including their level of specialization. A licensed certified social worker also has obtained significant training and supervision.

Nutrition

✔ There are several levels of specialization in the field of dietetics. The doctoral level nutrition practitioner may be a physician with board certification in nutrition or a registered dietitian (R.D.) with a doctoral degree. The specialist R.D. has earned a master's degree in nutrition and/or has 3 to 5 years of experience. The generalist R.D. holds a bachelor's degree in nutrition. In some states, these individuals are licensed by a state's board of dietetics. The dietetic technician (D.T.R.) holds an associate degree in nutrition and works under the supervision of a registered dietitian. The American Dietetic Association maintains a listing of registered dietitians throughout the United States [800-877-1600].

Exercise

✔ At this time there is no recognized registry or licensure of fitness professionals. You should look for instructors that are certified and experienced in working with clients with weight-management challenges. There are a number of certifications a fitness instructor may earn. The most credible are those from a not-for-profit, nationally recognized organization that follows recognized testing guidelines. ACE-certified Personal Trainers may work with clinically challenged clients only after obtaining approval and guidelines from the client's personal physician. Individuals certified by the ACSM as a Preventive and Rehabilitative Exercise Specialist usually have a master's degree and may work with clients with clinical challenges, but still under the guidance of the client's personal physician.

Therapist, Psychotherapist, Counselor, Nutritionist, Exercise Physiologist

✔ These titles are not protected and have no governing bodies. Anyone may use these titles freely as they do not reflect training, experience or adherence to a set of ethical principles. (Note: The title of Nutritionist is limited in some states.)

office visit about weight lost can boost your client's confidence and morale.

Beyond sending your clients to healthcare professionals, there also are some creative ways to develop your referral network. Newsletters are an excellent way to keep your name and services visible. Providing educational talks and "brown bag lunch" discussions, both on and off your worksite, can introduce you to a wide range of professionals and potential clients. You may even be able to secure a regular spot on a local morning TV news show where you can review principles of lifestyle changes. While you may not be paid to provide any of these services, these opportunities can provide a wealth of exposure.

Working in a Supporting Role.
Lifestyle and weight management consultants are a natural adjunct to healthcare interventions aimed at changing behaviors, and are likely to play an increasingly important role in preventative healthcare. However, when working with individuals who have been referred to you, always remain professional and bear in mind whose client they are. Work in concert with the referring professional and ensure that your recommendations complement the medical treatment the client is currently receiving. Consultants who "steal" clients from their referral sources will soon find their sources have dried up.

The time spent establishing and maintaining your referral network is both a professional responsibility and an effective marketing strategy. You'll find it is time well invested as these professionals may begin referring clients to

you. As a courtesy, always send a letter to the professional you are referring to, introducing the client and summarizing your reasons for referral. For instance, are you referring a client for an assessment, assessment and treatment, or are you seeking suggestions for management? Periodically send a follow-up letter indicating the client's progress toward reaching their goals. Keep all correspondence brief — ideally one page.

It is critical to obtain the client's written permission to both secure and release any information to other healthcare providers. Always advise the professional you are calling that you have obtained the client's consent to speak with them. Be prepared to fax or mail a copy of the client's consent form to professionals who wish to have it in their records before talking further with you.

Summary

As a lifestyle and weight management consultant, you offer an important service that encompasses principles of nutrition, exercise science and behavior modification to promote lifestyle change for a wide variety of clients. You have an ethical and professional responsibility to adequately screen clients for their suitability for treatment, assess relevant medical and psychological factors and fitness parameters, and refer to allied health professionals when indicated. In addition, the information that is gathered during the assessment phase provides an important foundation for establishing an individualized, safe and effective weight management program.

References

American Council on Exercise. (1991). *Personal Trainer Manual.* San Diego: American Council on Exercise.

American Psychiatric Association. (1994). *Diagnostic and Statistical Manual of Mental Disorders.* (4th ed.) Washington D.C.

American College of Sports Medicine. (1995). *ACSM's Guidelines for Exercise Testing and Prescription.* (5th ed.) Baltimore: Williams & Wilkins.

Brownell, K.D. (1994). *The LEARN Program for Weight Control.* (6th ed.) Dallas: American Health.

Brownell, K.D. & Wadden, T.A. (1992). Etiology and treatment of obesity: Understanding a serious, prevalent, and refractory disorder. *Journal of Consulting and Clinical Psychology,* 60, 505-517.

Bruce, B. & Wilfley, D. (1996). Binge eating among the overweight population: A serious and prevalent problem. *Journal of the American Dietetic Association,* 96, 58-61.

Drewnowski, A. (1990). *Toward safe weight loss: Recommendations for adult weight loss programs in Michigan. Final report of Task Force to Establish Weight Loss Guidelines.* E. Lansing: Michigan Health Council.

Fifth Report of the Joint Committee on Detection, Evaluation, and Treatment of High Blood Pressure (JNCV). (1993). *Archives of Internal Medicine,* 153, 154-183.

Foster, G.D. (1995). Reasonable weights: Determinants, definitions, and directions. In Allison, D.B. and Pi-Sunyer, F.X. (Eds.). *Obesity Treatment.* New York: Plenum.

Institute of Medicine. (1995). *Weighing the Options: Criteria for Evaluating Weight Management Programs.* Washington: National Academy Press.

Kirschenbaum, D.S. (1994). *Weight Loss Through Persistence.* Oakland: New Harbinger.

Kuczmarski, R.J., Flegal, K.M., Campbell, S.M. & Johnson C. L. (1994). Increasing prevalence of overweight among US adults: The National Health and Nutrition Examination Surveys, 1960 to 1991. *Journal of the American Medical Association,* 272, 205-211.

Spitzer, R.L., Devlin, M., Walsh, B.T., Hasin, D., Wing, R., Marcus, M., Stunkard, A.J., Wadden, T.A., Yanovski, S., Agras, S., Mitchell, J. & Nonas, C. (1992). Binge eating disorder: A multi-site field trial of the diagnostic criteria. *International Journal of Eating Disorders,* 11, 191-203.

United States Department of Agriculture (USDA) and U.S. Department of Health and Human Services (DHHS). (1990). *Dietary guidelines for Americans.* (3rd ed.) Washington D.C.: Government Printing Office.

Wadden, T.A., Sternberg, J.A., Letizia, K.A., Stunkard, A.J. & Foster, G.D. (1989). Treatment of obesity by very-low-calorie diet, behavior therapy, and their combination: A five-year perspective. *International Journal of Obesity,* 13-2, 39-46.

Williamson, D.F., Serdula, M.K., Anda, R.F., Levy, A. & Byers, T. (1992). Weight loss attempts in adults: Goals, duration, and rate of weight loss. *American Journal of Public Health,* 82, 1251-1257.

Winner, K. (1991). *A Weighty Issue: Dangers and Deceptions of The Weight Loss Industry.* New York: Department of Consumer Affairs.

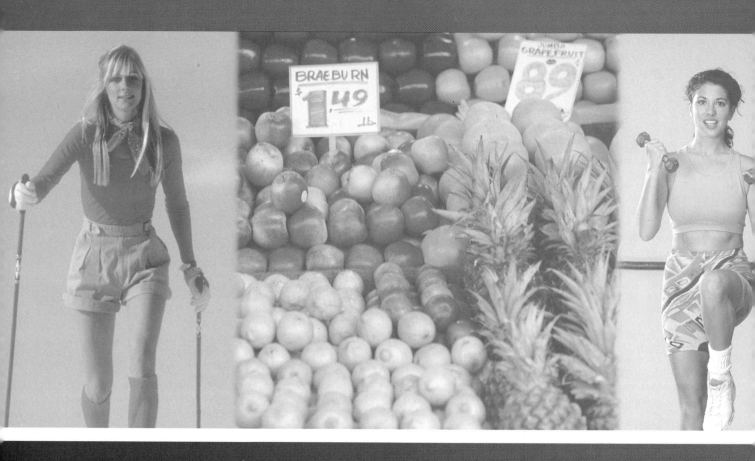

CHAPTER SEVEN

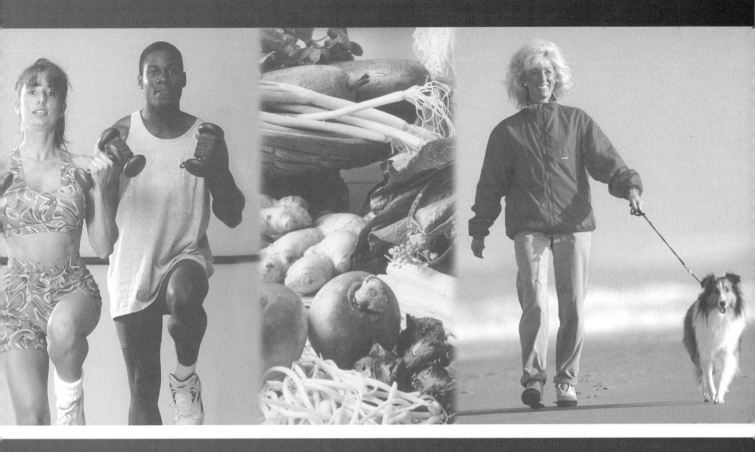

Applied Exercise Science

Daniel Kosich

Daniel Kosich, Ph.D., is president of EXERFIT Consulting, senior consultant to IDEA, co-exercise science editor for Shape *magazine and technical advisor for* New Woman *magazine. He is the author of* GET REAL: A Personal Guide to Real-Life Weight Management, *and has developed numerous fitness and nutrition education programs for fitness center personnel and the general public.*

Introduction

Because the balance between energy expenditure and energy intake ultimately determines whether an individual will lose, maintain or gain weight, understanding the factors that influence energy balance is essential for anyone who works with weight-management programs. The implication is quite straightforward. If energy intake exceeds energy expenditure (a positive energy balance), weight gain occurs. If expenditure is greater than intake (a negative energy balance), weight loss occurs; if they're equal, weight is maintained. Sounds simple, but, like most aspects of human physiology, ultimate energy balance involves many factors.

Energy Balance

Energy balance can be thought of as **calorie** balance. In this chapter, energy and calorie are used synonymously. The balance is simply the relationship between the number of calories consumed in one's diet and all of the calories expended through the costs of just being alive and awake, usually referred to as **resting metabolic rate (RMR)**, plus all the calorie costs of performing daily physiological "tasks" and physical activities. These include the energy required to digest dietary nutrients, as well as the energy needed for such activities as walking, sitting and climbing stairs to name a few.

The RMR (which includes **basal metabolic rate, BMR**) usually accounts for about 60 percent to 75 percent of daily expenditure. Obviously, it "costs" a lot of energy to maintain cardiac function, neural function and repair of the body's cells and structures, even in the absence of physical activity. The RMR is directly related to **fat-free mass**: the greater the fat-free mass, the higher the RMR. RMR is a more common measurement than BMR, and is taken early in the morning after an overnight fast and at least eight hours of sleep. The sleep is at home and the measurement is in the lab. BMR is measured immediately upon awakening, following eight hours of sleep and a 12-hour fast, but it requires an overnight stay at the lab, so it is less practical than an RMR measurement. BMR registers at approximately 10 percent lower than RMR.

Many weight-management clients are surprised to learn that most adult women have an RMR of at least 1,200 kcal/day and most men have an RMR of 1,500 kcal/day. In many cases, the values for both genders are several hundred kcal/day higher. These values are often used as suggestions for the absolute minimum daily dietary intake requirements in weight-management attempts.

The costs of digestive processes (referred to as the **thermic effect of a meal**) account for about 10 percent of daily energy expenditure. **Adenosine triphosphate (ATP)** is required to break apart the relatively huge molecules of **protein** and **complex carbohydrates** into the building blocks of **amino acids** and simple sugars, respectively, so that they can be transported across the wall of the small intestine. Large fat molecules also must be enzymatically broken down, but typically require less energy than proteins and complex carbohydrates. The many important aspects associated with caloric intake is discussed in detail in Chapter 9. With regard to energy intake, this chapter focuses on the impact of severe calorie restriction, including **weight cycling** (lose, regain, lose, regain . . .), which commonly results from repeated low-calorie diets.

The costs of activity (the thermic effect of activity) account for about 15 percent to 30 percent of total daily energy output. Obviously, the greater the amount of physical activity, the greater this expenditure becomes. In practical terms, only about 15 percent of total daily energy expenditure comes from activity in a sedentary individual. For a highly active person, this number jumps to 30 percent or more.

While there are several factors affecting energy expenditure, physical activity is by far the best way to substantially increase one's daily caloric expenditure. Let's briefly review how the body produces energy and its effect on **energy balance**.

Energy Production

When a muscle contracts and exerts force, the energy used to drive the contraction comes from adenosine triphosphate (ATP). How quickly and efficiently a muscle cell produces ATP determines how much work the cell can do before it fatigues. While there is some ATP stored in a muscle cell, the supply is limited.

Therefore, muscle cells must produce more ATP in order to continue working. Muscle cells replenish the ATP supply using three distinct biochemical pathways or series of chemical reactions: the **aerobic energy system**, the **anaerobic glucose system** and the **anaerobic creatine phosphate system**.

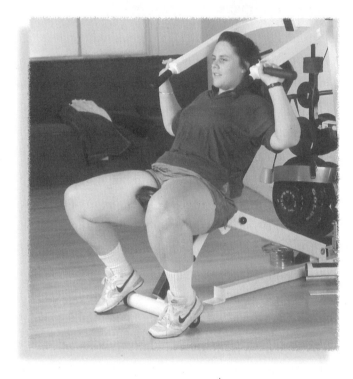

Resistance training is an excellent way to minimize the reduction in lean body mass that often accompanies weight loss.

Aerobic and Anaerobic Energy Systems

"Aerobic" means "with oxygen." The aerobic energy system for producing ATP is dominant when adequate oxygen is delivered into the cell to meet energy production needs, such as when the muscle is at rest. Most cells, including muscle cells, contain structures called **mitochondria**, the site of aerobic energy (ATP) production. The greater the number of mitochondria in a cell, the greater the cell's capability to produce aerobic energy.

Two other energy systems serve as the primary sources of ATP when an inadequate supply of oxygen is available in the cell to meet its energy needs. In the absence of sufficient oxygen, muscles rely on the anaerobic ("without oxygen") systems, which provide a rapidly available source of ATP. This is useful, for instance, when a muscle needs to generate force quickly, such as when a person lifts a heavy weight. The anaerobic systems also predominate when rhythmic, large muscle movements, like running or cycling, are performed at an intensity (oxygen cost) greater than an individual's **functional aerobic capacity** (sub-anaerobic threshold pace). The anaerobic production of ATP occurs inside the cell but outside the mitochondria.

It is important to note that the aerobic and anaerobic systems are always working. Energy production doesn't work like an on/off switch. It is a matter of predominance. When adequate oxygen is not available in the mitochondria of a cell to meet ATP needs, the anaerobic systems kick into high gear to assist the aerobic system. The aerobic system does not shut off.

Most cells, such as those in the heart, brain and other organs, have little or no anaerobic capability. Therefore, these cells must be continuously supplied with oxygen. If the oxygen supply is cut off, such as when a blood clot forms where a coronary artery has become clogged, the area of the heart muscle (myocardium) beyond the blockage suffers a **myocardial infarction**, or heart attack. If enough of the myocardium is involved, the result is a fatal heart attack. Blockage of an artery into the brain can lead to a **stroke**.

Unlike the heart and the brain, skeletal muscles, such as the triceps and quadriceps, have a significant anaerobic capability. **Fats** (**fatty acids**) and carbohydrates (glucose) are the

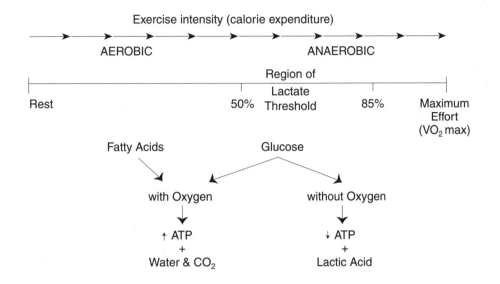

Figure 7.1
Energy production and relative intensity in an exercising muscle.

two substances (substrates) used to produce most of the ATP supply. Proteins, comprised of various combinations of amino acids, are not a preferred energy source; in an adequately nourished client, proteins play a minor role in energy production. However, when a diet does not supply sufficient carbohydrate calories, the body is capable of using protein that is stored in tissues like muscle to produce the energy it needs. This process, known as **gluconeogenesis**, always occurs to a limited extent, but it is not healthy to rely on it for substantial energy production.

Gluconeogenesis, combined with abnormal fat metabolism, results in **ketosis**. We will look at its impact later in this chapter.

As illustrated in Figure 7.1, when the cardiorespiratory system is able to supply adequate oxygen to the mitochondria of muscle cells, both fatty acids and glucose are used to produce ATP. In other words, at rest, most of the needed ATP is produced aerobically, using both fatty acids and glucose. Keep in mind that oxygen use (VO_2) is directly related to caloric expenditure. For every liter (l) of oxygen used, approximately five **kilocalories (kcal)** of energy

are expended. (One kilocalorie is the amount of heat needed to raise one liter of water one degree centigrade.) As VO_2 increases, caloric expenditure also increases. Exercise intensity, oxygen cost and calorie expenditure can be thought of as equivalent expressions.

The body expends about 1 to 1.5 kcal per minute at rest (VO_2 = 0.2 to 0.3l O_2/min). An individual's actual resting caloric expenditure is related to a number of factors, with **lean body mass** being a significant component. About 50 percent to 60 percent of this 1 to 1.5 kcal/min comes from fatty acids, even in an untrained person. In a well-trained endurance athlete, fatty acids provide as much as 70 percent of the resting caloric expenditure.

There are many myths surrounding energy expenditure, for example: 1) one must "use up" the muscle's sugar supply before fat can be used; or, 2) it takes 20 minutes of exercise before fat begins to be used for energy production. Fat is used for energy even while we are sleeping, albeit in small volume.

As exercise intensity increases, the cardiovascular system makes every attempt (through increased heart rate and stroke volume, and increased oxygen extraction in the active muscle

During aerobic exercise, the body uses oxygen and fatty acids and glucose to produce ATP. For every liter of oxygen used, approximately 5 calories of energy are expended.

fibers) to elevate its delivery of oxygen into the mitochondria of exercising muscles to produce enough ATP aerobically. As long as sufficient oxygen is available, the aerobic system continues to predominate, even though calorie expenditure per minute can increase substantially above the resting rate. Keep in mind that the primary by-

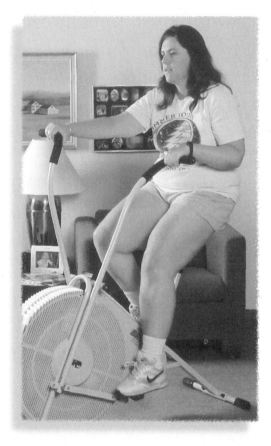

products are water and carbon dioxide, which typically do not lead to muscle fatigue.

At some point in increasing intensity (determined both by a client's level of aerobic fitness and by genetics) there is not enough oxygen available in the mitochondria of the exercising muscles to meet energy needs, so the anaerobic systems are called on to rapidly produce ATP. The intensity at which adequate oxygen is no longer available is typically referred to as the lactate threshold or **anaerobic threshold**. In most situations, lactate and anaerobic thresholds occur

at the same exercise intensity (Wilmore & Costill, 1994).

As illustrated in Figure 7.1, this threshold is reached somewhere in the range of 50 percent to 85 percent of maximum effort. At intensities above the threshold, the aerobic system does not stop functioning — it is merely incapable of producing enough ATP to meet energy demands at that pace. The anaerobic systems provide the energy necessary above and beyond the aerobic capability. As depicted in Figure 7.1, **VO₂ max** is reached when the anaerobic systems are also working at maximum capability. The primary source of anaerobic ATP production is **glucose**.

Glucose is carried in the blood and stored in muscles and the liver as **glycogen**, a large molecule made up of chains of glucose. Individual glucose molecules can be quickly broken off glycogen to enter the energy pathway.

A second source of anaerobic ATP production is **creatine phosphate**, a molecule that can be broken apart quickly to help produce ATP. However, the body has an extremely limited supply of creatine phosphate and ATP. Even in a well-trained athlete there is only enough of this secondary fuel to last for about 10 seconds of maximal effort.

When an exercising muscle relies primarily on the anaerobic systems (intensities between the threshold and maximal effort) to meet its energy needs, the by-products (lactic acid accumulation, heat, hydrogen ions) lead to rapid muscle fatigue. Effort at that intensity can be maintained for only a few minutes at most.

To summarize, as long as a muscle cell meets its energy needs aerobically, it relies on fatty acids and glucose to produce ATP. The by-products of aerobic ATP production are water and carbon dioxide (CO_2). Both are relatively easy for the body to eliminate, so aerobic energy production does not lead to rapid muscle fatigue. When the anaerobic systems become highly active, the accumulation of by-products leads to a rapid fatigue.

As noted, water is a by-product of the aerobic system. We lose a lot of it every day in order to regulate internal temperature. This is why it's important to drink a sufficient amount of water each day. Both aerobic and anaerobic systems produce heat, which must be "transported" to the skin where it can be dissipated to the environment in the form of sweat. At rest, the production of water is low enough that the sweat evaporates before reaching the surface of the skin (insensible perspiration). If a client doubts that they are sweating even at rest, have them put a plastic bag on part of their arm for several minutes. When you remove it, they will be able to see the condensed moisture.

As intensity increases, so does heat production and water loss. The greater the intensity of exercise and/or the longer the duration, the greater the need for additional water.

It is not uncommon for those pursuing weight loss to minimize water intake, thinking, perhaps, that it will keep them from retaining water. Quite the opposite is true. Adequate hydration is essential for maintaining fluid balance. Inadequate water intake can actually be a factor in water-retention problems. You should encourage clients to consume at least six glasses of water per day. In addition, they should be advised to consume 8 ounces in the half-hour before exercise, 3 to 4 ounces every 10 minutes or so during exercise, and another 8 ounces in the 30 minutes after exercise. In addition to temperature regulations, adequate hydration is important for replenishing glycogen stores in muscle cells, since each gram of glycogen is stored along with 4 grams of water.

Believe it or not, all this chemistry is directly related to energy balance and weight management. Understanding how energy is used will allow you to help your clients make better food choices to fuel their body's particular needs and meet their weight-loss goals.

Losing Body Fat

A well-nourished body's primary energy reserve is its fat stores. This fat is stored as **triglycerides** in adipose cells around the body, as well as in skeletal muscle fibers. Relatively little carbohydrate (glycogen) is stored, and protein is not a preferred source of energy. This means that energy balance fluctuations have the greatest effect on body fat. The balance can be expressed in specific numbers. Recall that there are approximately 3,500 kilocalories (kcal) in 1 pound of fat. This implies that in order to lose 1 pound of fat,

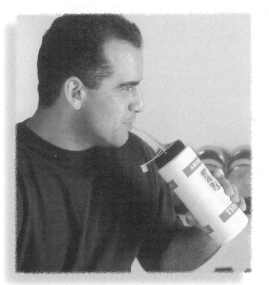

3,500 more kilocalories must be burned than are consumed. In other words, to lose 1 pound of fat per week there must be a negative balance of 3,500 kilocalories per week. For most people, generating this negative energy balance is best accomplished by increasing caloric expenditure and modestly reducing caloric intake.

The greater the intensity or duration of the exercise, the greater the amount of water that is lost. Therefore, it is essential that your clients drink plenty of water before, during and after exercise.

This is where an understanding of the effects of the aerobic and anaerobic energy systems becomes critical. Referring to Figure 7.1, you will see that fat (fatty acids) is used as part of the aerobic energy system, not the anaerobic systems. Many advertisements, and even some fitness instructors, have erroneously said that "aerobic exercise is essential for fat loss because fat is only burned aerobically." But as you look at Figure 7.1, an important consideration with regard to ultimate fat loss is the by-products of the systems, not the substrates used. Simply put, the aerobic system predominates as long as there is adequate oxygen and glucose in the muscles being used because the by-products do not cause fatigue. When the anaerobic systems become dominant, fatigue quickly follows.

The key to maximizing fat loss is to maximize caloric expenditure, not to try and burn a particular type of fuel (such as fat). For those with a low aerobic fitness level the implications are clear. For example, in an untrained adult, an exercise intensity of about 5 kcal/minute (a VO_2 of approximately 1 liter O_2/min) will likely put him near the lactate threshold. He could certainly work harder, but only for a short time. If his goal is to generate a substantial negative energy balance, he clearly needs to sustain aerobic exercise. But not because fat is burned aerobically; rather, because if he works anaerobically, the exercise duration will be short and the total energy expenditure will be limited.

For example, if he works at 5 kcal/min for 30 minutes, he will expend 150 kilocalories during the session. If he does this three times per week, he will generate a negative energy balance of only 450 kcal/week. This would mean seven to eight weeks before the 3,500 kcal/pound of fat could be achieved.

But if he tried to work at a greater intensity, he would tire within a few minutes, expending even fewer calories. If he can increase to 60 minutes per day, or exercise for 30 minutes six times a week, the negative balance would double. But 1 pound of fat loss a month can still be frustrating. It's easy to see why untrained clients with limited time, who depend solely on exercise for fat loss, can become frustrated.

If the same individual eliminated 200 to 300 kcal/day from his diet, he would add 1,400 to 2,100 kcal/week to his negative energy balance. His rate of weight loss would increase to about 1 pound every 10 to 14 days. The temptation to drastically restrict dietary calories is understandable.

Even when his level of fitness is dramatically improved three to four months after beginning a training program, research suggests that the maximum effective rate of weight loss is 1 to 2 pounds per week. For example, the client who was limited to sustained exercise at 5 kcal/minute can now work comfortably (aerobically) at 12 kcal/minute. If he works out four days/week for 45 minutes/session, and he cuts 200 kcal/day (1,400 kcal/week) from his diet, he will be at about a negative 3,500 kcal balance, which is equivalent to 1 pound of weight loss.

$$\begin{array}{r} 12 \text{ kcal/min} \\ \times\ \underline{45 \text{ min/session}} \\ 540 \text{ kcal/session} \end{array}$$

$$\begin{array}{r} 540 \text{ kcal/session} \\ \times\ \underline{4 \text{ sessions/week}} \\ 2{,}160 \text{ kcal/week} \end{array}$$

Notice that none of the calculations make reference to the number of calories coming from fat. The percentage of energy produced from fat during an exercise session is important only in that it represents the predominance of the aerobic energy system. The physiological advantage of being able to use more fat for ATP production — at any given subthreshold intensity — is that it spares the muscles' store of glycogen.

"Fat burns in the flame of glucose," meaning that fat can only enter the mitochondrial energy pathways when there is enough of the end-product of glucose **catabolism** — pyruvic acid — along with oxygen, also present in the muscle cell. One of the key physiological adaptations of improved aerobic fitness is an enhanced capacity to utilize stored fat for ATP production.

Functionally, it means that the lactate threshold is not reached until a much higher absolute intensity (caloric expenditure) is reached. This allows for more intense, as well as longer duration, aerobic exercise. Thus, more total calories can be expended during each exercise session.

Even though the percentage of total energy provided by fat catabolism decreases as exercise intensity increases, the key to weight management is the total volume of fat used, which is directly linked with total caloric expenditure. So, the statement: "aerobic exercise is essential for fat loss because fat is only burned aerobically" should actually read "aerobic exercise is essential, especially in the untrained, because it can be sustained long enough to expend a significant number of total calories."

Anaerobic exercise is not without benefit. For the untrained individual it is simply ineffective. However, elite athletes, such as 400-meter sprinters whose training and performance emphasize anaerobic predominance, certainly maintain a lean body composition. This is directly related to the total number of calories they burn during training, not the percentage contribution of the energy substrates.

Another factor that has an impact on the expenditure side of the energy balance equation is the greater-than-RMR metabolic rate following a bout of exercise. This increased oxygen requirement in the recovery phase is referred to as **excess post-exercise oxygen consumption (EPOC)**. This oxygen need, historically referred to as oxygen debt, includes the equivalent of the oxygen deficit accumulated at the outset of the bout (O_2 debt), plus additional oxygen for factors such as respiratory muscle recovery, elevated enzyme activity and reloading of oxygen on the **myoglobin** molecule (Costill, 1994).

The two elements that likely have the most significant impact on EPOC are the intensity and duration of the exercise bout. While the exact caloric expenditure of EPOC is difficult to predict, generally the longer and/or more

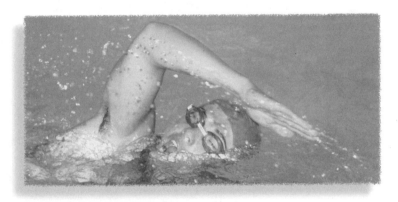

intense the session, the greater the EPOC (Costill, 1994). However, a highly conditioned individual exercising at 75 percent of VO_2 max for an hour will undoubtedly have a greater EPOC than when he was in poor condition and exercised at the same relative intensity.

It has been reported that aerobic exercise can increase the post-exercise metabolic rate for up to 17 to 24 hours; heavy resistance training may lead to an even longer increase in EPOC (Wilmore, 1995).

This presentation of energy systems is clearly a brief, simplified abstract of a complex set of biochemical pathways. The primary intent is to dispel the

The key to maximum fat utilization and weight loss is to maximize total calorie expenditure through physical activity.

Table 7.1
Estimated Calorie Costs
of Selected Activities

Activity	kcal/ pound-minute
Basketball	0.06
Bicycling	
7 mph	0.03
10 mph	0.05
Running	
7.5 mph (8 min/mi)	0.09
10 mph (6 min/mi)	0.12
Sitting	0.011
Sleeping	0.009
Standing	0.012
Swimming,	
crawl stroke, 3mph	0.13
Tennis	0.05
Walking, 3.5 mph	0.03
Weight training	0.05
Wrestling	0.09

e.g. 120-pound woman running at 8 minutes/mile,
kcal/minute = 10.8

These estimated values are not accurate in all situations.
For example, the amount of resistance used in weight
training could dramatically alter the actual kcal
cost/pound-minute.

Adapted from Costill & Wilmore, 1994.

notion that the key to maximizing fat metabolism is to work at a relatively low intensity, since the percentage of fat's contribution is inversely related to intensity. The real key to maximum fat utilization and, ultimately, weight loss is to maximize total caloric expenditure. Table 7.1 gives the approximate energy expenditure for several daily and fitness activities.

Because of the variety of individual responses to energy balance, many weight-management experts recommend that programs for the general public place less emphasis on detailed arithmetic predictions of expected weight loss and ultimate goals, and more emphasis on simply getting

clients to substantially increase caloric expenditure.

In addition, keep in mind that the calculated predictions for expected rates of weight loss are theoretical estimates. A number of factors (e.g., age, activity level, genetics) affect individual weight loss. For example, research suggests that the body adapts to reduced calorie intake by slowing its metabolism. The reasons are not totally clear, but may involve metabolic adjustments described by the so-called **set-point theory** (Bray, 1975). While still controversial, several studies do support this theory. If it is valid, the actual negative energy balance caused by reduced calorie intake would be less than in the examples given. Also, if weight loss includes a loss of lean tissue, which it usually does, RMR is reduced, thereby attenuating the overall impact of caloric expenditure.

As a consultant, you need to understand the implications of energy system predominance during exercise. However, without sophisticated equipment to accurately measure energy expenditure, and without client dedication to keeping detailed dietary records to calculate energy intake, calorie calculations are merely estimates. Ultimately, these estimates may lead to more frustration and a sense of failure, rather than motivating clients toward lifestyle change.

With these concepts of energy balance as a foundation, let's turn our attention to the components of a fitness program as they apply to weight management.

Fitness Program Components

Aerobic (cardiorespiratory) and resistance training are the components of an activity/exercise program that have the greatest impact on energy balance. Because there is little increase in oxygen demand (caloric expenditure) above resting levels, flexibility exercise may appear to have little impact on body weight. But taking a five-minute stretch break instead of reaching for a candy bar when faced with a stressful situation can certainly have an impact on energy balance.

Any type of fitness training — whether it be aerobic training, strength training or flexibility training — is based on the **principles** of **overload** and **specificity**. Overload implies that in order to train one of the body's systems, such as the cardiopulmonary or the skeletal muscle system, that system must be made to work harder than it is accustomed to working. Specificity suggests that the optimal overload for aerobic improvements is different than the overload that is best for strength improvements. The flexibility overload is also unique. To optimize the effects of each specific overload, the fitness-training program is built on four elements: 1) the correct type of activity; 2) the appropriate intensity; 3) sufficient duration; and 4) adequate frequency.

Cardiorespiratory (Aerobic) Fitness

The overload necessary to cause significant improvements in cardiorespiratory performance is an increased **venous return** sustained for a prolonged period. In other words, the exercise(s) must cause a sustained increase in the amount of blood returning to the heart.

Type of Exercise. The type of exercise is related to the principle of specificity of training. For maximum effectiveness, and lowest risk of injury, aerobic exercises need to be rhythmic and continuous, and involve the large muscle groups. Generally, the hip flexors and extensors (iliopsoas and rectus femoris) and the knee flexors and extensors (hamstrings, quadriceps) should be involved. Low-impact activity, such as walking, cycling, low-impact aerobic dance, step aerobics and stair climbing are generally recommended for those who need to lose weight.

Activities combining upper- and lower-extremity movements, such as cross-country skiing, rowing and swimming, can lead to high levels of aerobic capacity. However, for those with physical challenges, such as spinal cord problems that prohibit lower-extremity movement, exercises using large upper-body muscles, such as upper-body ergometry, will clearly enhance aerobic fitness.

Rhythmic, large muscle movements are essential for a significant increase in blood flow back to the heart. The rhythmic squeezing action of the large muscles against the veins within these muscles is called the muscle pump. This muscle pump leads to a significant increase in venous return, which is required for effective aerobic conditioning.

Intensity of Exercise. The intensity element is critical. The realities of aerobic and anaerobic energy production make it clear that exercising at too great an intensity for a client's level of fitness leads to reliance on the anaerobic systems, rather than the aerobic systems. Research shows that optimum exercise intensity for cardiorespiratory fitness improvement is in the range of about 50 percent to 85 percent of maximum oxygen consumption. This corresponds to about 60 percent to 90 percent of maximum heart rate. The ranges are broad to allow for varying levels of fitness as well as genetic factors. The higher a client's level of fitness, the higher the appropriate exercise intensity. Recent research also shows that untrained individuals will begin to improve aerobic fitness at relative intensities as low as 40 percent of VO_2 max (approximately 50 percent HR max).

This more modest intensity enables the beginner to experience the benefits of aerobic exercise without feeling that exhaustive effort is essential.

Heart rate during exercise can provide an excellent monitor of intensity. Keep in mind that many factors will cause an increase in heart rate and that an elevated heart rate is not necessarily an indication of an effective aerobic training pace. However, if the increased heart rate is accomplished by the correct type of activity, the cardiovascular training potential is substantial. Monitoring a **target heart rate (THR)** training zone can provide an excellent indication of correct exercise intensity if it is determined by using a **submaximal graded exercise test**, and reassessed as fitness level improves. If, on the other hand, the THR is calculated by estimating maximal heart rate from the 220 minus age formula, there can be substantial error. (See Chapter 9 for more information on calculating THR.)

Clients also can monitor intensity by learning to recognize the response to exercise at, or above, the lactate threshold.

Exercising above this threshold leads to hyperventilation, lactate buildup and rapid fatigue.

Some clients find the **Rating of Perceived Exertion (RPE)** scale to be an effective way to monitor intensity (ACSM, 1995). (See Chapter 9 for more details on using the RPE scale.)

The "talk test" is another easy method for monitoring exercise intensity. The client should be able to carry on a comfortable conversation while exercising. If breathing is difficult, the intensity is too high to be sustained for very long.

Recognizing the onset of muscle fatigue (sometimes experienced as a "burning" sensation) associated with the rapid buildup of lactate (when the lactate threshold is exceeded) is another

way for clients to know it is time to slow down a bit.

Compliance with exercise is critical for long-term weight loss success (Grilo, 1995). Exercising at a reasonably comfortable intensity helps many individuals develop a positive attitude toward their exercise program. Recognizing that health benefits accrue with an intensity of just 40 percent of VO_2 max, you can encourage an untrained client to focus on "a comfortably vigorous" intensity, rather than specific thresholds such as a target heart rate training zone. One study (Goodrick, 1994) also suggests that teaching clients to self-regulate intensity, rather than constantly supervising their intensity, may increase long-term compliance.

Duration of Exercise. Aerobic exercise must last for at least 10 to 20 minutes per session to lead to substantial fitness improvements over time. Once a client reaches the proper intensity, the activity must be sustained for the minimum time to cause adequate aerobic overload. Recent research suggests that two 10-minute sessions will lead to the same improvements as one 20-minute session if they are done at the same relative intensity. Some clients find it more convenient to fit two 10-minute sessions into a day than to find a 20-minute time block.

Because aerobic training is related to the oxygen cost of activity, there is an inverse relationship between intensity and duration. If intensity is increased, the duration can be decreased with similar training effect. Conversely, if the intensity is decreased, the duration must be increased to achieve the same training effect. For example, working for 30 minutes at a 10 kcal/minute pace (30 x 10 = 300 kcal), will have approximately the same training effect as working for 60 minutes at 5 kcal/minute (60 x 5 = 300 kcal). The key to weight management is to have your client achieve the

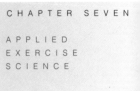

maximum caloric expenditure per exercise session.

Interval training is an increasingly popular method of training (LaForge & Kosich, 1995). There are two types of interval training: 1) performance interval training — a very high-intensity effort designed to enhance competitive performance in a specific sport; and 2) fitness interval training — a modest-to-vigorous intensity effort designed to improve general fitness. Interval training has been used for many years by competitive athletes. In performance training, interval training may involve periods of maximal or near-maximal effort followed by short periods of rest. This can lead to significant performance benefits due to an increased tolerance to the buildup of lactic acid. Only well-trained athletes should do performance intervals. Because of the high intensity of performance intervals, an untrained person is at increased risk for injury, not to mention quick fatigue.

However, fitness intervals should be encouraged even for those just beginning a weight-management program. In fitness interval exercise, the client periodically increases intensity throughout a workout. The intervals are not rigidly defined as in performance interval training. Most importantly, the increase in intensity is capped when the lactate threshold is reached. At this point, the intensity is decreased. Figure 7.2 illustrates how fitness interval exercise might apply in a general fitness or weight-management program.

Frequency of Exercise. Cardiorespiratory training is ideally done at an appropriate intensity and continued for sufficient duration at least three days per week. While training three days per week may be sufficient for aerobic improvement, the energy balance considerations are paramount in a weight management program.

Daily activity, if at all possible, is recommended. A reasonable goal would ultimately be to add 300 to 500 kilocalories to daily energy expenditure. These goals certainly include activities of daily living, such as gardening or

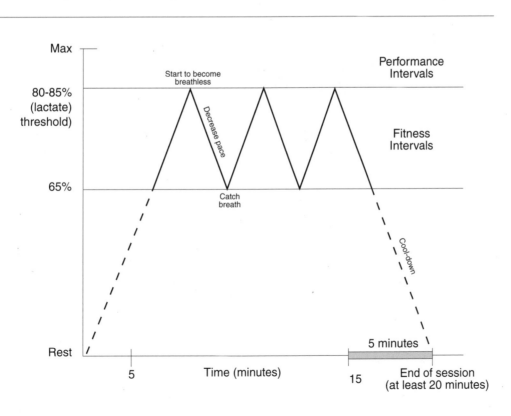

Figure 7.2
How fitness interval training might apply to a general fitness or weight-management program.

carrying groceries, as well as structured exercise sessions.

In general, the greater the frequency, the more rapid the improvements. Still, it is important to allow adequate rest and recovery to minimize the risks associated with overtraining. Most experts encourage even competitive athletes to take at least one day per week for rest or a low-intensity recreational activity, such as a round of golf.

Warm-up and Cool-down

Both a warm-up and a cool-down period are an essential part of any exercise session (not just aerobic exercise). Warming up accomplishes important

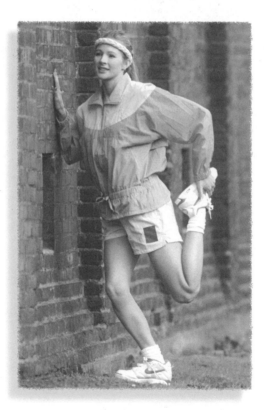

An adequate warm-up, which includes light aerobic activity and flexibility exercises, reduces both the potential for fatigue and the risk of exercise-related injuries.

changes that reduce the risk of injury, as well as make the exercise session more comfortable. First, it causes an actual increase in the temperature of the muscle and connective tissues, reducing the risk of soft tissue injury. It also allows the cardiovascular system to redirect blood flow from the abdominal area to the active muscles (where the

need for oxygen is increasing in response to exercise). This blood shunt is accomplished when arteries that supply blood to the gut constrict and the arteries that deliver blood to the active muscles dilate. Heart rate will quickly rise to near maximum in an attempt to supply adequate oxygen if a minimum of three to five minutes of warm-up is not done, especially if a relatively intense pace is attempted too soon. Cool down to 18 to 20 beats per 10 seconds (108-120 bpm) to allow the system to reverse the blood shunt. Beginning exercisers may require a longer cool-down period.

It is often difficult to emphasize the importance of an adequate warm-up and cool-down to a client. The best approach to both is to work at a much lower intensity in whatever activity the client is using for training. Examples include slow cycling for cycling, walking for jogging, and slow swimming for swimming. An adequate warm-up and cool-down not only reduce the potential for fatigue, they also reduce the risk of exercise-related injuries.

Immediately after the cool-down period is an ideal time for the client to perform stretching and flexibility exercises, since it is best for muscles to be warm in order to increase flexibility.

Strength Training

Not long ago, aerobic exercise was thought by many to be the most important and effective type of exercise in weight-management programs. Strength training was not seen as a very important or effective adjunct to aerobic exercise. However, there is now strong evidence that combining strength training with aerobic exercise may be more effective than aerobic exercise alone (Westcott, 1993). This is likely due to the increase in lean body mass that typically results from a strength-training program, which helps to maintain, or even increase, RMR in clients who are not restricting calories. Even in those who significantly restrict calorie intake, strength training may attenuate the loss of lean mass (Ballor, 1994). The degree to which changes in lean body mass affect caloric expenditure is not clear. But the many benefits of strength training, in addition to the potential weight-management benefits, suggest that it is an important component of an exercise program.

It is important to realize that it is common for two equally successful strength athletes to have very different training routines. Research has not identified one best strength-training protocol. However, there are some well-accepted general principles that will lead to substantial improvements if used regularly. Strength-training programs are designed by manipulating the elements used in aerobic training: type, intensity, frequency and duration.

Types of Strength Overloads

Achieving the overload that leads to strength improvement is quite simple. First, the client must resist the movement of the target muscle. Second, to continue the strength gain, the resistance must progressively increase. To strengthen the biceps group, resist elbow flexion. To strengthen the middle trapezius and rhomboids, resist scapular retraction, and so forth. To effectively design a strength-training (resistance) program, a working knowledge of functional **kinesiology** and **biomechanics** is essential for both safety and effectiveness.

For many years, strength-training programs have been described as being **isometric, isotonic or isokinetic**, based on the type of muscle contraction involved during the exercise. (The prefix "iso" means "same.")

Isometric (same length) refers to exercises that develop high-intensity contractions in the muscle with no change in muscle length. Generally, isometric exercises call for a maximal effort against an immovable object, like a wall or desk. Isometric training clearly increases muscle strength but, unfortunately, only in a narrow range of the joint angle where the contraction occurs. There is also the likelihood of a client performing a **Valsalva maneuver** (breath holding) during isometric exercise. This can be risky for a hypertensive client. (Valsalva should be avoided in any general strength-training program, regardless of the type of exercise used.)

Isotonic (same tone or tension) refers to exercises that use a given amount of external resistance that is challenged throughout the entire range of motion. However, it is not correct to assume that the tension in the muscle is constant throughout the range of motion. The actual amount of force generated by a muscle will change throughout the movement because of the biomechanics at the joint or joints involved. For example, even though a 10-pound dumbbell is obviously a constant weight throughout a biceps curl, the biceps does not generate a constant 10 pounds of force throughout its entire contraction.

Because of this fact, many experts now suggest that strength exercises using a fixed amount of external resistance be referred to as "dynamic constant external resistance" training, not isotonic training. Exercises performed using machines with a shaped cam can be called "dynamic variable external resistance." These descriptions accurately suggest that even though the free weight is constant, or the pin on the machine stays in the same plate throughout the movement, the amount of force generated by the overloaded muscles changes throughout the movement.

Isokinetic (same speed) refers to a type of resistance exercise that causes the exercising muscles to generate a maximum amount of force throughout the entire range of movement, maintaining a constant speed of movement at the same time. While true isokinetic training leads to significant strength gains, machines can be expensive and their use is generally limited to medical and research facilities.

Isokinetic and dynamic resistance exercises are performed with either **concentric** or eccentric muscle contractions, or both.

Concentric (shortening) movements are often referred to as the positive phase of a lift. **Eccentric** (lengthening) movements, on the other hand, are referred to as the negative phase. There are a few types of apparatus that challenge only the concentric phase of a muscle's movement. However, most types of strength-training equipment challenge both concentric and eccentric movements. Strength exercises do not require expensive equipment to be effective (Kosich, 1995).

General Recommendations. With regard to the type of strength-training activity, the most important consideration is what will be used to provide the resistance. Free weights, machines, elastic resistance, water resistance and body weight can all be used to challenge muscles to become stronger.

The intensity and duration of strength training are key elements of your client's exercise program. They are generally measured as the amount of resistance applied to the muscle's contraction before the muscle temporarily fatigues. For instance, **one repetition maximum (1RM)** resistance is the amount of resistance that can be moved through the range of motion one time before the muscle is temporarily fatigued. Eight RM is the resistance that can be moved for eight repetitions before the muscle temporarily fatigues.

Intensity recommendations for general fitness strength training are from 8 to 15 RM of each exercise to achieve optimum strength gains. It is important to reach the point of temporary failure to optimize strength gains.

The number of sets of each exercise performed is another consideration. Several studies have shown that one set of 8 to 15 RM will lead to essentially the same strength gains as two or three sets. However, other experts feel that while one set will lead to substantial gains in the untrained individual, additional strength gains will be made by performing multiple sets as strength increases. If multiple sets are performed, rest at least one to two minutes between sets. For many people, however, the gains achieved by performing one set are remarkable and the time saved is an important factor (Westcott, 1993).

Strength exercises ideally should be performed two to three times per week on non-consecutive days.

In summary, the general recommendations are to do one to three sets of 8 to 15 RM, two to three times per week. In a carefully designed strength program, 10 to 12 exercises can target all the major muscle groups. Therefore, an effective strength workout can be accomplished in 20 to 25 minutes.

Clearly, there are many fitness enthusiasts and strength athletes who follow protocols much different than the one just outlined. The most important factor in any strength-training program is to ensure your client's safety by instructing proper form and technique for every exercise. Then, if more advanced techniques are employed, be certain the client is physically ready and your knowledge base is sufficient.

Flexibility Training

Flexibility is defined as the range of motion of a joint. Therefore, flexibility training is designed to maintain or increase the range of motion in a specific area, such as the low back, the hamstrings or the shoulder girdle. Unfortunately, there is not an abundance of research regarding the most effective stretching techniques.

Flexibility training has little physiological impact on the issues related to weight management, but stretching exercises can dramatically reduce muscle tension and stress. While stretching may not directly impact energy balance on the expenditure side of the equation, it could acutely reduce the potential for eating behaviors triggered by a negative response to a stressful situation.

There are a multitude of stretching techniques (Alter, 1988) and some (as with strength techniques) require more skill and a higher level of flexibility to perform them safely. Overstretching the tissues — tendons and ligaments — associated with maintaining joint integrity, can potentially lead to destabilization at the joint. Therefore, you must understand the elements of specific overload that appear to be safest and most effective for general fitness.

To stretch a muscle, it is necessary to put the related joint(s) in opposition to the movement(s) it causes. As with developing effective strength programs, a working knowledge of functional kinesiology is important for performing safe and effective stretches.

With regard to the need for a warm-up prior to stretching, it depends on the purpose and intention of the stretch. If the purpose is to release muscle tension or experience the calming effect of a gentle stretch, there is no need for a warm-up. However, if the intention of the stretch is to increase the range of motion of a particular joint, a warm-up is essential. If this is the case, have the client perform the stretches after an aerobic workout, or after five to 10 minutes of rhythmic, large muscle movements to increase

core temperature.

In either situation, the lowest risk stretch is to slowly move to the point where a gentle tension or tightness is felt in the muscle(s) being stretched. Do not stretch to the point of pain, in either the muscle or the joint. Hold the stretch in this static position for about 10 seconds, being sure not to hold the breath. Some research suggests that four sets of 10- to 15-second stretches can lead to significant improvements in flexibility. Stretching can be done every day, and a minimum of four to five times per week is advised. All the major

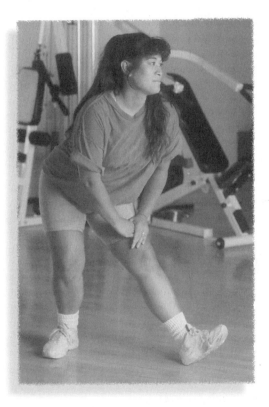

muscles can be stretched in about 10 minutes.

The more rapidly the muscle is stretched, the greater the risk of injury to the muscle and/or connective tissues. Slow, well-controlled stretches that take the muscle just to the point where tension is felt pose relatively little risk. Rapid, ballistic ("bouncing") stretches are not appropriate for general flexibility programs.

While stretching does not have a significant physiological impact on the issues related to weight management, it can dramatically reduce muscle tension and stress.

Physical Activity: Health vs. Fitness

G rowing evidence suggests that there is some distinction between the characteristics of exercise required to yield health benefits and those required for achieving improvements in physical fitness (Haskell, 1995).

The potential health benefits of regular exercise are well-documented. For instance, regular aerobic exercise has a number of significant health benefits, both for those who are apparently healthy and for those who suffer from

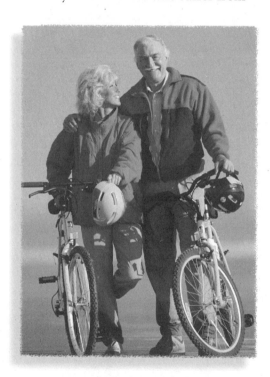

Some individuals, particularly older adults or at-risk individuals, may reap greater benefits from low-to-moderate activities than from higher-intensity ones.

various health problems, including being overweight.

Weight-bearing exercises, such as jogging, brisk walking and strength training, have been shown to help strengthen the skeletal system. This not only reduces the risk for developing osteoporosis, but also slows or stops the progress of existing conditions for which physicians recommend exercise.

Since aerobic exercise training increases the sensitivity of the cells to insulin, it is usually part of the

treatment program for diabetics whose blood sugar is well controlled. Less insulin, or other medication, is often required to regulate blood sugar levels effectively in diabetics who exercise regularly. In several reported cases, type II diabetics medicated with drugs other than insulin were able to significantly reduce, or eliminate, medications by maintaining a healthy body weight, exercising regularly and eating appropriately.

Aerobic exercise is often part of the therapy for reducing the risk of coronary artery disease in high-risk individuals, as well as for those who have suffered a heart attack. Four primary risk factors for developing coronary artery disease are: 1) lack of adequate aerobic exercise, 2) high blood pressure (**hypertension**), 3) smoking and 4) high blood cholesterol.

Aerobic exercise can significantly reduce these risks for several reasons. First, many of those with high blood pressure also are overweight. Aerobic exercise definitely assists in reducing excess body fat as well as lowering blood pressure in those with hypertension. Second, many smokers find that regular aerobic exercise provides a great incentive to quit smoking. Third, regular, brisk aerobic exercise often leads to an increase in the level of **high-density lipoprotein (HDL)**, or "good" cholesterol. Appropriate aerobic exercise is now recommended by the Arthritis Foundation as an integral part of therapy for those with arthritis. It certainly helps maintain aerobic fitness, as well as a healthy body weight. However, appropriate strength and flexibility exercises also are recommended to maintain muscle strength and joint range of motion. Contact your local chapter of the Arthritis Foundation for more information.

Strength exercise not only helps maintain balance between opposing muscle groups, but also plays a key role in helping maintain the calcium integrity of skeletal bones at highest risk for developing osteoporosis. Some studies also suggest that regular strength training may have a beneficial effect on both blood pressure and blood lipids (Westcott, 1993).

Historically, the guidelines for exercise for both health benefits and improved fitness have been the same, with an emphasis on the need for reasonably vigorous activity to achieve the best results. What is emerging is a recognition that "moderate intensity" exercise, especially for the deconditioned, can lead to significant improvements in health without accompanying improvements in fitness. Table 7.2 illustrates the distinction between relatively moderate and vigorous aerobic exercise.

The implications, especially for elderly or at-risk individuals, is encouraging. Those who opt for low-to-moderate forms of activity in favor of performing vigorous exercise may be able to improve their health without the anxiety or risk associated with higher-intensity exercise. This, combined with the evidence that shorter bouts of exercise (10 minutes) repeated two or three times during the day will have the same effect as one 20- or 30-minute session, may provide the incentive for previously sedentary individuals to become more active. It also may be an important consideration for those who find it difficult to commit to exercise for 20 minutes at a time.

Since many of these individuals are likely dealing with weight-management issues, the significance should be clear. Whatever they can do to increase caloric expenditure will be of benefit. Because the additional calorie output will be modest, becoming moderately active probably will not result in notable weight loss. However, in the significantly overweight, a loss of even 10 to 15

Table 7.2
Aerobic Exercise Intensity

Intensity	% max heart rate	% max VO$_2$
Very low	< 30	< 25
Low	30 - 49	25 - 39
Moderate	50 - 69	40 - 59
Vigorous	70 - 89	60 - 84

Adapted from Haskell, 1995.

pounds can lead to an improvement in health (Foreyt & Goodrick, 1994).

Long-term Weight Management

Even though billions of dollars are spent every year on weight-management products, and approximately one-third of American women and one-fourth of American men are on a diet on any given day, the weight of the average American adult has increased 10 pounds in the past decade (Foreyt, 1994). The statistics are just as gloomy for American youth. Obviously, something is wrong.

Thousands of people — young and old, male and female — have lost weight; in some cases several times. But the fact remains that most people who lose weight will regain it within, at most, a couple of years. The key to effective weight management is clearly establishing lifestyle habits that promote healthy weight management. One important habit is patience. While our culture often encourages an attitude of quick fixes and overnight make-overs, the reality is that most changes, such as the physiological changes in fitness and **body composition**, take time. As a consultant, you have a tremendous opportunity to help clients develop more realistic expectations.

Rate of Change: Fitness and Body Composition

Expectations for change should be measured in weeks and months, not hours and days. John Foreyt, Ph.D., suggests that it takes most people at least six months of persistent effort to transform a change into a lifestyle habit. This certainly applies to the exercise, dietary and behavioral elements of adapting to a healthy weight management lifestyle.

Fitness. The rate of change in factors such as aerobic fitness and muscular strength are directly related to the intensity, duration and frequency with which the appropriate overloads are applied. In other words, the greater the amount of effort, the more rapidly changes will occur.

If a client performs 30 minutes of aerobic exercise at a vigorous intensity, at least three days per week, it is reasonable to expect her to begin to notice improved performance between the fourth and sixth week. By the 12th to 16th week, she will have a significantly improved aerobic capacity, perhaps by as much as 15 percent to 20 percent. If she continues to train at a vigorous intensity for six months, the rate of change will decrease, but she will probably be able to exercise for extended periods at a pace that six months prior would have been exhaustive in a few minutes.

As with aerobic improvements, the rate of strength improvement is directly related to the amount of work done. Training with one set of 8 to 15 RM, three days per week, may yield noticeable improvements within two to three weeks. At eight weeks she will be significantly stronger, and by the 12th week she could be as much as 20 percent stronger.

The degree of change in factors like muscle size has a definite genetic component. Two people doing exactly the same program will likely show different rates of change, as well as different total adaptations.

Keep in mind that the degree of change is influenced by the client's level of fitness at the beginning of the program.

Similarly, the higher the level of fitness, the more difficult it becomes to continue to make improvements. This is called "hitting a plateau." It is perfectly acceptable to maintain a consistent program when a client reaches a reasonable fitness goal.

Athletes, on the other hand, are constantly striving for any training challenge that might improve their performance.

Flexibility improvements occur more rapidly than either aerobic or strength changes if the stretches are done four to six days per week. Improved range of motion in a "tight" muscle can be expected within a week.

Body composition. Anatomically, the body is composed of five distinct parts: **adipose tissue** (fat), muscles, organs, bones and everything else. With reference to weight (fat) management, exercise physiologists have historically described the body as consisting of just two components: fat weight and lean body mass. Lean body mass is sometimes mistakenly thought of as only muscle, but actually represents everything but fat—blood, bones, connective tissue, organs, etc. So, the phrase **"fat-free mass"** is often used instead of lean body mass.

Most techniques that assess body composition ultimately predict a percentage of total body weight carried as fat — body fat percentage. What remains are the muscles, bones and organs, not just muscles (lean mass). Chapter 4 presents a detailed discussion of the many factors that influence body composition and the various methods to determine it.

How rapidly does body-fat percentage

change? How rapidly does fat-free mass change? It depends.

Changes in body-fat percentage are directly related to energy balance. As long as dietary intake is sufficient (generally thought to be no less than 1,200 kcal/day for women and 1,500 kcal/day for men), generating a negative energy balance should result in a decrease in the amount of body fat. The best way to reduce body-fat percentage is to significantly increase daily caloric expenditure through exercise, and eat a sensible diet. Encourage clients to be especially patient in seeing changes in body composition. Significant changes are usually noticeable between the sixth and eighth week of a balanced program. A reasonable goal for body-fat percentage in most healthy adults who are not significantly overweight is between about 17 percent to 24 percent for women and 12 percent to 17 percent for men. An increase in muscle mass as a result of strength-training exercise accounts for the vast majority of an increased fat-free mass. But there also will be more connective tissue, maybe a little more blood volume and increased bone density. This is why the more recent two-component model for body composition makes more sense.

Men tend to show a greater increase in muscle cell size (hypertrophy) than women. But this is not always the case. For example, some women have a higher natural level of the testosterone hormone than others. Under the stress of intense strength-training overload, those men and women with higher testosterone levels will likely show the greatest **hypertrophy**. It is not possible to predict the exact rate of change.

Approaches to Achieving a Healthy Body Weight

The three most common approaches to achieving and maintaining a healthy body weight are: 1) dieting alone; 2) exercise alone; or 3) a combination of dieting plus exercise. It is important to examine the research to carefully distinguish between the short-term and long-term effects of these approaches. There is no question that significantly reducing calorie intake will lead to an initial weight loss. However, it is believed that within a relatively short period (two to three weeks) the body adjusts its RMR downward in response to the decreased caloric intake (Foreyt & Goodrick, 1994). As the RMR decreases, the effect of dieting on creating a negative energy balance is attenuated, slowing or halting further weight loss, even though the restricted diet continues.

The magnitude of calorie restriction appears to be important (Thompson, 1994). Drastic reductions (more than 700 kcal/day) may lead to more profound metabolic adaptations than a modest reduction. (This is discussed in more detail in Chapter 4).

There are obvious concerns with low-calorie dieting, some physiological and others related to program compliance.

Physiologically, a number of studies have shown that weight loss can include a decrease in lean mass, which explains at least part of the decrease in RMR. But a significant loss of lean tissue, except in the significantly overweight, is not the desired outcome of a weight-management program.

Another concern with low-calorie dieting is the risk of an inadequate intake of nutrients and carbohydrates. It is unlikely that diets providing fewer than 1,200 to 1,500 kilocalories per day (unless on a nutrient formula taken under medical supervision) can supply an adequate amount of several vitamins and minerals (Katch & McArdle, 1991). Calcium, iron and folic acid are notable examples, especially for women.

Lastly, very few people stay with a low-calorie diet for prolonged periods.

Rigid attempts to control intake simply do not work for most people (Foreyt & Goodrick, 1994). When caloric intake increases, even rising to more appropriate levels, without an accompanying increased energy output, a positive energy balance is created and the lost weight is regained. Recall that more than 90 percent of those who attempt weight loss with dieting alone have regained all (or more) of the lost weight within two to three years.

There is no doubt that, physiologically and psychologically, the most effective long-term weight-management

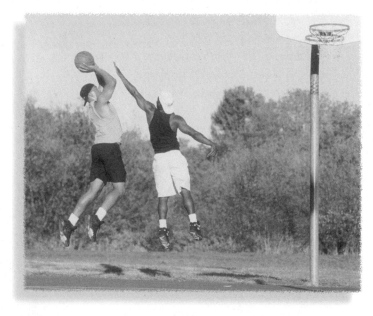

Explain to your clients that the key to sticking to an exercise program is to make it a part of their lifestyle. Activities such as a pick-up game of basketball or playing with their kids are two great ways to incorporate exercise into their lives.

lifestyles are those that include adequate activity and a sensible diet.

Foreyt (1995) reported a fascinating study done at Baylor Medical School. Three groups — diet alone, exercise alone, diet-plus-exercise — were followed over a three-year period. The diet group was restricted to 1,200 kcal/day for women and 1,500 kcal/day for men. The exercise group added about 300 kcal to their daily pre-study energy expenditure. The diet-plus-exercise group combined the protocols.

As expected, at three months, both the diet and the diet-plus-exercise groups had lost significantly more

weight than the exercise group. At 12 months, the diet and diet-plus-exercise groups had still lost more weight than the exercise group. But both of these groups had regained weight since the three-month measurement. At 24 months, the only group that continued to show a significant weight loss, primarily as body fat, was the exercise group. Additionally, total weight lost was greater than the 12-month measurement. Both the diet and diet-plus-exercise groups had regained weight back to at least pre-study levels. In analyzing follow-up inquiries, the researchers pose an interesting proposition. Not surprisingly, they conclude that most people cannot sustain a rigid, restricted diet for prolonged periods. In the diet-only group, the significant weight loss in the first three months had reversed by the 12-month measurement. Subjects were not adhering to the dietary protocol.

The intriguing suspicion, however, is that if a client combines a rigid, restricted diet with a moderate exercise program, when adherence to the diet falters, adherence to the exercise program also falters. Perhaps, they suggest, the diet and exercise are perceived as equal parts of a too-rigid lifestyle. While the hypothesis needs more study, it is clear that few people can sustain a rigid lifestyle approach for long.

The researchers also reported that subjects in the exercise group were eating a healthier, lower-fat, higher-carbohydrate diet by the end of the study.

Their recommendations: Emphasize becoming more active, while continually reinforcing the positive effects. De-emphasize rigid dietary control and focus on the benefits of making an attempt to consume fewer fats and more carbohydrates.

Obviously, calorie intake is important. Low-fat and non-fat foods (ice cream, cookies, etc.) still have calories, so a client needs to know that just because a food is low in fat does not mean that it can be consumed in un-limited quantities.

You must be aware of the numerous other approaches to weight manage-ment. Surgical procedures, drug inter-vention, supplements and spot-reduc-ing devices continue to be of public interest.

Surgical Procedures. Currently the most common form of cosmetic surgery is the surgical removal of fat using a technique known as **liposuction**. This technique is used to remove small am-ounts of fat from such areas as under the chin, above the elbows, around the knees and small areas on the lateral hip and buttocks area. The technique is not recommended for removal of large am-ounts of body fat.

As with any surgical procedure, there are risks during and after surgery. Some who have undergone the procedure re-port positive results; others regret hav-ing undergone it because of bruising, nerve loss or scarring.

If a client is considering liposuction, you should make the following recom-mendations:

1. Get more than one opinion from board-certified plastic surgeons or gyne-cologists who are qualified to perform the procedure.

2. Clearly understand both the potential risks and benefits that may result.

3. Speak with several of the surgeon's former patients to see whether they are pleased with the results and if their situ-ations were similar.

4. Understand that adopting a life-style of adequate activity and sensible eating is still a critical requirement, even if the surgery is performed.

Drug Intervention. There are cur-rently two drugs approved by the Food and Drug Administration for treating obesity in the U.S. Fenfluramine, ap-proved in 1973, appears to act on the hypothalamus to suppress the appetite. Phentermine is used to counter the side-effects of depression often report-ed by those taking fenfluramine. There is significant debate regarding the effi-cacy of such treatment for obese indi-viduals who do not seem to respond to energy balance manipulation.

Supporters contend that, for some, obesity is a genetically based disease, and that medical intervention is, there-fore, appropriate. They can cite abun-dant data showing that those who take the medication show significant weight loss. Pharmaceutical companies contin-ue to aggressively pursue obesity med-ication research.

Those who question the efficacy of drug intervention cite the fact that since the U.S. Food and Drug Admin-istration limits treatment to 12 weeks, most of the subjects who demonstrate weight loss regain the weight when the treatment is discontinued. Further, as with any medication, there are side effects, some of which may not yet be apparent.

Many scientists also question the suggestion that the evolutionary pro-cess could create such a prevalent "obesity gene" in a culture where obesi-ty has become a major health problem in less than a century's time. Their con-tention is that the problem is clearly one of too many calories consumed and too few calories expended — the ener-gy balance equation in action. Con-tinued research is needed to clarify these theories.

Supplements. Claims that particular supplements will lead to increased mus-cle mass and/or decreased body-fat per-centage are plentiful. One example is chromium picolinate, which claims to increase muscle mass, raise RMR and subsequently lead to decreased body-fat percentage. Currently, there are no well-designed, independent studies that substantiate this claim.

Spot Reducing. Although not as common as a decade ago, some products and devices still claim that they can selectively reduce **subcutaneous** fat in specific anatomical regions. While the turnover rate of free-fatty acids may vary in different **adipose** cells due to variable hormone-sensitive receptor density, fat mobilization appears to be a system-wide response. There continues to be no clinical evidence to support the efficacy for spot-reducing claims (Wilmore & Costill, 1994).

Weight Cycling

Weight cycling is the repeated process of weight loss followed by weight gain, often referred to as the "yo-yo" effect. It has been reported in the popular press, as well as in professional literature, as leading to several negative physiological, medical and psychological consequences.

Weight cycling is most common in those who use restricted calorie diets to lose weight, then subsequently regain it when calorie intake increases. However, athletes, such as wrestlers, also may be chronic weight cyclers. Weight cycling has been reported to reduce lean body mass, increase body-fat percentage, chronically lower RMR, impair glucose tolerance and increase blood pressure. It also has been reported to cause negative effects on mood and self-esteem.

However, a recent multi-center study concluded that the majority of claims for the long-term effects of weight cycling were not substantiated when reviewing the vast majority of clinical studies (National Task Force on the Prevention and Treatment of Obesity, 1994). Given this, there are several implications for you as a lifestyle and weight management consultant.

Keep an open mind. What may appear to be widely supported and well-documented claims may not accurately reflect the majority of scientific evidence.

For instance, the task force reviewed 12 clinical studies examining the effect of weight cycling on total body fat: one showed that weight cycling increased total body fat; 11 reported that weight cycling had no impact on total body fat.

In all, 43 studies on the effects of weight cycling in humans or animals conducted between 1966 and 1994 were evaluated. Similar results occurred when evaluating potential consequences. The majority in each case reported no negative effects.

Recognize, however, that a consensus of the Task Force does not mean weight cycling does not cause individually negative responses. It simply suggests that a great deal more research is needed in this area. There is no question, for instance, that individuals have reported significant frustration related to their repeated lack of success in weight management.

At this point in time, the most important implication appears to be that, in general, the health risks associated with obesity — hypertension, type II diabetes, cancer, heart disease, joint problems, etc. — outweigh the reported risks of continuing to attempt to lose weight. In other words, encourage clients to keep trying. Sometimes it takes several attempts before a client is ultimately successful.

Environmental Concerns

You should be aware of the effect of selected environmental conditions on exercise performance.

Altitude. Because there is less oxygen in the air at progressively higher altitudes, even well-trained athletes need to work at reduced intensity levels until they become acclimated to higher altitudes. It generally takes about two weeks to acclimate to altitudes up to about 8,000 feet, but can take up to four to five weeks to adapt to altitudes higher than 12,000 feet. Noticeable improvements, however, are generally observed within four to five days.

Because there is less oxygen in the air at higher altitudes, the heart will beat faster in order to deliver adequate oxygen to the muscles, even at rest. During exercise, the heart rate may be as much as 50 percent higher than normal, so pay particular attention to the onset of **hyperventilation** when beginning an exercise program at a higher altitude. Lower intensity to allow the client to complete the session without being exhausted.

There are a number of potential problems associated with exercise at a high altitude, including headache, **insomnia**, irritability, weakness, dizziness and **dehydration**. (Drinking plenty of fluids is essential.) Be sure to report any symptoms to a physician to reduce the risk of more severe complications. It might seem reasonable to assume that training at higher altitudes would enhance aerobic capacity upon returning to lower altitudes. While it may be true in the short-term, the changes the body makes to enhance oxygen delivery at higher altitudes are lost within three to four weeks of return to lower altitudes.

Heat. When we exercise in a hotter-than-normal environment, blood vessels near the skin open to facilitate the transfer of body heat to the environment so that the body's internal temperature can be maintained. This causes a reduction in both **venous return** and **stroke volume**. At any intensity, heart rate will be higher than usual as the cardiorespiratory system attempts to maintain cardiac output to meet the oxygen needs of the muscles.

Because sweating is one of the body's most effective means of regulating internal temperature, exercising in hot, humid conditions is especially stressful to the unacclimated person. In order for sweat to dissipate heat, it must evap-

orate. When humidity is high, sweat does not evaporate. So even though your client may be sweating profusely, there is still a risk of severe heat problems.

The main concerns with exercising in heat and humidity are replenishing water and allowing the maximum amount of sweat evaporation. To replenish water, drink at least 3 to 6 ounces every 10 to 15 minutes during exercise — the cooler the water the better, because cooler water empties more rapidly than warm water into the intestines where it can be absorbed. Drink 8 ounces of

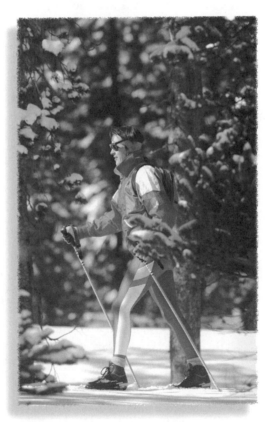

When exercising in the cold, remind your clients to dress in layers and to replenish body fluids by drinking plenty of water.

water 20 to 30 minutes before exercise, and another 8 to 10 ounces of water in the 30 minutes following the exercise session. To allow evaporation of sweat, wear lightweight clothing. Light colors — white is best — reflect heat better than dark colors. Wear a light-colored hat to prevent heat absorption through the top of the head. Never wear rubberized or waterproof garments that prevent the evaporation of sweat. Such practices could lead to severe heat stress. Experts recommend 100-percent cotton garments, rather than synthetics, for exercising in the heat, although there are now a number of specialized fabrics on the market that wick perspiration away from the body. Be sure to have your clients use sunscreen to reduce the risk of sunburn and skin cancer.

Cold. It surprises some to learn that replenishment of body fluids is just as important when exercising in a cold environment as it is when exercising in the heat. Not only is water lost as vapor in exhaled air, but the kidneys increase urine production in the cold. Exercising in the cold generally produces enough body heat so that few problems occur during the exercise session. However, risks become apparent when exercise is stopped and the possibility of losing too much body heat increases.

The easiest way to make sure the body doesn't overheat during exercise, or lose too much heat during a rest period, is to dress in layers. As body temperature increases during high-intensity exercise, successive layers of clothing can be removed to allow heat to dissipate. Layers can be replaced during rest or periods of low-intensity effort to help maintain body heat.

Be certain that the layers near the client's skin are made from fabrics such as wool, polypropylene or any of the newer synthetic materials that wick moisture away from the skin. During a period of rest or low-intensity effort, a layer of wet clothing next to the skin will cause the body to lose heat. If the day is windy, the outer layer should provide wind protection to reduce the chilling effects felt during a rest period. It is important to wear a hat when exercising in the cold, especially during periods of rest, since a significant amount of heat can be lost through the scalp.

Pollution. We all recognize that air pollution is a significant problem in many areas. Exercising outdoors when pollution levels are high should clearly be avoided. This is particularly important for clients with respiratory problems (ACSM, 1991). Other recommendations:

1. Try to exercise in the early morning hours when pollution levels are typically lowest.

2. Avoid walking, jogging and cycling along roadways with heavy traffic. The increased ventilation rate that comes with exercise will significantly increase the amount of car exhaust a client is breathing.

3. Pay attention to the air pollution index reports, which are increasingly becoming a part of weather reports in metropolitan areas.

Summary

Your opportunities as a lifestyle and weight management consultant are immense. Weight-control problems are an increasingly notable health risk for all ages and genders.

Helping your clients make sensible, realistic lifestyle changes to accomplish appropriate weight-management goals will enhance their lives significantly.

It is imperative that you continue to remain a student of literature in the areas that affect body weight, not just exercise science. As the controversy regarding the effects of weight cycling illustrates, new and important information emerges continually.

Healthy weight management involves more than just exercise and sensible eating. It also involves attitude and perspective. As a consultant, an awareness of the highly variable individual responses to both physical and psychological issues is absolutely essential, and compassion and understanding are paramount.

References

Alter, M. (1988). *The Science of Stretching.* Champaign: Human Kinetics.

American College of Sports Medicine. (1995). *Guidelines for Exercise Testing and Prescription.* (5th ed.) Philadelphia: Lea & Febiger.

American Council on Exercise. (1996). (Cotton, R.T., Ed.) *Personal Trainer Manual.* (2nd ed.) San Diego: American Council on Exercise.

American Heart Association. (1992). *Circulation,* 86-1.

Ballor, D. & Poehlman, E. (1994). Exercise enhances fat-free mass preservation during diet-induced weight loss: A Meta-analytical finding. *International Journal of Obesity,* 18, 35-40.

Bray, G. & Gallagher, T. (1975). Manifestations of hypothalamic obesity in man: a comprehensive investigation of eight patients and a review of the literature. *Medicine,* 54, 301-330.

Brownell, K. (1989). *The LEARN Program for Weight Control.* Dallas: American Health Publishing.

Costill, D. & Wilmore, J. (1994). *Physiology of Sport & Exercise.* Champaign: Human Kinetics.

Foreyt, J. & Goodrick, G. (1994). *Living Without Dieting.* Houston: Warner Books, Harrison Publishing.

Foreyt, J. & Goodrick, G. Impact of behavior therapy on weight loss. *Journal of the American Dietetic Association,* 95-1, 118- 119.

Goodrick, G., et al. (1994). Exercise adherence in the obese: self-regulated intensity. *Medicine, Exercise, Nutrition and Health,* 3, 335-338.

Grilo, C. (1995). The role of physical activity in weight loss and weight loss management. *Medicine, Exercise, Nutrition and Health,* 4, 60-76.

Haskell, W. (October, 1995). More vs. Less. *IDEA Today,* 13-9, 40-47.

Katch. F. & McArdle, W. (1991). *Nutrition, Weight Control and Exercise.* (3rd ed.) Philadelphia: Lea & Febiger.

Kosich, D. (1995). *GET REAL: A Personal Guide to Real-Life Weight Management.* San Diego: IDEA Press.

LaForge, R. & Kosich, D. (1995). Fat Burning: Just the Facts. *IDEA Today,* 13-1, 65-70.

LaForge, R. & Kosich, D. (1994). Interval Exercise. *IDEA Personal Trainer,* Nov/Dec, 18-24.

McArdle, W., Katch, F. & Katch, V. (1991). *Exercise Physiology: Energy, Nutrition and Human Performance.* 3rd ed. Philadelphia: Lea & Febiger.

National Academy of Sciences. (1995). *Weighing the Options: Criteria for Evaluating Weight-Management Programs.* Washington, D.C.: National Academy Press.

National Task Force on the Prevention and Treatment of Obesity. (1994). Weight Cycling. *Journal of the American Medical Association,* 272-15, 1196-1202.

Nieman, D. (1995). *Fitness and Sports Medicine: A Health-Related Approach.* 3rd ed. Palo Alto, CA: Bull Publishing.

Sharkey, B. (1990). *Physiology of Fitness.* 3rd ed. Champaign: Human Kinetics.

Stunkard, A. & Wadden, T. (1992). *Obesity: Theory and Therapy.* 2nd ed. New York: Raven Press.

Westcott, W. (1993). *Be Strong: Strength Training for Muscular Fitness for Men and Women.* Dubuque: Brown & Benchmark.

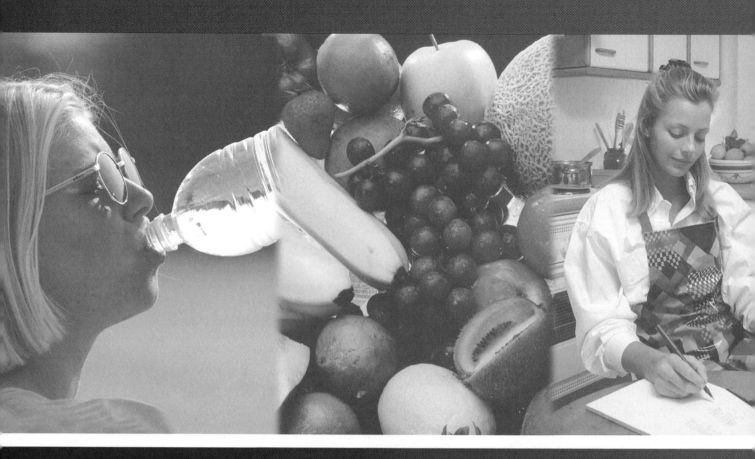

CHAPTER EIGHT

IN THIS CHAPTER:

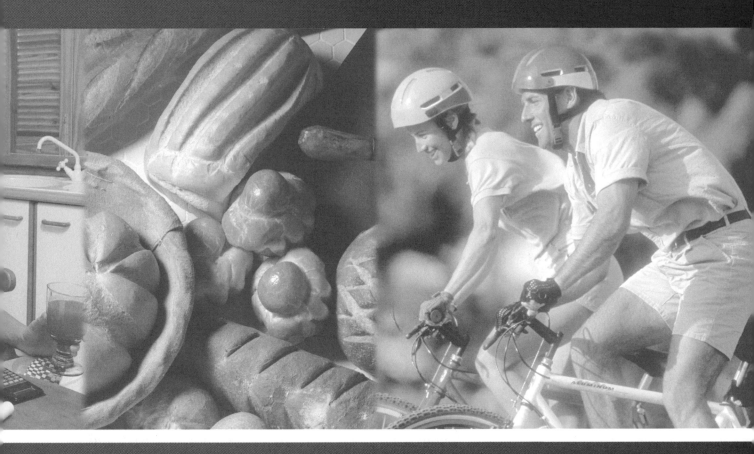

BASIC Nutrition

Eileen Stellefson

Eileen Stellefson, M.P.H., R.D., is the associate director of the
Weight Managment Center at the Medical University of South
Carolina in Charleston. She is both a nutrition specialist for
eating disorder patients and an instructor in the Department
of Psychiatry and Behavioral Sciences.

Introduction

Following a healthy meal plan is essential for effective weight control. Unfortunately, your clients probably learned about diet plans from magazines, books and/or weight control programs that promise quick fixes. Dieting is a $31 billion business that sells more misinformation than sound advice. This chapter will provide you with the knowledge you need to help your clients follow a well-balanced diet for overall good health, and for achieving and maintaining a healthy weight.

Variety, balance and moderation are the keys to a healthy diet. No one needs to follow a perfect diet every day to be healthy or to control weight. Trying to eliminate all foods that are considered "bad" from your client's diet may leave them feeling deprived, and can lead to overindulgence at a later date. The goal in helping people lose weight is for them to follow an overall healthy diet.

Nutrients

The science of **nutrition** is fairly new. It has only been in this century that people have formally studied how food affects health. We know that there are at least 40 specific **nutrients** that satisfy three basic functions: the need for **energy**, the need for tissue growth and repair, and the need to regulate **metabolic functions** that are constantly occurring in the body. Nutrients are divided into categories based on their chemical structure and function.

Water

The most important nutrient, water is second only to oxygen as a substance necessary to sustain life. It is the most abundant substance in the body, accounting for 50 percent to 70 percent of the body's weight.

All tissues contain varying amounts of water. It makes up 75 percent of muscle tissue, but only 25 percent of fat. The body weight of lean individuals is comprised of a relatively high percentage of water. Conversely, the body weight of individuals with a high percentage of body fat is made up of a considerably lower percentage of water.

The body uses water for just about all of its functions, as every cell in the body relies on water to carry out its activities. Water transports nutrients to and removes wastes from the cells, as well as helps to regulate body temperature. Failure to consume adequate water results in fatigue, faulty regulation of body temperature and an increased risk of **heat exhaustion** and **heat stroke**. Less active clients should be advised to drink eight glasses of fluid (preferably water) per day, and those who engage in moderate-to-strenuous activity should drink more. Clients need to learn that thirst should not be used as an indicator of when their body needs fluid. By the time they feel thirsty they will be well

on their way to becoming **dehydrated**. Have your clients consume 8 ounces in the half-hour before exercise, 3 to 4 ounces every 10 minutes or so during exercise, and another 8 ounces in the 30 minutes after exercise, whether they are thirsty or not.

Vitamins

Vitamins are organic substances that are essential to life and play a key role in energy production, growth, maintenance and repair. They are only needed in small amounts, but must be obtained from the diet as the body cannot manufacture them. There are 13 vitamins needed by humans. They provide no calories and, therefore, cannot be used for fuel.

Vitamins are divided into two categories: **water soluble** and **fat soluble**. Vitamins A, D, E and K are fat-soluble vitamins that are absorbed with the help of fats, and are stored in fat. There are eight water-soluble vitamins: the B vitamins and vitamin C. Table 8.1 outlines the functions of vitamins as well as common food sources.

Minerals

Minerals are inorganic substances that must be included in the diet to maintain a number of vital functions and body processes, such as the regulation of heart beat, transportation of oxygen to every cell, formation of **hemoglobin,** the building of bones and teeth, and muscle contraction. Minerals that are required in amounts greater than 100 milligrams per day may be referred to as major minerals and include calcium, phosphorous, sodium, chloride and magnesium. Minor minerals needed in smaller amounts, also referred to as trace minerals, include iron, zinc, copper, iodine, manganese, molybdenum, arsenic, boron, nickel and silicon. The various functions and sources of these minerals are summarized in Table 8.2.

Table 8.1
Vitamin Facts

Vitamin	U.S. RDA*	Best Sources	Functions
A (carotene)	5,000 IU/day	yellow or orange fruits and vegetables, green leafy vegetables, fortified oatmeal, liver, dairy products	formation and maintenance of skin, hair and mucous membranes; helps you see in dim light; bone and tooth growth
B_1 (thiamine)	1.5 mg/day	fortified cereals and oatmeals, meats, rice and pasta, whole grains, liver	helps body release energy from carbohydrates during metabolism; growth and muscle tone
B_2 (riboflavin)	1.7 mg/day	whole grains, green leafy vegetables, organ meats,	helps body release energy from protein, milk and eggs, fat and carbohydrates during metabolism
B_6 (pyridoxine)	2 mg/day	fish, poultry, lean meats, bananas, prunes, dried beans, whole grains, avocados	helps build body tissue and aids in metabolism of protein
B_{12} (cobalamin)	6 mcg/day	meats, milk products, seafood	aids cell development, functioning of the nervous system and the metabolism of protein and fat
Biotin	0.3 mg/day	cereal/grain products, yeast, legumes, liver	involved in metabolism of protein, fats and carbohydrates
Folate (Folacin, folic acid)	0.4 mg/day	green leafy vegetables, organ meats, dried peas, beans and lentils	aids in genetic material development; involved in red blood cell production
Niacin	20 mg/day	meat, poultry, fish, enriched cereals, peanuts, potatoes, dairy products, eggs	involved in carbohydrate, protein and fat metabolism
Pantothenic Acid	10 mg/day	lean meats, whole grains, legumes, vegetables, fruits	helps release energy from fats and carbohydrates
C (absorbic acid)	60 mg/day	citrus fruits, berries and vegetables— especially peppers	essential for structure of bones, cartilage, muscle and blood vessels; helps maintain capillaries and gums and aids in absorption of iron
D	400 IU/day	fortified milk, sunlight, fish, eggs, butter, fortified margarine	aids in bone and tooth formation; helps maintain heart action and nervous system
E	30 IU/day	fortified and multi-grain cereals, nuts, wheat germ, vegetable oils, green leafy vegetables	protects blood cells, body tissue and essential fatty acids from harmful destruction in the body
K	**	green leafy vegetables, fruit, dairy and grain products	essential for blood clotting functions

* For Adults and Children over four. IU = international units; mg = milligrams; mcg = micrograms.
** There is no U.S. RDA for vitamin K, however the Recommended Dietary Allowance is 1 mcg/kg of bodyweight.

Table 8.2
Mineral Facts

Mineral	U.S. RDA	Best Sources	Functions
Calcium	1,000 mg/day	milk and milk products	strong bones, teeth, muscle tissue; regulates heart beat, muscle action and nerve function; blood clotting
Chromium	No RDA	corn oil, clams, whole grain cereals, brewer's yeast	glucose metabolism (energy); increases effectiveness of insulin
Copper	2 mg/day	oysters, nuts, organ meats, legumes	formation of red blood cells, bone growth and health, works with vitamin C to form elastin
Iodine	150 mcg/day	seafood, iodized salt	component of hormone thyroxine, which controls metabolism
Iron	18 mg/day	meats and organ meats, legumes	hemoglobin formation, improves blood quality, increases resistance to stress and disease
Magnesium	No RDA	nuts, green vegetables, whole grains	acid/alkaline balance; important in metabolism of carbohydrates, minerals and sugar
Manganese	No RDA	nuts, whole grains, vegetables, fruits	enzyme activation; carbohydrate and fat production; sex hormone production; skeletal development
Phosphorus	1,000 mg/day	fish, meat, poultry, eggs, grains	bone development; important in protein, fat and carbohydrate utilization
Potassium	No RDA	lean meat, vegetables, fruits	fluid balance; controls activity of heart muscle, nervous system, kidneys
Selenium	50-200 mcg/day provisional RDA	seafood, organ meats, lean meats, grains	protects body tissues against oxidative damage from radiation, pollution and normal metabolic processing
Zinc	15 mg/day	lean meats, liver, eggs, seafood, whole grains	involved in digestion and metabolism; important in development of reproductive system; aids in healing

Source: American Institute for Cancer Research.

A note about minerals: They may compete in the intestine for **absorption**. Excessive intake of a single mineral (usually through a large supplemented dose) can restrict the absorption of a competing mineral.

The Caloric Nutrients

Proteins, **carbohydrates** and **fats** are the three nutrients that provide calories. These calories are used by the body to sustain life by helping to maintain body temperature, and facilitating the

Table 8.3

Protein Complementarity Chart

How to Get Complete Proteins Without Meat

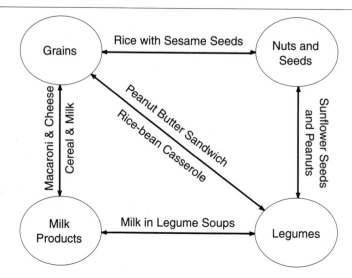

Grains	Brown rice, whole wheat, corn meal, rye, millet, barley oats, buckwheat
Legumes	All dry beans and peanuts: soybean, kidney, black bean, black-eye, aduzki, lima, garbanzo, lentil, split pea, dahl, navy bean, pinto, mung, etc. Tofu is a legume.
Seeds and Nuts	Seeds: sunflower, pumpkin, squash, sesame, chia Nuts: almonds, cashews, walnuts, filberts, brazil, pine, pistachios
Dairy Products	Complete protein in and of themselves as they are animal foods — therefore, will complement any food with protein.

Adapted from *Diet for a Small Planet* by Frances M. Lappé. Reprinted with permission.

growth and repair of all organs and tissues. Many people believe carbohydrate calories to be "good" calories and fat calories to be "bad" calories. In reality, though, they both serve a vital purpose in our diet. One reason fat calories are considered bad is that Americans eat too many of them, which can result in excess body fat and weight. Fat is a very concentrated source of energy and contains more than twice the calories of protein or carbohydrates.

1 gram protein = 4 calories
1 gram carbohydrate = 4 calories
1 gram fat = 9 calories
1 gram alcohol = 7 calories

Alcohol also provides calories, but is not considered a nutrient since it does not contribute to the growth, maintenance or repair of body tissue. Alcohol can be converted to fat when total caloric intake exceeds caloric expenditure, and it also can be damaging to tissues if consumed in excessive amounts for long periods of time.

Protein

Proteins are organic substances containing carbon, oxygen, hydrogen and nitrogen. Each protein molecule is made up of subunits called **amino acids**. Twenty different amino acids are found in the body, 11 of which it is able to manufacture on its own. The remaining nine amino acids are considered essential and must be consumed through our diet. Meat, fish, poultry and dairy products contain all of the **essential amino acids** and are, therefore, considered **complete proteins**. Vegetables, grains and nuts do not provide all of the essential amino acids by themselves; however, these **incomplete protein** foods can be combined to get all of the essential amino acids. Table 8.3 demonstrates how various foods can be combined to create complete proteins.

Protein is the body's major building material. The brain, muscles, skin, hair and **connective tissue** are all composed primarily of protein.

Protein is needed to make the **enzymes** and hormones that regulate such body processes as water balance, and also are critical components of the **antibodies** that fight foreign organisms. Finally, protein can be used as a source of energy, but only when the diet is limited in carbohydrates and fats.

The average American diet, often dominated by such foods as steak and eggs, is comprised of too much protein. Because many high-protein foods also are high in fat and calories, this type of diet may encourage weight gain. Still, many people view a high-protein diet as a means of losing weight. The dangers of this type of diet are discussed in detail later in this chapter.

Carbohydrates

To this day, some people avoid eating carbohydrates for fear that they are "fattening." This belief arose from fad diets of the 1970s when people eliminated carbohydrate foods from their diet and lost weight very rapidly. But the lost pounds came mostly from water, not fat. It's no surprise that, when they began to eat carbohydrate foods again, their lost weight returned just as rapidly as it left.

Carbohydrates are divided into two types: complex and simple. **Complex carbohydrates** (or starches), such as bread, rice, cereal and potatoes, take longer for the body to break down. These foods also can provide fiber and other vitamins and minerals. Simple sugars, which are rapidly digested and absorbed, are found in foods such as fruit and milk, which provide vitamins and minerals. Most simple sugars consumed by Americans, however, come in the form of soft drinks, cakes, cookies and candy, and provide little more than calories.

Most people should now recognize that carbohydrates are the body's best

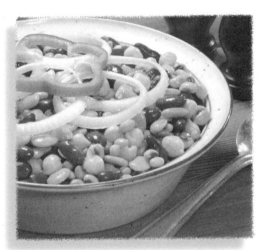

Dietary protein does not have to come from animal sources. Legumes such as nuts and beans are an excellent source of protein, especially when combined with grains.

source of energy. As carbohydrate foods make their way through the digestive system, they are broken down into a more usable form of energy called **glucose** — the only form of carbohydrate that the body can use directly for energy, and the only energy source used by the brain and nervous system. Glucose can be stored in the liver and muscles where it is transformed to **glycogen** and used as an energy source during exercise.

Fat

For many years, researchers have repeatedly established a link between a high-fat diet and heart disease.

Unfortunately, the implications of these findings have led to a nationwide fear of fat, making it the most misunderstood of all essential nutrients. Fat is a source of energy, supplying the **fatty acids** necessary for many of the body's activities. Linoleic acid, for example, is an **essential fatty acid** that must come from the diet and is needed to ensure proper growth in children and to make hormones and **cell membranes**. This essential **polyunsaturated fat** is found in vegetable oils, nuts, seeds and wheat germ. Fats also are essential for carrying the fat-soluble vitamins into the body, and they serve to enhance the flavor, aroma and texture of foods.

Only a small amount of fat — as little as one tablespoon a day of polyunsaturated fat — is needed to meet the basic nutritional needs. While experts recommend that we eat more than this, they also recommend that we limit our fat intake to no more than 30 percent of our total calories, since fat promotes satiety. People who are trying to lose weight do not need to limit their fat intake to less than 20 percent of total calories.

Fat and Cholesterol

For years, people were taught that they simply needed to eat less **cholesterol** to reduce **serum cholesterol**. It was then found that the amount and type of fat eaten influenced blood cholesterol levels more than the amount of dietary cholesterol consumed. Food companies and health professionals discuss fats in terms of "good" fats and "bad" fats because the two types affect cholesterol carriers in different ways. Good fats are the polyunsaturated and **monounsaturated fats**, and bad fats are the **saturated fats**. In reality, most dietary fats contain varying amounts of all

Figure 8.1
A comparison of dietary fats.

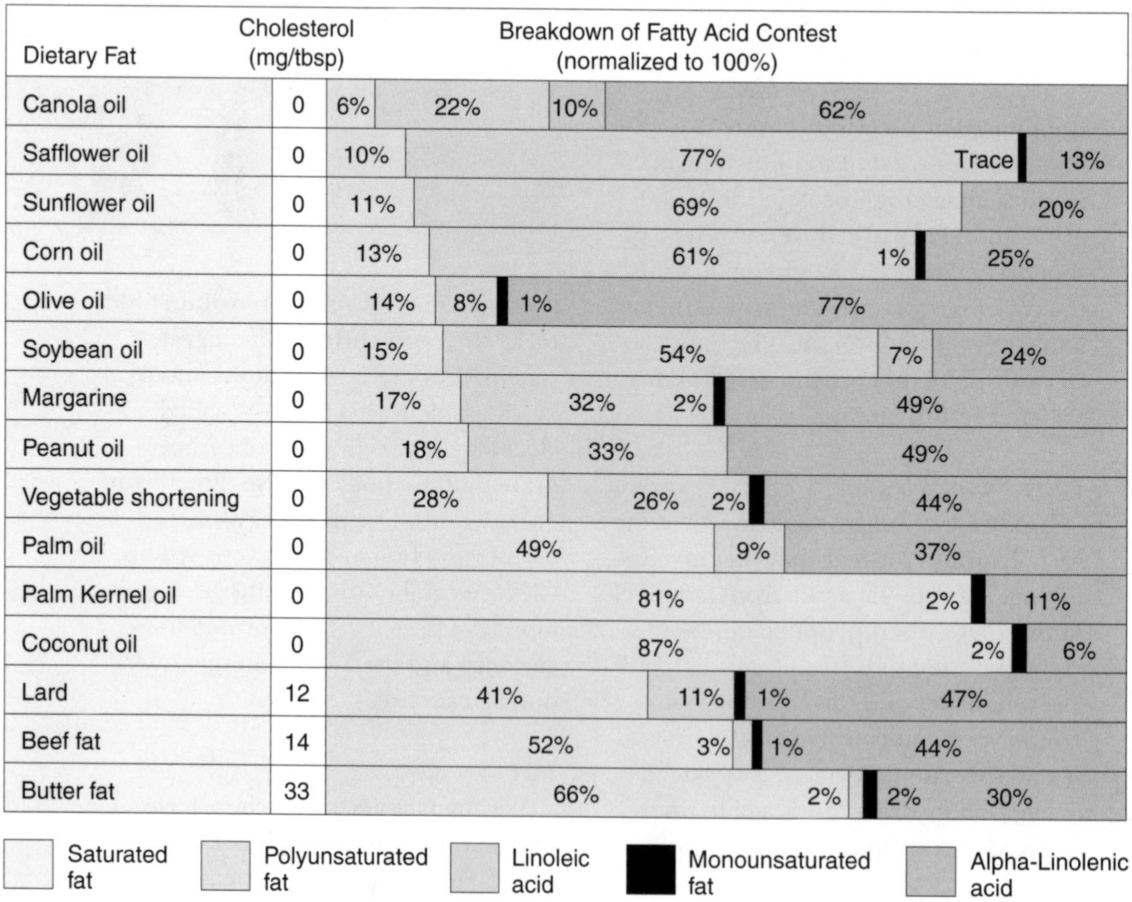

Dietary Fat	Cholesterol (mg/tbsp)	Breakdown of Fatty Acid Contest (normalized to 100%)				
Canola oil	0	6%	22%	10%	62%	
Safflower oil	0	10%	77%		Trace	13%
Sunflower oil	0	11%	69%		20%	
Corn oil	0	13%	61%	1%	25%	
Olive oil	0	14%	8%	1%	77%	
Soybean oil	0	15%	54%	7%	24%	
Margarine	0	17%	32%	2%	49%	
Peanut oil	0	18%	33%	49%		
Vegetable shortening	0	28%	26%	2%	44%	
Palm oil	0	49%	9%	37%		
Palm Kernel oil	0	81%	2%	11%		
Coconut oil	0	87%	2%	6%		
Lard	12	41%	11%	1%	47%	
Beef fat	14	52%	3%	1%	44%	
Butter fat	33	66%	2%	2%	30%	

☐ Saturated fat   ☐ Polyunsaturated fat   ☐ Linoleic acid   ■ Monounsaturated fat   ☐ Alpha-Linolenic acid three types (Figure 8.1). Clients should be advised to choose a diet that contains less than 10 percent saturated fat, from 10 percent to 15 percent monounsaturated fat, and 10 percent polyunsaturated fat.

Saturated fats generally come from animal sources (meats, dairy) and are solid at room temperature. Other non-animal sources of saturated fat include tropical oils such as coconut and palm kernel oil. Saturated fats interfere with the removal of cholesterol from the blood.

Polyunsaturated fats come from plant sources and are liquid at room temperature. Examples include corn, safflower and sunflower oils. They tend to lower cholesterol in the blood by lowering the level of **low-density lipoproteins (LDLs)**, those responsible for depositing cholesterol onto the artery walls. One drawback to polyunsaturated fats is that they also lower the level of **high-density lipoproteins (HDLs)**, the so-called good cholesterol.

Monounsaturated fats also are liquid at room temperature and are found in peanut, canola and olive oils. These fats reduce total blood cholesterol by lowering the LDL fraction while keeping the HDL stable.

The National Cholesterol Education Program recommends keeping blood cholesterol levels at less than 200 mg/dl, with HDL and LDL levels of greater than 35 mg/dl, and less than 130 mg/dl, respectively. It is important that clients know not only their total cholesterol, but also their HDL, which is responsible for carrying cholesterol from the artery to the liver for removal.

Fiber

Fiber, the indigestible part of a carbohydrate, makes up the cell wall of all plant foods. While not a nutrient, fiber is an important element of a healthy diet. Fibers are grouped into two categories: soluble and insoluble. Soluble fibers are composed of cellulose and add bulk to the diet. Insoluble fibers form gels in water and are composed primarily of pectin and guar gums. Both types are important because of their distinct health benefits. Studies suggest that soluble fiber may help reduce blood cholesterol and blood glucose in some people, while insoluble fiber is important for proper bowel function and can reduce symptoms of chronic constipation, diverticular disease and hemorrhoids.

Most fiber-containing foods have a combination of both types of fibers. Wheat products are high in insoluble fiber whereas citrus fruits, oats, legumes and barley are high in soluble fiber. Eating a high-fiber diet (25 to 35 grams of fiber per day) may help to reduce the risk of heart disease, cancer, diabetes and diverticular disease. High-fiber foods also can be helpful with weight control efforts since fiber swells with water, giving people a more satisfied feeling. Also, soluble fiber lingers in the stomach, helping one feel full.

For best results, teach clients to add fiber to their diets gradually to avoid possible stomach upset, **bloating**, flatulence and diarrhea. It also is important to drink plenty of water when adding fiber to the diet because it acts like a sponge and attracts water to it, which makes its passage through the digestive system easier. Adding more than 35 grams of fiber to the diet is not recommended since excessive fiber intake may actually interfere with the absorption of some minerals.

Dietary Guidelines

The Dietary Guidelines issued by the U.S. Department of Agriculture and the Department of Health and Human Services, were revised in 1995 to reflect our better understanding of

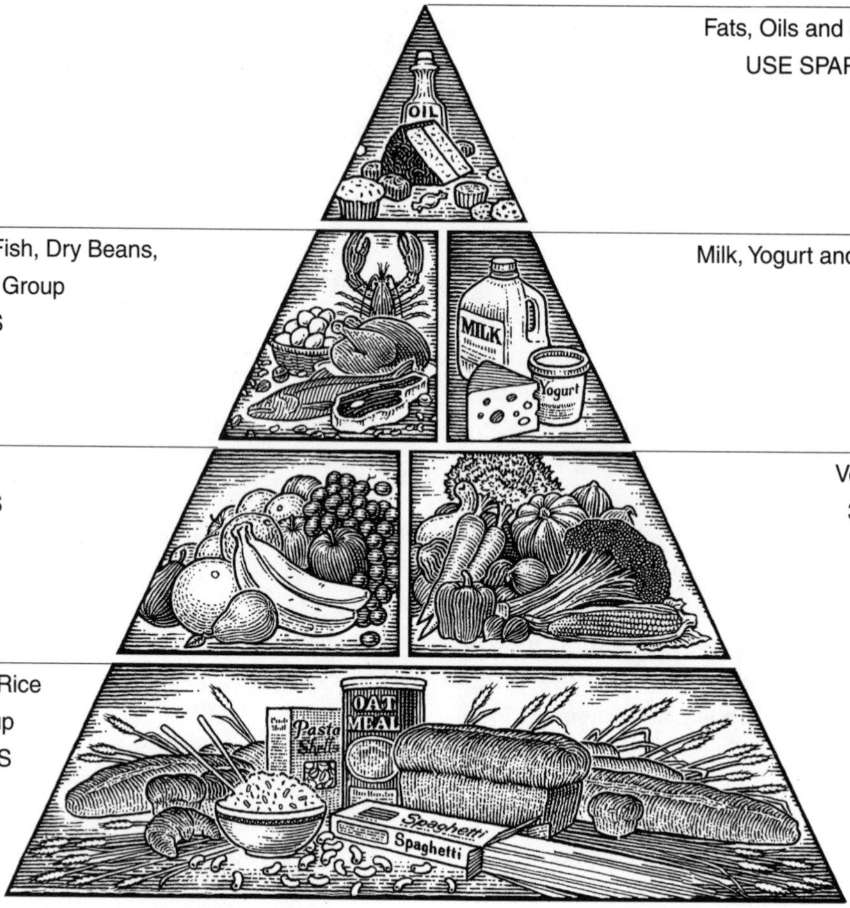

Fats, Oils and Sweets
USE SPARINGLY

Meat, Poultry, Fish, Dry Beans,
Eggs and Nuts Group
2-3 SERVINGS

Milk, Yogurt and Cheese Group
2-3 SERVINGS

Fruit Group
2-4 SERVINGS

Vegetable Group
3-5 SERVINGS

Bread, Cereal, Rice
and Pasta Group
6-11 SERVINGS

Use the Food Guide Pyramid to help you eat better every day ... the Dietary Guidelines way. Start with plenty of Breads, Cereals, Rice and Pasta; Vegetables; and Fruits. Add two to three servings from the Milk group and two to three servings from the Meat group.

Each of these food groups provides some, but not all, of the nutrients you need. No one food group is more important than another — for good health you need them all. Go easy on fats, oils and sweets, the foods in the tip of the Pyramid.

Source: U.S. Department of Agriculture

Figure 8.2
The Food
Guide
Pyramid.

the effects of such things as dietary fat and alcohol on our health. The purpose of these guidelines is to help people choose and prepare foods that will decrease their risk of diet-related **chronic diseases** such as **heart disease**, **stroke**, **high blood pressure**, **diabetes**, **osteoporosis** and certain cancers. The guidelines are based on the current state of knowledge of diet and disease.

The 1995 edition of the Dietary Guidelines are as follows:

1. Eat a variety of foods. As mentioned earlier in the chapter, there

are more than 40 nutrients that are essential to good health. The best way to get adequate amounts of these nutrients is to consume a variety of wholesome foods.

2. Balance the food you eat with physical activity to maintain or improve your weight. Excess weight is a known risk factor for many chronic diseases. We know that genetics and environment each play a role in determining one's weight, and that to lose weight, one must consume fewer calories than one is expending through a combination of

a sensible diet and regular exercise.

3. Choose a diet low in total fat, saturated fat and cholesterol. Genetics, overweight and a diet high in total fat, saturated fats and cholesterol, all contribute to elevated blood cholesterol levels, an important risk factor for heart disease. A diet composed of less than 300 mg cholesterol and 30 percent calories from fat per day (with less than 10 percent calories from saturated fat) is recommended.

4. Choose a diet with plenty of vegetables, fruits and grain products. The recommended diet should be made up of 55 percent to 60 percent carbohydrates, with the majority coming from complex carbohydrates. A diet high in these foods provides many vitamins, minerals, fiber and newly discovered elements called phytochemicals, which may reduce the risk of some diseases. Complex carbohydrates also are quite filling and may help with weight control by providing volume without the caloric density of foods high in fat.

In general, Americans do not eat enough fruits and vegetables. The National Cancer Institute, along with grocery stores and local government agencies, has promoted the Five-A-Day campaign for several years now to encourage Americans to eat at least five servings of fruits and vegetables each day.

5. Choose a diet moderate in sugars. Although there is no evidence that sugar causes weight gain, diabetes or hyperactivity, it provides little more than calories to our diet. A diet containing an excess amount of sugar may contain an excess number of calories and can result in weight gain.

6. Choose a diet moderate in salt and sodium. A small amount of sodium is essential to health, but the typical American diet contains much more than is actually needed. A high-sodium diet can aggravate high blood pressure,

Table 8.4
How to Use the Daily Food Guide Pyramid

What Counts as One Serving?

Breads, Cereals, Rice and Pasta
    1 slice of bread
    ½ cup of cooked rice or pasta
    ½ cup of cooked cereal
    1 ounce of ready-to-eat cereal

Vegetables
    ½ cup of chopped raw or cooked
       vegetables
    1 cup of leafy raw vegetables

Fruits
    1 piece of fruit or melon wedge
    ¾ cup of juice
    ½ cup of canned fruit
    ¼ cup of dried fruit

Milk, Yogurt and Cheese
    1 cup of milk or yogurt
    1½ to 2 ounces of cheese

Meat, Poultry, Fish, Dry Beans, Egg and Nuts
    2½ to 3 ounces of cooked lean meat,
       poultry or fish
    Count ½ cup of cooked beans, or 1 egg,
       or 2 tablespoons of peanut butter as 1
       ounce of lean meat (about ⅓ serving)

Fats, Oils and Sweets
    Limit calories from these, especially if you
       need to lose weight

The amount you eat may be more than one serving. For example, a dinner portion of spaghetti would count as two or three servings of pasta.

especially in those predisposed to the disease. Sources of sodium include table salt, monosodium glutamate (MSG), baking soda, baking powder, canned foods and soups, processed meats and convenience foods such as frozen dinners.

7. If you drink alcoholic beverages, do so in moderation. Alcoholic beverages are high in calories and low in nutrients, and contribute to excess weight and body fat. Alcohol may increase appetite and decrease resistance to other

Table 8.5

How Many Servings Do You Need Each Day?

	Women and Some Older Adults	Children, Teen Girls, Active Women, Most Men	Teen Boys and Active Men
Calorie Level*	about 1,600	about 2,200	about 2,800
Bread Group	6	9	11
Vegetable Group	3	4	5
Fruit Group	2	3	4
Milk Group	2-3**	2-3**	2-3**
Meat Group	2, for a total of 5 ounces	2, for a total of 6 ounces	3, for a total of 7 ounces

* These are the calorie levels if you choose low-fat, lean foods from the five major food groups and use foods from the fats, oils and sweets group sparingly.

** Women who are pregnant or breast feeding, teenagers and young adults to age 24 need three servings.

foods, and chronic consumption damages the liver, brain, heart and other vital organs. The newly revised guidelines reflect the possible benefits of moderate alcohol intake, such as a reduced risk of heart disease. This research is still very controversial. It is always best to guide your clients to discuss appropriate alcohol intake with their physician. Pregnant women should avoid alcoholic beverages because of the risk of birth defects.

What is a Healthy Food Plan?

The **Food Guide Pyramid** (Figure 8.2) was developed by the U.S. Department of Agriculture and is supported by the Department of Health and Human Services. It puts the dietary guidelines into practice by outlining the amounts and types of foods people should eat to help decrease their risk of chronic diseases. It is not a rigid **prescription**, but a general guide.

At the base of the pyramid is the bread, cereal, rice and pasta group. There should be more servings consumed per day from this group than any other. As discussed earlier, these foods contain carbohydrates, which our body needs in the greatest amount. To get the recommended amount of fiber in the diet, choose at least three servings of high-fiber foods such as whole wheat bread or brown rice.

The next level of the pyramid represents the fruits and vegetables groups. Again, these are carbohydrate-rich foods that also contain other essential nutrients such as vitamins A and C, folate, iron, magnesium, potassium and **phytochemicals** (elements in fruits and vegetables believed to be beneficial).

The third level of the pyramid is the protein level. As shown, we need fewer servings of these foods than of carbohydrates. The meat group supplies iron and zinc, while the milk group provides the needed calcium.

The fourth level is the fats, oils and sweets. These foods can be included in a healthy diet, but in very small amounts.

Although your clients may feel that the recommended servings for certain food groups are excessive for accomplishing weight loss, you should point

Table 8.6

1,800-Calorie Sample Meal Plan

Breakfast	Calories
⅓ cantaloupe	90
1½ cup oatmeal	240
¾ cup skim milk	60
Lunch	
1½ cup pasta	240
¾ cup lean meat sauce	165
1½ cup green salad	65
3 Tbsp. reduced-calorie Italian dressing	
diet drink	—
Snack	
1½ cup skim milk	120
9 wheat crackers	120
Supper	
4½ oz. chicken	160
½ cup rice	12
¾ cup carrots	35
1½ cup green salad	65
3 Tbsp. reduced-fat French dressing	
¾ cup fruit	90
unsweetened tea	—
Snack	
¾ banana	90
1½ cup fat-free yogurt	150

Table 8.7

**Calorie and Nutrient Values
for Sample Servings of Food Groups**

Group	Carbohydrates (grams)	Protein (grams)	Fat (grams)	Calories
Bread	15	3	1	80
Fruit	15	-	-	60
Milk				
skim	12	8	0-1	90
2% fat	12	8	5	120
whole	12	8	8	150
Meat (per ounce)				
very lean	-	7	1	35
lean	-	7	3	55
medium fat	-	7	5	75
high fat	-	7	8	100
Vegetables	5	2	-	25
Fat	-	-	5	45

out that serving sizes are very modest (Table 8.4). The Food Guide Pyramid, depending on the number of servings eaten, is appropriate for individuals consuming as few as 1,200 calories to as many as 3,000 calories. (Table 8.5). To keep calories low, help your clients choose the minimal number of servings and make sure these choices are low in fat. For higher calorie needs, more servings or slightly higher-fat choices may be in order.

The Food Guide Pyramid in Practice

Many clients complain that following a healthy meal plan does not leave them feeling full or satisfied. Eating the recommended number of servings from the Food Guide Pyramid can provide the body with all the nutrients it needs. For weight control, the foods should be divided into at least three evenly spaced meals each day with foods from every level of the pyramid consumed at each meal (Table 8.6). Eating enough at regular intervals should help prevent hunger that may result in overeating later. Also, by eating a combination of protein, carbohydrates and fats in the portions suggested by the pyramid, digestion and absorption of food occurs at a slower rate, helping one to feel full for a longer period of time.

Calories

The much-maligned **calorie** is merely a way of measuring the potential heat in the food we eat. The formal definition of a calorie is the amount of energy expended in raising the temperature of one gram of water one degree Celsius. The simple rule of losing weight still applies: To lose one pound of body fat, one must burn an extra 3,500 calories

Table 8.8
Reducing Calories at Lunch

Original Meal	Lower Calorie Meal	Calories Saved
2 oz. bologna	2 oz. skinless chicken	78
2 slices white bread	2 slices wheat bread	0
1 Tbsp. mayo	1 Tbsp. low-cal mayo	51
1 cup whole milk	1 cup 2% milk	30
1 slice chocolate cake	2 fig bars	135

Table 8.9
Recipe Ingredient Alternatives

For	Use	Calories Saved
1 cup whole milk (155 calories)	skim milk (86 calories)	69
½ cup butter (810 calories)	diet margarine (400 calories)	410
1 Tbsp oil (120 calories)	non-stick spray (0 calories)	120
½ cup mayonnaise (788 calories)	reduced-fat mayo (320 calories)	468
½ cup sour cream (246 calories)	plain yogurt (72 calories)	174
4 oz. cream cheese (396 calories)	low-fat cream cheese (240 calories)	156
1 cup evaporated milk (336 calories)	evaporated skim milk (200 calories)	136

beyond what they are consuming. This can be accomplished either through eating less, exercising more, or the recommended combination of reducing food intake and increasing the amount of exercise. Table 8.7 lists the calories and grams of carbohydrates, protein and fat for a reference serving of each of the food groups. Table 8.8 provides an example of calories saved at a lunch by making some substitutions.

There are several formulas for determining the caloric needs of your clients. Here's an easy formula to follow: To estimate caloric requirements, take the target weight of your client in pounds and multiply by 10 for light activity, 15 for moderate activity, and 20 for heavy activity. Subtract 100 calories for clients age 35 to 44, subtract 200 calories for clients age 45 to 54, subtract 300 calories for clients age 55 to 64 and subtract 400 calories for clients age 65 and above. This should give you a daily calorie level appropriate for weight loss, but should not be less than 1,200 calories per day.

Fat and Calories

People seem to assume that 30 percent calories from fat means either 30 percent of the volume of food eaten or 30 grams of fat. However, since fat is calorically dense (9 calories per gram), 30 percent of the calories from fat would take up far less than one-third the volume of food, and having 30 grams of fat a day would be far less than the recommended amount. For example, if your client is following a 1,200 calorie diet, they would consume 40 grams of fat to equal 30 percent of calories. (30 percent x 1,200 calories = 360 calories; 360 calories divided by 9 fat calories/gram = 40 grams of fat)

Recent studies have indicated that fat calories are more easily converted to body fat than carbohydrate or protein calories because fat requires less energy to be converted to **triglycerides** (the storage form of fat). However, a person still would have to consume somewhere in the range of 3,500 excess calories to gain one extra pound of fat tissue, and these excess calories can come from any of the caloric nutrients. There are some studies showing that those who consumed a diet in excess of the 30 percent calories from fat had a more difficult time losing weight, but no studies to date have shown that consuming less than 30 percent calories from fat is more advantageous for weight loss.

Reducing High-fat Foods

In teaching your clients how to reduce their fat intake, you must take into consideration both the seen and unseen fats in foods. Visible fats are easier to recognize and, therefore, reduce or eliminate. These fats include the fat or skin surrounding meat, butter, margarine, sour cream, salad dressing, mayonnaise and oils. "Invisible" fats include the marbled fat in meat, the fat in milk and dairy products and the fat added to baked products and combination dishes. In today's grocery stores, many shelves contain nothing but reduced-fat and non-fat food items. Over the years, these foods have become tastier as manufacturers spend a large percent of their budget on developing good taste without the fat. Unfortunately, as taste goes up, and guilt goes down, people tend to eat too many calories from these fat-free foods and are losing the battle to control their weight. Table 8.9 provides some tips on how to lower fat content when cooking.

Preventing and Treating Obesity

There is no doubt about it. Your clients must eat fewer calories than they expend to lose weight. The most appropriate way to reduce calorie intake is to use the Food Guide Pyramid. Use Table 8.5 to determine the appropriate number of servings your client should consume from each food

Table 8.10
Grocery Shopping Guide

Fruits and Vegetables
    Fresh: all acceptable
    Canned and frozen: avoid those with
        added fat

Breads, Cereals and Grains
    Choose those with
        2 grams fat or less per serving

Crackers and Chips
    Choose those with 4 grams fat
        or less per ounce

Cookies
    Choose those with less than
        4 grams fat per ounce

Soups
    Choose those with 2 grams fat
        or less per serving

Meats
    Choose lean cuts; trim all fat and remove
        skin before cooking; use fish and poultry
        more frequently than red meat; use
        ground beef or turkey that is 91-99%
        fat free

Lean Meat Choices
    Beef: round, loin, sirloin, chuck arm
    Pork: tenderloin, center loin, ham
    Veal: all cuts except ground
    Lamb: leg, loin, fore shanks
    Poultry: light meat without the skin

Lunch Meats
    Choose those with less than
        4 grams fat per ounce

Frozen Entrees
    Choose those with less than
        8 grams fat per serving

Dairy
    Milk: choose skim, 2 percent, 1 percent
    Low fat cheese: choose those with less
        than 6 grams fat per ounce
    Yogurt: choose those with less
        than 2 grams fat per cup
    Light sour cream: choose those with
        less than 2 grams fat per ounce

Fats
    Margarine: choose reduced-fat
        or those in tub
    Oils: choose canola, olive, corn,
        sunflower, safflower
    Mayonnaise and salad dressings:
        try reduced-fat varieties

Table 8.11

The First Step in Eating Right Is Buying Right:
A Guide to Choosing Low-fat, Low-cholesterol Foods

Variety is the spice of life. Choose foods every day from each of the following food groups. Choose different foods from within groups, especially foods low in saturated fat and cholesterol (the Choose column). As a guide, the recommended daily number of servings for adults is listed for each food group. But you'll have to decide on the number of servings you need to lose or maintain your weight. If you need help, ask a dietitian or your doctor.

	Choose	Go Easy on	Decrease

Meat, Poultry, Fish and Shellfish *(up to 6 ounces a day)*	Lean cuts of meat with fat trimmed:
	  beef — round, sirloin, chuck, loin
	  lamb — leg, arm, loin, rib
	  pork — tenderloin, leg (fresh), shoulder (arm or picnic)
	  veal — all trimmed cuts except ground
	  poultry without skin
	  fish, shellfish
			"Prime" grade
			Fatty cuts of meat:
			  beef — corned beef brisket, regular ground, short ribs
			  pork — spareribs, blade roll
			Goose, domestic duck
			Organ meats, like liver, kidney, sweetbreads, brain
			Sausage, bacon
			Regular luncheon meats
			Frankfurters
			Caviar, roe

Dairy Products *(2 servings a day; 3 servings for women who are pregnant or breast feeding)*	Skim milk, 1% milk, low-fat buttermilk, low-fat evaporated or nonfat milk Low-fat yogurt and low-fat frozen yogurt Low-fat soft cheeses, like cottage, farmer and pot Cheeses labeled no more than 2 to 6 grams of fat per ounce	2% milk Whole milk Yogurt Part-skim ricotta Part-skim or imitation hard cheeses, like part-skim mozzarella "Light" cream cheese "Light" sour cream	Whole milk: regular, evaporated, condensed Cream, half-and-half, most nondairy creamers and products, real or nondairy whipped cream Cream cheese Ice cream Sour cream Custard-style yogurt Whole-milk ricotta High-fat cheeses, like Neufchatel, Brie, Swiss, American, mozzarella, feta, cheddar, Muenster
Eggs *(no more than 3 egg yolks a week)*	Egg whites, Cholesterol-free egg substitutes	Egg yolks	
Fats and Oils *(up to 6 to 8 teaspoons a day)*	Unsaturated vegetable oils: corn, olive, peanut, rapeseed (canola oil), safflower, sesame, soybean Margarine or shortening made with unsaturated fats: liquid, tub, stick, diet Mayonnaise, salad dressings made with unsaturated fats Low-fat dressings	Nuts and seeds Avocados and olives	Butter, coconut oil, palm kernel oil, palm oil, lard, bacon fat Margarine or shortening made with saturated fats Dressings made with egg yolk

continued on next page

Table 8.11 continued

	Choose	Go Easy on	Decrease
Breads, Cereals, Pasta, Rice, Dried Peas and Beans *(6 to 11 servings a day)*	Breads, like white, whole wheat, pumpernickel and rye breads; pita; bagels; English muffins; sandwich buns; dinner rolls; rice cakes Low-fat crackers, like matzo, bread sticks, rye krisp, saltines, zwieback Hot cereals, most cold dry cereals Pastas, like plain noodles, spaghetti, macaroni Any grain rice Dried peas and beans like split peas, black-eyed peas, chick peas, kidney beans, navy beans, lentils, soybeans, soybean curd (tofu)	Store-bought pancakes, waffles, biscuits, muffins, cornbread	Croissants, butter rolls, sweet rolls, Danish pastry, doughnuts, Most snack crackers, like butter crackers, those made with saturated fats Granola-type cereals made with saturated fats Pasta and rice prepared with cream, butter or cheese sauces; egg noodles
Fruits and Vegetables *(2 to 4 servings of fruit and 3 to 5 servings of vegetables a day)*	Fresh, frozen, canned, or dried fruits and vegetables		Vegetables prepared in butter or cream sauces
Sweets and Snacks *(avoid too many sweets)*	Low-fat frozen desserts, like sherbet, sorbet, Italian ice, frozen yogurt, popsicles Low-fat cakes, like angel food cake Low-fat cookies, like fig bars and gingersnaps Low-fat candy, like jelly beans, hard candy, licorice Low-fat snacks, like plain popcorn, pretzels Nonfat beverages, like carbonated drinks, juices, tea, coffee	Frozen desserts, like ice milk Homemade cakes, cookies and pies using unsaturated oil sparingly Fruit crisps and cobblers Potato and corn chips prepared with unsaturated vegetable oil	High-fat frozen desserts, like ice cream High-fat cakes, like most store-bought, pound and frosted cakes Store-bought pies Most store-bought cookies Most candy, like chocolate bars Potato and corn chips prepared with saturated fat Buttered popcorn High-fat beverages, like frappes, milkshakes, floats and eggnogs

Prepared by the National Heart, Lung and Blood Institute.

group. Your client should eat ordinary foods found in the grocery store. There is no need to have them buy special foods or drinks for the purpose of weight loss, since it does not allow the client to practice new **lifestyle behaviors**. Also, it is likely that when that food or drink is unavailable, the old behaviors, as well as the lost weight, will return.

Grocery Shopping

Once a product is in the house, it is much more difficult to avoid it or eat it in moderate amounts. Teach your clients that the best way to avoid eating certain foods is to limit their access to them. This strategy works best at the point of purchase — the grocery store. If it isn't part of a healthy eating plan, your clients don't have to buy it.

Almost every food item now has a low-fat counterpart, and it may be easier for some people to try low-fat foods before attempting fat-free versions. A low-fat product often has as good a taste as the original without all the fat. Still, the taste of the fat-free product may take some getting used to. Tables 8.10 and 8.11 list suggestions for healthy shopping.

Food Labels

For several years now, the USDA has required that nearly all packaged food products have a nutrition label. (Exceptions include foods manufactured by very small businesses, single nutrient items such as sugar and extremely small packages). This is good news for your clients as they look to make educated food choices in the grocery store.

The new food label includes a "Nutrition Facts" section that provides consistency and detail, and helps in understanding the value of the food eaten

Choosing whole grain breads and cereals can help your clients feel more satisfied and meet their daily fiber requirement.

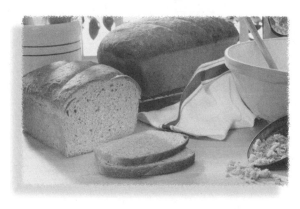

(Figure 8.3). Real-life serving sizes are now more the rule than the exception. The **Percent Daily Value** has replaced the Percent **Recommended Dietary Allowance (RDA)** on the new label. The Percent Daily Value helps your clients know whether an item has a significant amount of a particular nutrient based on

a 2,000-calorie diet. This would need to be adjusted if one's intake was more or less than this amount. For example, if a label reads 10 grams of fat, it would provide 15 percent of the recommended amount for a 2,000-calorie diet. For a 1,500-calorie diet, it would provide 20 percent of the Daily Value. If health claims or nutrient claims are found on the front of the label, they must meet strict definitions as determined by the federal government (Table 8.12).

Eating Out

More than likely, your clients will be eating out at least occasionally. Restaurants can pose a problem because they are looked at as "special" occasions in which the customer (your client) does not want to make healthy food choices. Fortunately, though, restaurants are more accommodating than ever before. A 1988 National Restaurant Association Survey found that nearly 90 percent of table service restaurants will alter food preparations on request. And fast-food restaurants have recently made changes and added new items to accommodate the health-and diet-conscious person.

Encourage your clients to pay special attention to descriptions on restaurant menus. They are appealing, but certain ingredients may mean they are high in fat (Table 8.13). The most dangerous restaurant feature for many dieters is the buffet or loaded salad bar. If the buffet is ordered, then careful planning is needed to choose a meal that will provide nutritional balance without excess calories. Tables 8.14 and 8.15 list some of the best choices to make when eating out.

Vegetarian Eating

A growing segment of the health-conscious population is choosing a vegetarian lifestyle, and as long as care is taken in food selection, vegetarian eating can provide all of the protein and other

Serving Size

Is your serving the same size as the one on the label? If you eat double the serving size listed, you need to double the nutrient and calorie values. If you eat one-half the serving size shown here, cut the nutrient and calorie values in half.

Calories

Are you overweight? Cut back a little on calories! Look here to see how a serving of the food adds to your daily total. A 5' 4", 138-lb active woman needs about 2,200 calories each day. A 5' 10", 174-lb active man needs about 2,900. How about you?

Total Carbohydrate

When you cut down on fat, you can eat more Carbohydrates. Carbohydrates are in foods like bread, potatoes, fruits and vegetables. Choose these often! They give you more nutrients than sugars like soda pop and candy.

Dietary Fiber

Grandmother called it "roughage," but her advice to eat more is still up-to-date! That goes for both soluble and insoluble kinds of dietary fiber. Fruits, vegetables, whole-grain foods, beans and peas are all good sources and can help reduce the risk of heart disease and cancer.

Protein

Most Americans get more than they need. Where there is animal protein, there is also fat and cholesterol. Eat small servings of lean meat, fish and poultry. Use skim or low-fat milk, yogurt and cheese. Try vegetable proteins like beans, grains and cereals.

Vitamins and Minerals

Your goal here is 100% of each for the day. Don't count on one food to do it all. Let a combination of foods add up to a winning score.

Total Fat

Aim low: Most people need to cut back on fat! Too much fat may contribute to heart disease and cancer. Try to limit your calories from fat. For a healthy heart, choose foods with a big difference between the total number of calories and the number of calories from fat.

Saturated Fat

A new kind of fat? No — saturated fat is part of the total fat in food. It is listed separately because it's the key player in raising blood cholesterol and your risk of heart disease. Eat less!

Cholesterol

Too much cholesterol — a second cousin to fat — can lead to heart disease. Challenge yourself to eat less than 300 mg each day.

Sodium

You call it "salt," the label calls it "sodium." Either way, it may add up to high blood pressure in some people. So, keep your sodium intake low — 2,400 to 3,000 mg or less each day. (The American Heart Association recommends no more than 3,000 mg sodium per day for healthy adults)

Daily Value

Feel like you're drowning in numbers? Let the Daily Value be your guide. Daily Values are listed for people who eat 2,000 or 2,500 calories each day. If you eat more, your personal daily value may be higher than what's listed on the label. If you eat less, your personal daily value may be lower. For fat, saturated fat, cholesterol and sodium, choose foods with a low % Daily Value. For total carbohydrates, dietary fiber, vitamins and minerals, your daily value goal is to reach 100% of each.

Nutrition Facts

Serving Size ½ cup (114g)

Servings Per Container 4

Amount Per Serving

Calories 90	Calories from Fat 30

	% Daily Value*
Total Fat 3g	**5%**
Saturated Fat 0g	0%
Cholesterol 0mg	0%
Sodium 300mg	13%
Total Carbohydrate 13g	4%
Dietary Fiber 3g	12%
Sugars 3g	
Protein 3g	

Vitamin A	80%	●	Vitamin C	60%
Calcium	4%	●	Iron	4%

*Percent Daily Values are based on a 2,000 calorie diet. Your daily values may be higher or lower depending on your calorie needs:

	Calories	2,000	2,500
Total Fat	Less than	65g	80g
Sat Fat	Less than	20g	25g
Cholesterol	Less than	300mg	300mg
Sodium	Less than	2,400mg	2,400mg
Total Carbohydrate		300g	375g
Fiber		25g	30g

Calories per gram:

Fat 9 ● Carbohydrate 4 ● Protein 4

(More nutrients may be listed on some labels)

mg = milligrams (1,000 mg = 1 g)
g = grams (about 28 g = 1 ounce)

Figure 8.3

How to read the new food label.

Source: American Heart Assocation

Table 8.12
Nutrient Content Claims

Low — A product has a low enough amount of a nutrient to allow frequent intake without concern about going over dietary recommendations. It is used in combination with: sodium, calorie, fat, saturated fat and cholesterol

low sodium: no more than 140 mg sodium per standardized serving size

low calorie: no more than 40 calories per standardized serving size

low fat: no more than 3 g fat per standardized serving size

low saturated fat: no more than 1 g saturated fat per standardized serving size

low cholesterol: no more than 20 mg cholesterol per standardized serving size

Very Low or Less — A product has no more than 35 mg per standardized serving size (refers to sodium only)

Reduced or Less — A product has at least a 25% reduction in a nutrient compared to the regular product

Light (or Lite) — A product has ⅓ fewer calories or 50% of the fat found in a comparable product

Good Source — A product has 10% to 19% of the daily value for a nutrient

High, Rich In, or Excellent Source — A product has at least 20% of the daily value for a nutrient

More — A product has at least 10% more of a desirable nutrient than does a comparable product

Lean — Refers to meat or poultry products with less than 10 g fat, less than 4 g saturated fat, and less than 95 mg cholesterol per standardized serving size and per 100 g

Extra Lean — Refers to meat or poultry products with less than 5 g fat, less than 2 g saturated fat, and less than 95mg cholesterol per standardized serving size and per 100 g

Free — A product has virtually none of a nutrient. It is used in combination with: calorie, sugar, sodium, salt, fat, saturated fat and cholesterol

Requirements for Health Claims

According to government requirements, foods must meet three criteria to carry a health claim:

1. not exceed specific levels for total fat, saturated fat, cholesterol and sodium. These are the main nutrients that health professionals suggest consumers limit in their daily diets.

2. contain at least 10% of the daily value, before supplementation, for any one or all of the following: protein, dietary fiber, vitamin A, vitamin C, calcium and iron. These are the nutrients that health professionals suggest consumers get adequate amounts of in their daily diets.

3. meet nutrient levels that are specific for each approved health claim. (See "Allowable Health Claims")

Allowable Health Claims

The diet and health areas where health claims are allowed include:
Calcium and osteoporosis
To make a claim in this area, a food serving must have at least 20% of the daily value for calcium.

Sodium and high blood pressure (hypertension)
To make a claim in this area, a food must meet the requirement for "low sodium" (no more than 140 mg per standardized serving).

Dietary fat and cancer
To make a claim in this area, a food must meet the requirement for "low fat" (no more than 3 g per standardized serving).

Dietary saturated fat and cholesterol and risk of coronary heart disease
To make a claim in this area, a food must meet requirements for "low saturated fat" (no more than 1 g per standardized serving), "low fat" (no more than 3 g per standardized serving), and "low cholesterol" (no more than 20 mg per standardized serving).

Fruits and vegetables and cancer
To make a claim in this area, a food must be a fruit or vegetable, must meet the requirement for "low fat" (no more than 3 g per standardized serving), and be a naturally "good source" (10% to 19% of the

continued on next page

Table 8.12 continued

daily value) of one or more of the following: vitamin A, vitamin C, dietary fiber.

Fiber-containing grain products, fruits and vegetables and cancer
To make a claim in this area, a food must contain grain products, fruits or vegetables. It must also meet the requirement for "low fat" (no more than 3 g per standardized serving) and be a naturally "good source" (10% to 19% of the daily value) of dietary fiber.

Fiber-containing fruits, vegetables and grain products and risk of coronary heart disease
To make a claim in this area, a food must contain grain products, fruits or vegetables. It must also meet the requirement for "low fat" (no more than 3 g per standardized serving), "low cholesterol" (no more than 20 mg per standardized serving), and be a naturally "good source" of soluble fiber

Source: Food and Drug Administration

Table 8.13

Descriptive Words Used in Restaurants Indicating High-fat Choices

Alfredo	Beurre Blanc	Fried
Au gratin	Breaded	Hollandaise
Batter Dipped	Creamy	Parmigiana
Béarnaise	Crispy	Puffed
Bechamel	En croute	Tempura
Escalloped	Flaky	

Descriptive Words Indicating Low-fat Choices

Baked	Broiled	Roasted
Smoked	Steamed	Marinara
Flame-cooked	Poached	Grilled

nutrients essential for good health. As long as a variety of plant proteins are consumed on a regular basis, the body will have an adequate supply of all of the essential amino acids. It is best to combine plant proteins as shown in Table 8.3 to ensure consumption of these amino acids. Vegetarians need to be careful to get enough iron and zinc by eating a variety of foods containing these nutrients.

Weight-loss Programs

While many people try to lose weight on their own, some prefer the support and assistance offered by an organized program. Programs such as Overeaters Anonymous, TOPS and Weight Watchers are offered in most communities. Weight-loss clinics offered at hospitals, medical centers, physician and dietitian offices also are available. Although you may provide knowledge and skills to your clients regarding proper diet and exercise, you may need to refer certain people to one of these programs to enhance their success rate. However, it is important to recognize that programs that offer miracle or painless cures for weight problems are part of a $31 billion business, which includes methods that not only make it impossible to achieve permanent weight loss, but can be both dangerous and detrimental to one's health as well. What follows is a rundown of some of the more popular (albeit not the safest) weight-loss methods of recent years.

Fad Diets

Prolonged, unbalanced diets that include only one or two foods, or that eliminate entire food groups can lead to severe nutritional deficiencies. It is impossible to lose 10 pounds of fat in 10 days as many promoters of fad diets claim. What is lost is water and important muscle tissue, with only a small percentage of the weight loss coming from fat.

Fad diets do not touch on the behaviors and emotional ties associated

Table 8.14

Best Choices When Eating Out

Appetizers and Soups
Choose fresh fruits, fruit juices, broth-based soups and boiled or steamed fish.

Entrees
Choose meats that are broiled, roasted or baked. Select low-fat meat such as seafood, chicken, turkey (without skin), veal, and beef such as london broil or tenderloin. Ask to have meats cooked without butter. Ask about ingredients when uncertain about their description on the menu.

Vegetables
Choose vegetables that are plain (without sauces). Limit or avoid sour cream and butter.

Salads
Ask that dressing be served on the side. Avoid high-calorie ingredients such as croutons, bacon, cheese and avocado. Use vinegar or lemon juice as a dressing.

Sandwiches
Ask that spreads be served on the side. Use mustard, lettuce, tomatoes and toasted bread to improve sandwiches without adding calories. Choose lower calorie fillings such as lean beef, chicken, turkey and tuna (unless high in mayonnaise).

Beverages
Try having ice water or club soda with meals. Have coffee or tea without added cream or sugar. Limit yourself to one alcoholic beverage.

Oriental Restaurants
Choose steamed dishes, stir-fried dishes, vegetable-based dishes, vegetable-based soups, steamed rice. Avoid deep-fried and/or batter-dipped foods, fried rice, sauces and gravies.

Italian
Choose lean veal, chicken or fish. Choose tomato-based marinara, marsala and cacciatore sauces on pasta. Avoid sausages, meatballs and meat sauces, cream or butter sauces, breaded or fried meats and vegetables, buttery garlic bread.

Mexican
Choose grilled meat and vegetable dishes like fajitas. Choose tostadas, taco salad without the shell, rice, beans, tomato and chili sauces. Avoid fried meat dishes, high-fat side dishes such as sour cream or guacamole, large amounts of cheese, "smothered" dishes, fried chips.

Indian
Choose Tandoori chicken and fish dishes as well as those using a low-fat yogurt curry sauce. Choose vegetables prepared without ghee (clarified butter), lentils or seekh kabob.

Greek
Choose plaki (fish with tomatoes, onions and garlic), shish kabob, rice and pita bread.

Japanese
Choose tofu dishes and "yakimono" (broiled) dishes. Avoid deep-fried foods such as tempura.

Steakhouse
Choose small portions of lean cuts of beef such as london broil, filet mignon, sirloin or round steak. Have visible fats removed before broiling.

---

with eating and never help to establish better eating habits.

High-protein Diets

High-protein diets severely restrict carbohydrates and can deplete glycogen from the muscles, induce water loss, and can result in complications such as **ketosis** (a condition characterized by increased levels of blood acids), potassium and calcium depletion, muscle weakness and, possibly, kidney problems. These diets became popular because the water loss associated with them showed up on the scale — people thought they were losing pounds at an amazingly rapid rate. It was fortunate that many people could not sustain this type of regimen on their own, or there would have been several deaths

Table 8.15

Discover Nutrition Anytime, Anywhere

Does eating on the run put a detour in your healthy eating plans? Consider your options before grabbing those empty calories. Make your best choice based on what's available. Here are some suggested food choices to get you on the road to good nutrition ... anytime, anywhere!

Fast Food
    Small hamburger
    Baked potato
    Salad / reduced-fat
        dressing
    Grilled chicken sandwich
    Roast beef sandwich
    Roasted chick
    Baked fish
    Taco
    Fajita

Salad Bar
    Raw vegetables
    Chick peas / kidney beans
    Fresh fruit
    Cottage cheese
    Diced ham
    Marinated mushrooms /
        beets
    Bean salad
    Reduced-calorie dressing

Cafeteria
    Salad / reduced-fat
        dressing
    Pasta with tomato sauce
    Yogurt
    Chili

Breakfast/Brunch
    Cereal
    Bagel
    English muffin
    Fresh fruit or juice
    Waffle
    Pancakes
    Blueberry or bran muffin
    Yogurt

Vending Machine
    Pretzels
    Raisins / dried fruit
    Fruit juice
    Trail mix
    Crackers with
        peanut butter
    Fig bar cookie
    Gingersnaps

Mall
    Soft pretzel
    Frozen yogurt
    Stuffed baked potato
    Vegetable pizza slice
    Plain popcorn
    Tostada chips with salsa

Deli
    Turkey breast, smoked
        turkey, ham or roast beef
        on whole wheat bread
    Sub roll, or pita
    Grilled chicken salad
    Vegetable soup
    Vinegar-based coleslaw

Source: National Center for Nutrition and Dietetics of The American Dietetic Association and its Foundation.

attributed to high-protein diets. Examples of this diet fad include the Atkins Diet, Stillman Diet and Scarsdale Diet, all very popular in the 1970s and still around today. Unfortunately, the popular Cambridge Diet, a high-protein liquid diet, did result in several deaths due to the inadequate quality and quantity of protein, as well as too little potassium.

Fasting

Fasting is not recommended because it causes the body to go into ketosis and encourages the loss of minerals and lean body tissue. Water and muscle are lost very quickly, and the weight loss that goes along with them may be encouraging to the person using this method. Unfortunately, health and energy is also lost as **metabolism** slows and **electrolyte** imbalances occur.

Diet Pills

Your clients will likely ask you about the status of diet pills. Much research is currently being conducted on prescription medication for obesity. Two of the most popularly prescribed medications are fenfluramine and phentermine. While fenfluramine appears to act on a body-control system called the **serotonin** system, phentermine acts on the **sympathetic nervous system**. It appears that the combination of these drugs may be more effective than the single use of either. These medications have not been approved for long-term use in obesity treatment; however, many physicians are now prescribing them for their overweight patients.

Diet pills purchased over the counter consist of amphetamines, **diuretics**, herbs and mineral supplements, and have been shown to be ineffective for long-term weight loss. They also may promote such side effects as nervousness, sleeplessness and irritability.

Diuretics and **laxatives** should never be used for weight loss because of the dangerous potential for electrolyte imbalances and cardiac problems.

Other non-prescription diet pills may contain Ma Huang, a botanical source of the stimulant ephedrine. The Food and Drug Administration has issued warnings regarding pills containing Ma Huang because of the many reports of adverse reactions including increased blood pressure and heart rate, heart attack and stroke.

Chromium

One of the hottest weight-loss supplements to hit the shelves in the '90s is chromium. Marketers of chromium supplements, most often packaged as chromium picolinate, claim that this supplement "melts away fat" by increasing metabolism. It also is pitched as having muscle-building properties, and as a source of increased energy. There is currently no scientific evidence that chromium supplements aid in weight loss, improve muscle mass or increase one's energy. And, because side effects often do not show up right away, there may be dangers from taking these supplements that have yet to be revealed. Chromium is a mineral needed in the body in minute amounts. It helps insulin metabolize blood sugar and also may aid in the control of blood lipids. The Recommended Dietary Allowance for chromium has not been set, but the presumed safe and adequate range is

50 to 200 micrograms. This is easily achieved by eating whole grains, peas, cheese, mushrooms and brewers yeast. Expensive supplements provide far more chromium than is needed by the body.

Fallacies about Weight Control

1. "Drinking water helps you lose weight faster." Although water is essential to life and may make one feel full, there is no truth that water helps one "get rid of fat" any faster than the tried-and-true way of eating fewer calories than are expended.

2. "To lose weight, all I have to do is cut out fat." Although fat is the most calorically dense nutrient, it is only when a reduction in fat results in a reduction in total calories that this statement holds true. Many people are gaining weight even while eating the many fat-free products now available. How can this be? The recent National Health and Nutrition Examination Survey (NHANES), revealed that although Americans are eating less fat, they are eating more calories and aren't losing any more weight than they were before.

3. "You must eat all of your food before 8 p.m. to lose weight." Americans are a society of couch potatoes, both on weekends and at night. A person has often completed 100 percent of their needed food intake by supper, but will sit in front of the television at night and munch hundreds more calories. The problem isn't the time, it's the additional calories. If a person eats supper or a snack after 8 p.m., and it is part of their meal plan, then they will still be successful in losing weight. The body's metabolism continues to run 24 hours per day.

Special Dietary Needs

Whatever the special needs of your clients, they most likely will want to follow the dietary guidelines discussed in this chapter. It is important, however, that you are aware of the physiological changes and dietary modifications needed by those with chronic diseases associated with **obesity** (see Chapter 10). Remember, you should refer any of your clients that have a clinical challenge back to their physician for clearance to take part in a weight management program. Their initial food plan should be developed by a licensed or registered dietitian. Your role in these cases should be determined by your client's physician and may be as a support person for the dietitian's plan (see Chapters 3, 6 and 10).

Cardiovascular Disease

Cardiovascular disease is the number one cause of death in America, and is often the result of **atherosclerosis**, or the buildup of fatty deposits within the artery wall. This buildup, called plaque, causes the arteries to lose their **elasticity** and restrict the passage of blood. If a blood clot develops, blood ceases to flow through the arteries. If this clot affects the flow of blood to the heart, a **myocardial infarction**, or heart attack, results. If the clot affects the blood flow to the brain, a stroke results. Following a low-cholesterol, low-fat diet is one of the best defenses against cardiovascular disease.

Hypertension

Blood pressure measures the force of blood against artery walls as the heart pumps it through the body. The **systolic,** or top number, is the force of the blood against the artery walls when the heart beats. The diastolic, or bottom number, is the force of blood on the artery walls when the heart relaxes between beats. High blood pressure, or **hypertension,** results when blood pressure rises above normal limits (greater than 140/90). Hypertension is known as the silent killer because it damages

the heart, kidneys and nervous system without ever causing pain. Known risk factors include family history, overweight, excessive alcohol intake and a poor diet.

It is estimated that 40 percent of people with hypertension are sensitive to sodium in the diet. The only way to determine whether someone is sensitive to sodium is to have them reduce their intake of it to see if their blood pressure is reduced. It is advised that all people diagnosed with hypertension initially follow a low-sodium diet (Table 8.16) that has been developed by a licensed or registered dietitian. Weight reduction has also been found to be effective in reducing blood pressure. When dietary changes and weight loss do not normalize blood pressure, medication is usually prescribed.

Diabetes Mellitus

Diabetes mellitus is a disease in which insulin, the hormone secreted by the pancreas that transports glucose from the blood to the cells, is either not present (insulin-dependent diabetes) or unable to remove the normal level of glucose from the blood (non-insulin-dependent diabetes). When someone has the **genetic predisposition** for non-insulin-dependent diabetes, excess weight may cause insulin resistance, impeding the hormone from doing its job (see Chapter 10). Weight loss is the number-one treatment strategy for non-insulin-dependent diabetes, since most people afflicted with this disease are overweight. As little as a 10 percent reduction in total body weight may improve insulin performance. In a smaller percentage of adults, a modified diet is not enough to normalize blood glucose and either oral medication or insulin injections are needed. If any of your clients have diabetes, consult an expert before helping them with a weight-reduction plan.

Table 8.16

Foods to Eat or Avoid on a Moderate Low-sodium Diet

	Not Allowed	Allowed
Milk	Buttermilk, mineral water, chocolate drinks, certain sodas (read label)	Regular and skim milk (up to 2 cups per day), cream, yogurt, coffee, tea
Meat	All dried, salted, smoked or canned meat such as bacon, ham, bologna, salami, sausage and kosher meats	Beef, heart, liver, tongue, veal, chicken, pork, lamb, turkey, duck, rabbit
Fish	Frozen fish with salt added	Fresh fish, shrimp, lobster, unsalted tuna and salmon
Cheese	None except those listed in the next column	Unsalted cottage cheese or pot cheese, low-salt dietetic cheese
Eggs		Use as a substitute, 1 egg or 1 oz. meat
Butter and fats	Regular salad dressing (you can make your own)	Use sweet butter or margarine, unsalted oils and fats for frying, mayonnaise
Potatoes and pastas	Potato chips, instant potatoes	White and sweet potatoes, rice, spaghetti, noodles and macaroni
Breads and cereals	Baking powder biscuits and other hot breads unless low-salt, pretzels, self-rising flour mixes, regular crackers	White and whole wheat flour, unsalted matzos, cornmeal, low-salt cereals, cream of wheat, puffed wheat, puffed rice, shredded wheat, oatmeal
Fruits	Fruits with sodium added in preparation (read label)	Fresh, frozen and canned
Vegetables	Salted vegetables, including many canned and frozen vegetables	All vegetables prepared or packaged without salt
Dessert	Cakes, cookies, ice cream, sherbet, pastry, prepared mixes (read label)	Fruit, fruit ices, special low-salt dessert pudding and custard made with allowed milk and eggs, pie made without salt
Sweets	Molasses, chocolate	Sugar, honey, maple syrup, jelly and jam without added sodium, chewing gum, candy: gumdrops, marshmallows, sour balls
Miscellaneous	Baking powder and soda; bouillon cubes and broth; catsup; chili sauce; pickles; relishes; canned, frozen or powdered soup; worcestershire sauce; soy sauce; other meat sauces	Low-salt baking powder, bakers' compressed dry yeast, unflavored gelatin, unsalted nuts, coconut, seasonings, allspice, bay leaf, cinnamon, cloves, garlic, lemon juice, dry mustard, nutmeg, basil, paprika, oregano, parsley, vinegar, pepper, vanilla extract

Note: When in doubt, read the label. Problem-causing sources of sodium are salt, MSG, soy sauce, baking powder and soda or ingredients having sodium as part of their name.

Special Concerns for Women

In helping people lose weight, you may see a greater percentage of women than men. It is important to understand their special nutritional needs.

Osteoporosis

Osteoporosis is a condition in which bone mass decreases to the point of an increased risk of bone fracture. This condition is eight times more likely to occur in women than men, and often goes undiagnosed until a fracture occurs. (An X-ray cannot detect bone loss until more than 25 percent has deteriorated.) One of the risk factors for this disease is an inadequate supply of calcium in the diet. Bones and teeth contain 99 percent of the body's calcium. A **sedentary** lifestyle, excessive intake of alcohol, caffeine or phosphorous (soft drinks and meat) and cigarette smoking increase a woman's risk of developing this disease. Low **estrogen** levels, either occurring in post-menopausal women or in extremely thin, overexercising women, also leads to a loss of bone mass. Helping your clients achieve a moderate degree of exercise, and choose the appropriate number of servings from the dairy group, can help reduce their risk of osteoporosis. The current recommendations are as follows: three servings of dairy food per day up to age 25; two servings per day until **menopause;** and four servings per day following menopause.

You may be asked about calcium supplements. Remember, high doses of one mineral can interfere with the absorption of other minerals. It is best to encourage the consumption of calcium through a balanced diet since it is best absorbed with food. Clients should consult their physician before taking any supplement.

Iron-deficiency Anemia

Iron-deficiency **anemia** affects approximately 40 percent of women between the ages of 20 and 50. Iron deficiency is a problem because once iron levels drop, there is less hemoglobin available to supply oxygen to the tissues of the body. Symptoms of iron-deficiency anemia include reduced endurance, early and frequent fatigue and increased susceptibility to colds and viruses. A hemoglobin level below 12 mg/dl for women and 14 mg/dl for men is considered anemic.

Iron deficiency in women is often the result of inadequate dietary iron intake and menstrual blood loss. One of the easiest ways to get more iron in your

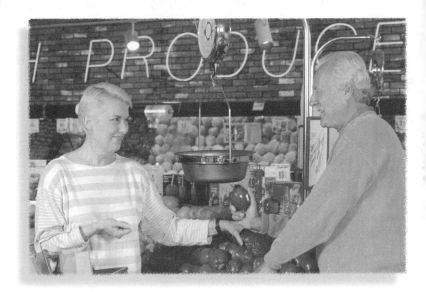

diet is to eat red meat. Because so many people have cut down on their red meat consumption without eating additional iron-rich foods, many women are consuming only one-half to three-fourths of the recommended intake of 15 mg per day. (Refer to Table 8.1 for dietary sources of iron.) Women who experience fatigue should consult their physician before taking iron supplements, since anemia can only be diagnosed through a blood test, and taking too much iron can be dangerous. Iron overload can cause deficiencies of copper

Both men and women can reduce their risk of many diseases, such as cancer, heart disease and stroke, by consuming plenty of fruits and vegetables every day.

and zinc, and may increase the risk of heart disease.

Eating Disorders

The increasing prevalence of eating disorders can be traced to biological, familial and societal influences. Eating disorders affect 10 times as many women as men, and society's preference for beautiful and slender women is likely part of the problem. It is important to know and recognize the signs of specific eating disorders.

If you suspect that a client meets any of the criteria, such as laxative use, large weight fluctuations, extreme distress in not losing weight faster, loss of menstrual cycle, puffiness in the face, **edema** or **compulsive exercise**, you must question them in greater depth, and empathetically refer them to an eating disorders specialist.

Summary

Whether trying to reduce the risk of a chronic disease, perform better in a sport or lose weight, the same nutrition principles apply. The diet business is overflowing with scams and promises of a quick fix. Unfortunately, your clients will find that there are no easy answers to the problems of disease and obesity. By helping them to eat a diet that is physiologically and psychologically filling, they will likely lose weight and feel better at the same time. This logical approach to weight management must be stressed as the only solution if long-term weight loss is to be achieved.

References

American Diabetic Association. (1995). The Exchange Lists for Meal Planning.

American Dietetic Association. (1994). Nutrition recommendations for people with diabetes mellitus. *Journal of the American Dietetic Association,* 4, 504-506.

American Heart Association. (1984). Special Report: Recommendations for the treatment of hyperlipidemia in adults. *Circulation,* 69, 103-114.

Committee on Diet and Health, Food and Nutrition Board, Commission on Life Sciences, National Research Council. (1989). *Diet and Health: Implications for Reducing Chronic Disease Risk.* Washington, D.C.: National Academy Press.

Food and Nutrition Board, Commission on Life Sciences, National Research Council. *Recommended Dietary Allowances.* (10th ed.) Washington D.C.: National Academy Press.

Goldstein, D.J., et al. (1994). Long-term weight loss: The effect of pharmacologic agents. *American Journal of Clinical Nutrition,* 60, 647-57.

Herbert, V. & Subak-Sharpe, G.J. (1995). *Total Nutrition: The Only Guide You'll Ever Need.* St. Martin's Press.

Human Nutrition Information Service. (1995). *Dietary Guidelines for Americans.* Washington, D.C.: U.S. Department of Agriculture.

Human Nutrition Information Service. (1992). *The Food Guide Pyramid.* Washington, D.C.: U.S. Department of Agriculture.

Keys, A., et al. (1950). *The Biology of Human Starvation.* Minneapolis: University of Minnesota Press.

National Cholesterol Education Program. (1988). The expert panel: Report of the national cholesterol education program expert panel on detection, evaluation and treatment of high blood cholesterol in adults. *Archives of Internal Medicine,* 148, 36-69.

Shils, M.E., et al. (1994). *Modern Nutrition in Health and Disease.* Philadelphia: Lea and Febiger.

St. Jeor, S.T. (1993). The role of weight managment in the health of women. *Journal of the American Dietetic Association,* 93, 1007-1013.

U.S. Department of Agriculture/Department of Health and Human Services. (1992). The Food Guide Pyramid. *HNIS, Home and Garden Bulletin,* Number 252.

U.S. Department of Agriculture/Department of Health and Human Services. (1995). Dietary Guidelines for Americans. *HNIS, Home and Garden Bulletin,* Number 232.

Brownell, K.D. (1989). *The Learn Program for Weight Control.* Dallas: American Health Publishing.

Brownell, K.D., et al. (1990). *The Weight Maintenance Survivor's Guide.* Dallas: Brownell and Hager Publishing.

Clark, N. (1990). *Nancy Clark's Sports Nutrition Guidebook.* Champaign: Leisure Press.

Fairburn, C.G. (1993). *Binge Eating: Nature, Assessment, and Treatment.* New York: Guilford Press.

Foreyt, J.P., et al. (1994). *Living Without Dieting.* Houston: Warner Books, Harrison Publishing.

Herbert, V., et al. (1995). *Total Nutrition: The Only Guide You'll Ever Need.* St. Martin's Press.

Tribole, E. (1992). *Eating on the Run.* Champaign: Leisure Press.

Newsletters/Journals

Healthy Weight Journal. Healthy Living Institute. 701-567-2646.

Nutrition Action Healthletter. Center for Science in the Public Interest. 202-332-9110.

Catalogues

Calorie Control Council
5775 Peachtree-Dunwoody Road
Suite 500-G
Atlanta, GA 30342
404-252-3663

Lowfat Lifeline
52 Condolea Court
Lake Oswego, OR 97035
503-636-1559

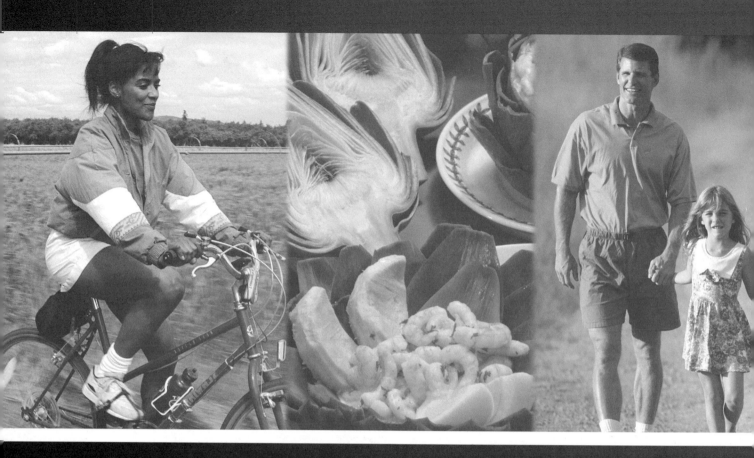

CHAPTER NINE

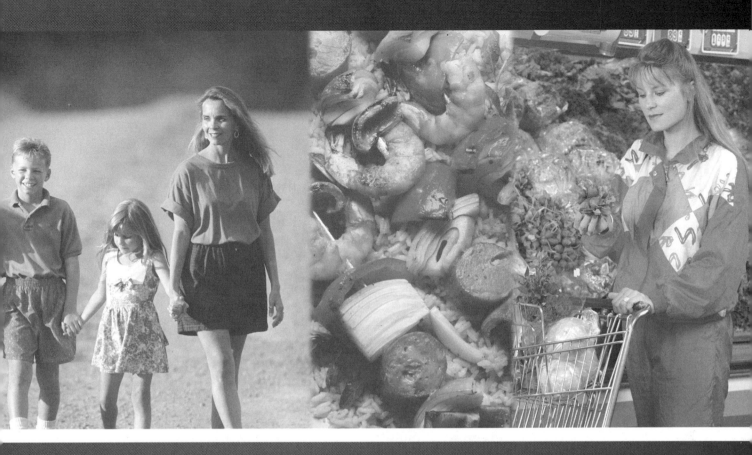

Implementation
PROGRAM PLANNING AND

Daniel Kosich
See Chapter 7
for author's biography.

Eileen Stellefson
See Chapter 8
for author's biography.

Claudia Plaisted
Claudia Plaisted, M.S., R.D., L.D.N.,
is a registered dietitian and nutrition
writer with 10 years of experience in
wellness nutrition and the treatment
of obesity and eating disorders.
She currently works at the Stedman
Nutrition Center/Center for Living
at Duke University Medical Center as
well as provides nutrition consultation
services to business and industry.

Meg Molloy
Meg Molloy, M.P.H., R.D., L.D.N., is president of
Strategies for Prevention, a health promotion/disease
prevention consulting business. She has over fifteen
years of experience in the health and nutrition field,
including designing nutrition and preventive health
programs in the areas of heart disease, diabetes,
weight control, eating disorders, and wellness and
sports nutrition. She is the author of Nutrition for
Health Living *and* Recipes for Health Living.

Introduction

A fundamental knowledge of the principles of applied exercise and nutrition, as well as related behavioral factors, is essential for you to be able to develop a client's weight management lifestyle program. You must recognize that each client is different and their long-term success depends on your ability to plan their programs accordingly. Rather than trying to fit all of your clients into the same "program mold," you must design and implement each client's program according to their individual needs.

In this chapter, you will learn the keys to developing appropriate exercise and nutrition plans for your clients. The behavioral elements of weight management discussed in Chapters 1, 2 and 3 also are considered, since it is important to recognize that a client's plan is an integrated, evolving matrix of exercise, nutritional and behavioral elements.

Goal Setting

One of the first steps in developing a client's program is to jointly establish reasonable, achievable goals. The client's number one goal is most often weight loss. However, you should be aware that achieving a healthy body weight (frequently a different weight than what a client has in mind) is contingent on reaching several other specific goals. The first challenge you face will probably be in persuading a client that the goal-setting process must focus on specific lifestyle changes involving exercise, eating and attitude rather than the preconceived weight they may have in mind.

One consistently effective way to approach goal setting is to utilize the SMART approach. This involves creating goals that are: Specific, Measurable, Action-oriented, Realistic and Timed.

The Goal-Setting Process in Action

Specific. "I want to lose weight," is not a specific goal, despite the fact that many of your clients will initially identify this as their one and only goal. You are responsible for helping them realize that such a general goal needs to be redefined in terms of the specific elements that will help them achieve it.

Here are some examples of specific goals:

1. "I will reduce my intake of dietary fat by 135 calories per day within two weeks of starting my new lifestyle."

2. "I will commit to aerobic exercise for at least 20 minutes, three days per week for the next three months."

3. "I will commit to sticking with my strength-training program at least two days per week for the next three months."

Measurable. Each specific goal must be measurable. One of the most valuable aspects of assessment is that a periodic reassessment allows you to give your clients feedback on their progress. This lets them know how close they are to reaching their goals. Reviewing a dietary record, for example, allows you to measure how close they are to their goal of cutting back on dietary fat calories. A weekly exercise record will determine whether or not they are sticking to their aerobic and strength-training programs.

Action-oriented. The "I want to lose weight" goal is too general and does not outline specific steps to take. On the other hand, reducing fat intake by 135 calories per day requires a client to read food labels to accomplish their goal.

Doing 20 minutes of aerobic exercise three days per week, and strength training two days per week are two specific actions the client may take to achieve their goal of long-term weight management.

Realistic. If a goal is not realistic, it is probably not achievable. Cutting back on dietary fat calories should be a realistic goal for most clients. Eliminating 135 fat calories per day means the client needs to find a way to eliminate just 15 grams of fat from their diet per day. This can be accomplished simply by substituting two glasses of skim milk for two glasses of two percent milk. The dietary record is by far the easiest way to help a client see how this goal can be accomplished.

Twenty minutes of aerobic exercise, three days per week is usually an achievable goal, even for the beginning exerciser. Since two 10-minute sessions will lead to the same benefits as one 20-minute session (Costill & Wilmore, 1994), clients with busy schedules can still accomplish this goal. However, setting an initial goal of 60 minutes, three days per week for a beginner is probably an unrealistic goal and not likely to be achieved.

Figure 9.1
Use this form to determine how well a specific goal meets the SMART guidelines.

Is it a SMART goal?

Goal: _____

Specific   How is the goal specific?

_____

_____

Measurable   How will achieving the goal be measured?

_____

_____

Action-oriented   What action(s) does the goal require?

_____

_____

Realistic   Is it a realistic goal based on history, program design, etc.?

_____

_____

Timed   What is the time frame for achieving the goal?

_____

_____

A 20-minute strength-training routine done twice a week is realistic for a client just starting a program. Longer, more frequent sessions increase the risk of non-compliance.

The key to establishing realistic goals is to make the lifestyle changes as small as possible within the guidelines for adequate overload (see Chapter 7). The more drastic the change, the more likely it becomes that a client will not adhere to the program. Over time, the specific guidelines for intensity, duration and frequency can be periodically adjusted. Foreyt and Goodrick (1994) suggest that it takes most people at least six months to adopt new habits.

Timed. The most effective goals have a specific time frame for accomplishment. "I will exercise for 20 minutes, three days per week," is a different goal than "I will exercise 20 minutes, three days per week, for the next three months." Setting a time frame can be a great motivator for a client because they have given themselves a deadline by which to complete their goal.

Clearly, goal setting is an on-going process. At the end of the first three months, establish a new goal for the next three months. Working with a client to develop SMART short-term goals sets the stage for achieving the long-term goal of living a healthy lifestyle to maintain a healthy body weight.

Figure 9.1 illustrates how to determine how well a specific goal meets the SMART guidelines.

Safe and Effective Weight Loss

The rate of weight loss expected by the client is often greater than what is recommended. It is important to explain to the client that a reduction of 3,500 calories, through a combination of diet and exercise, is necessary to lose 1 pound of fat. It is generally not possible to lose several pounds of fat per week.

The best way to achieve healthy weight loss is to combine regular exercise and sound nutrition, resulting in the following benefits:

1. Lean muscle tissue is better maintained and might even increase.

2. People experience positive changes in body shape.

3. People tend to have a more positive attitude since exercise usually enhances mood.

4. Physical activity is an essential component of the maintenance of the weight loss.

As discussed in Chapter 8, safe and effective weight loss does not require a calorie intake below 1,200 calories per day. The calorie deficit should be 500 to 1,000 calories less than what is needed for maintenance and should result in an average loss of 1 to 2 pounds per week. Weight loss averaging greater than 2 pounds per week is not recommended. Remember, fast weight loss is most likely caused by a loss of fluid, muscle and fat. Also, a restriction of more than 1,000 calories from one's typical intake can lead to feelings of deprivation that result in a return to old eating patterns.

Exercise Programming

Assessments are used to develop and implement cardiorespiratory (aerobic) and strength-training programs. As discussed in Chapter 7, comprehensive exercise programs identify the type, intensity, duration and frequency of activities that the client will pursue.

Using Assessment Data

The various assessments used to estimate cardiorespiratory, strength, flexibility and body composition status, as well as risk factors for cardiovascular disease, type II diabetes, etc., are discussed in detail in Chapter 6. From a program planning and implementation perspective, one of the most valuable uses of the assessment data is to establish a starting point. These assessments should not be used to compare one client to another. Classifying someone as "poor" or "fair" may reinforce a negative self-image, creating a demotivating effect. Assessment data should be used as an initial benchmark against which a client's progress is measured over time. For example, an individual who knows they are overweight doesn't necessarily want to know that they have 30 percent body fat. Taking a simple, repeatable series of circumference measurements (e.g., upper arm, chest, waist, hips, midthigh) will establish a baseline that can be used to measure change over time. You may use any of the formulas presented in Chapter 4 to estimate body-fat percentage for your own records. The client, however, initially only needs to know about their circumference values. Changes in their estimated body-fat percentage can be discussed later as a way to objectively demonstrate progress.

Cardiorespiratory (Aerobic) Program

Chapter 6 discusses the various cardiorespiratory fitness assessment protocols that can be used to estimate or measure aerobic fitness. (For a detailed discussion, see ACSM *Guidelines for Exercise Testing and Prescription*, 1995; Howley, 1992.) In order to achieve the

Figure 9.2
Ratings of perceived exertion.

RPE	New Rating Scale
6	0 Nothing at all
7 Very, very light	0.5 Very, very weak
8	1 Very weak
9 Very light	2 Weak
10	3 Moderate
11 Fairly light	4 Somewhat strong
12	5 Strong
13 Somewhat hard	6
14	7 Very strong
15 Hard	8
16	9
17 Very hard	10 Very, very strong
18	Maximal
19 Very, very hard	
20	

Source: Borg, G.V. (1982). Psychological basis of perceived exertion. *Medicine and Science in Sports and Exercise,* 14, 377-381.

most accurate results, you would need to use expensive equipment that is not readily available to you.

From a program development perspective, the most valuable application of the aerobic assessment is the educational benefit it can provide your clients. Specifically, it gives them the opportunity to experience the appropriate intensity level for aerobic exercise. The assessment does not have to predict VO_2 max, especially at the beginning of the program. It should reinforce the fact that, with an appropriate warm up and cool down, a cardiovascular workout at an effective aerobic intensity is invigorating rather than exhausting.

Intensity. It is important that you choose a method that is repeatable in

order to measure improvement over time. If possible, choose one that matches the type of aerobic activity the client will be doing. For example, if a client chooses walking, the baseline assessment can be performed on a treadmill. If cycling is preferred, the assessment can be done on a stationary ergometer.

The assessment does not have to be highly sophisticated. For example, when using a treadmill to assess the aerobic fitness of a client, you could:

1. Have the client warm up at a speed of 2 miles per hour (mph), 0 percent grade for three minutes.

2. Next, increase the speed to 3 mph, keeping the grade at 0 percent for the next two minutes.

3. Increase the grade 2 percent, every two minutes, while keeping the speed at 3 mph.

The goal is to use the assessment to teach the client to recognize when they are reaching their **anaerobic (lactate) threshold**: hyperventilation, lactic acid build-up in the muscles and a sense that the current pace cannot be maintained for much longer (see Chapter 7).

4. When the threshold is reached, lower the speed back to 2 mph and the grade to 0 percent for three to five minutes to allow the client to cool down. Throughout the assessment, focus on the client's acute responses to the rise in intensity:

✔ increasing rate and depth of ventilation (breathing)
✔ increasing heart rate
✔ changes in the client's perception of effort (rating of perceived exertion, or RPE)

Using a heart-rate monitor is one way to determine a training heart rate. For example, if the heart rate is 140 beats per minute (bpm) at the onset of hyperventilation, an appropriate training range would be 120 to 140 bpm, since 20 bpm less than the higher value is a good range for interval exercise (see Chapter 7). If the client is monitoring their own pulse, the range would be 20 to 23 beats per 10 seconds.

Many clients do not have access to a heart-rate monitor, or cannot accurately measure their pulse. Using the RPE scale (Figure 9.2) during the assessment is an another effective way to teach clients how to gauge their exercise intensity.

Research suggests that an RPE of 12 to 15 (using the 6 to 20 scale), or 3 to 5 (using the 0 to 10 scale), is an appropriate intensity for most individuals (Costill, 1994). The treadmill method outlined above can be used to match the client's RPE with the onset of labored breathing. When using the RPE scale be sure to have your clients rate the general feelings caused by the exercise rather than the exercise itself.

A similar assessment method can be devised using a cycle ergometer, measuring heart rate and/or RPE at the intensity that brings the client to the anaerobic (lactate) threshold.

If you are unable to actively demonstrate how to monitor intensity with your client, you can estimate their target heart-rate zone. This is easily done by first estimating their maximal heart rate using the formula: 220 minus age. From the maximal heart rate you can determine a target heart-rate range by calculating percentages: 40 percent to 60 percent for the deconditioned; 50 percent to 70 percent for the average exerciser; and 60 percent to 80 percent for those who are more fit. Keep in mind these percentages are merely an estimate and should be used in conjunction with the RPE scale to determine appropriate intensity.

The aerobic assessment is an effective way to teach your clients about interval exercise. Once you have deter-

Table 9.1

Options for a Cardiorespiratory Exercise Program

Outdoors	Indoors
Walk	Treadmill
Jog	Stair-stepper
Cycle	Group exercise (aerobics)
Cross-country ski	
	Rowing machine
Hike	
	Stationary cycle
Swim	
	Swim
In-line skate	
	Cross-country ski machine
Row	

mined their heart rate and/or RPE range, repeat a few intervals of increasing/decreasing intensity in order for the client to feel what it is like to "push their threshold." This also will help them clearly understand how to use their heart rate training range or RPE to monitor their intensity.

Goodrick (1994) suggests that teaching a client to recognize a "vigorous" aerobic exercise intensity enables them to self-regulate their intensity without constant cuing from an instructor. This can lead to an increased sense of confidence and self-efficacy, both significant factors in long-term exercise program compliance.

Using the "**talk test**" (as described in Chapter 7) to determine exercise intensity is advised for highly deconditioned clients for whom a 2 to 3 mph walking pace might prove too strenuous. The client should be able to carry on a comfortable conversation without having to take a breath between each word. It helps the client to understand the difference between the expected increase in the rate and depth of ventilation that occurs with exercise, and the **dyspnea** (labored breathing) that occurs above the anaerobic threshold. Simply teach the client to slow down or rest for a moment when the pace of aerobic exercise makes it impossible for them to put more than two words together without taking a breath. Then repeat intervals of increasing/decreasing intensity until that day's duration goal is reached.

Determining the appropriate intensity of aerobic exercise is clearly an essential element of the weight management client's exercise program. Whether you use a sophisticated method or a simple "talk test," it is a critical factor in enabling the client to exercise hard enough and long enough to maximize caloric expenditure.

Type. There are many activities that meet the guidelines for optimum aerobic benefits. Table 9.1 lists examples of various activities that can be used in a client's aerobic program.

Help your clients identify which activities they will most likely continue over time. Advise your client to alternate between two or three different activities as part of their aerobic program to prevent boredom and stay motivated.

While rhythmic, large muscle activities, such as walking, cycling and bench/step aerobics, typically lead to optimum aerobic benefits and calorie burning, other activities, such as tennis, racquetball and volleyball, also can burn a lot of calories. For the novice exerciser, however, these activities can quickly lead to anaerobic energy system predominance and rapid fatigue. A client who chooses activities requiring intermittent bursts of effort, such as tennis or racquetball, must be counseled to work at a modest pace in order to exercise for a longer duration and burn a significant number of calories. Monitoring intensity during these types of activities is generally more difficult than it is for rhythmic, large

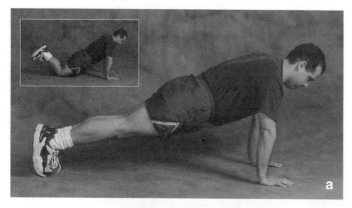

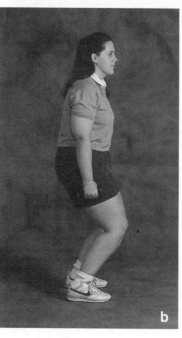

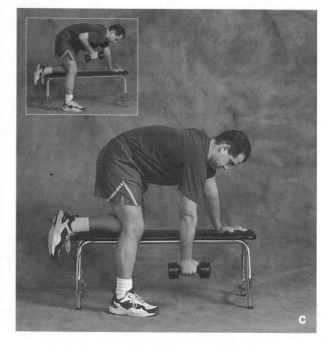

Figure 9.3
Examples of exercises that target specific muscle groups.

a. Push-up — chest and arms (Inset — modified version)

b. Squat — thighs

c. Bent-over row — upper back

muscle activities.

Duration. The guidelines for duration are discussed in detail in Chapter 7. With regard to program development and implementation, the inverse relationship between intensity and total caloric expenditure becomes important. This is because as intensity increases, the duration required to burn an equivalent number of calories per session decreases. A deconditioned client, however, generally will not be able to tolerate high-intensity exercise.

You can encourage your clients by letting them know that as their level of aerobic fitness improves and their intensity increases, they will burn more calories even if they exercise for the same length of time. Some of your clients may need to start with as little as five to 10 minutes of aerobic exercise, two to three times per day and gradually progress to 30 to 45 or more minutes, four to six times per week. Others may be able to start with 30 minutes, depending upon their initial level of fitness.

Frequency. The client should understand that the more often they commit to aerobic exercise, the greater their total weekly caloric expenditure will be. Your clients will experience the most benefits by exercising aerobically four or more times per week. They should be advised to take at least one day off from their exercise program. However, they should be encouraged to become more active in all aspects of their lives. Chapter 7 discusses guidelines for frequency in detail.

Strength Program

Currently, there is no consistent opinion on how to individually assess strength. Of course, there are tests to determine how many sit-ups or pull-ups can be performed in one minute or until muscle fatigue occurs. And we can determine how many pounds or kilograms of force can be generated by forearm flexors and extensors while squeezing a hand-grip dynamometer. But it is up to you to determine how to best utilize a muscle strength assessment to develop and implement a strength-training program for your client.

As with the cardiorespiratory assessment, the strength assessment should establish a baseline for measuring

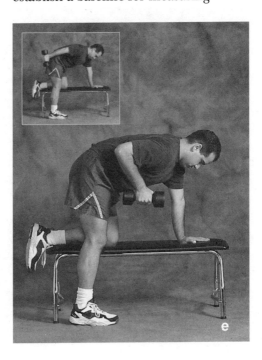

Figure 9.3 continued

d. Biceps curl

e. Triceps extension

Figure 9.3 continued

f. Lateral raise —
shoulders

g. Contralateral arm and
leg raise — back
(Inset — modified version

h. Rectus abdominus
crunch

i. Oblique crunch

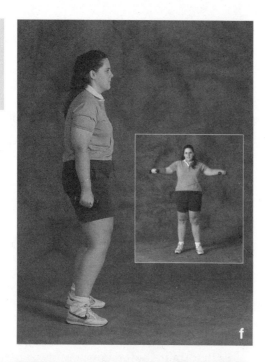

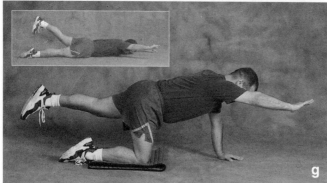

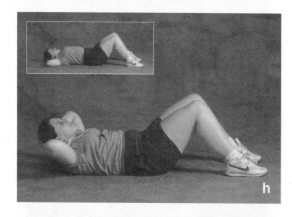

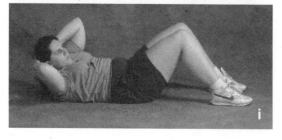

improvement while simultaneously teaching a client how to gain the maximum benefits from a strength-training program.

While there is a wide variety of opinions regarding the "optimum" guidelines for strength training, the American College of Sports Medicine (1995) recommends that the major muscle groups be trained two to three times per week with one to three sets of exercises. The weight should be sufficient to cause temporary muscle fatigue after about eight to 12 repetitions (8 to 12 RM). These guidelines can be used to design a strength assessment that will also serve as the initial strength-training program.

The major muscle groups include the shoulders (deltoids), upper back (latissimus, trapezius, rhomboids), chest (pectoralis), arms (biceps, triceps), thighs (quadriceps, hamstrings) and buttocks (gluteals). The most effective assessment uses equipment and exercises the client will be using in the training program, such as free weights, weight machines and elastic resistance.

There are many other muscles that ultimately can be strengthened. The initial complexity of the strength program depends on the client's level of experience and fitness. For the beginner, selecting 10 to 12 exercises that challenge the major muscles with 8 to 12 RM will enhance compliance. Including exercises that strengthen the abdominals and lower back also is recommended. It is not appropriate, however, to progressively increase the resistance to achieve 8 to 12 RM per set for these muscles. Because the abdominal and lower back muscles are responsible for stabilizing the trunk and pelvis (Ellison, 1995), more repetitions are recommended, especially for a beginner, since these muscles fatigue slowly.

Table 9.2 and Figure 9.3 a-i give

examples of several different exercises that target specific muscle groups. Clearly, there are many other exercises that may be used as well. Figure 9.4 is an example of a form that you can use for developing a strength-training program. (See the *ACE Personal Trainer Manual* for more examples of strength-training exercises).

During the initial assessment, particularly for the beginner, have the client perform one set of each exercise without any resistance in order to focus on proper form and technique. During the second set, estimate what resistance (weight) the client can lift for 12 repetitions without fatigue. If a third set is necessary, estimate what resistance will establish the 8 to 12 RM for that particular exercise.

This method of strength assessment teaches the client how to perform the initial exercises correctly, and establishes the 8 to 12 RM resistance. This same technique may be utilized as new exercises are added for variety and development.

Flexibility Program

While stretching exercises do not

Table 9.2
Strength Exercises by Muscle Group

Muscle Group	Exercise
Shoulder	Lateral raise Front raise Bent-over lateral raise
Upper back	Lat pull-down Bent-over row Seated row Shrugs
Chest	Push-ups Bench press Flyes
Arms	Biceps curl Triceps extension
Trunk	Contralateral arm and leg raise Abdominal crunches (rectus and obliques)
Legs and Buttocks	Squats Lunges (forward and reverse) Hip extension Quadriceps extension Bench stepping Hamstring curls Straight leg raise

Figure 9.4

A sample form for strength program development.

Strength Program Development Form

Muscle Group	Exercise	Weight	Repetitions
Shoulders			
Upper back			
Chest			
Arms			
Trunk			
Legs and Gluteals			

Note: Allow 1-2 minutes rest between sets.

significantly increase caloric expenditure, regular stretching is a crucial component of a client's exercise program. It is especially important to include stretching exercises for the chest, lower back, hamstrings, hip flexors and calf/achilles tendon (Figure 9.5). For more specific guidelines on flexibility training, see Chapter 7.

Table 9.3 summarizes the various elements of an exercise program, and should guide you in the development of cardiorespiratory, strength and flexibility programs for individual clients.

Tracking Progress

The value of using assessments in the development of a client's aerobic and strength-training programs is well established. To be successful, an assessment method must be easily reproduced to measure progress.

In most situations, you should allow at least six to eight weeks before reassessing aerobic parameters. The treadmill protocol described earlier can be repeated to measure improvement in aerobic fitness. When used correctly, reassessment is an excellent motivation-

al tool because the client is witness to the progress they have made by following their program.

Record Keeping

Many experts (Foreyt, 1994) believe that record keeping is an invaluable component of a client's weight-management program. This is particularly true during the first six months. However, since most people are pressed for time these days, record forms must be simple and easy to use. If these forms are complex, many clients will quickly lose the incentive to complete them.

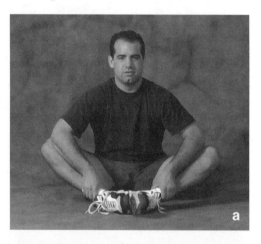

Figure 9.5
Examples of flexibility exercises that target specific muscle groups.

a. Adductor stretch

b. Hamstring stretch

c. Gastrocnemius stretch (Inset — soleus stretch)

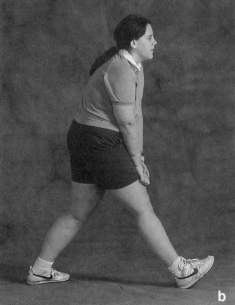

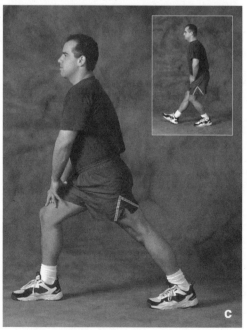

Table 9.3

Elements of an Exercise Program

	Intensity	Type	Duration	Frequency
Cardio-respiratory	Heart rate at onset of hyperventilation RPE ~12-14 (3-5) "Talk test" Interval exercise	Rhythmic, Large muscle	≥10 min/session ≥15-20 min/day the longer the better	≥3 times/week
Strength	8-12 RM for each exercise (exceptions: abdominals, lower back)	Free weights Machines Elastic Body weight Water	1-3 sets	2-3 times/week (non-consecutive days)
Flexibility	Point of tension in muscle(s) being stretched, not pain	Static Dynamic	4 sets of 10-15 seconds/stretch	3-5 times/week

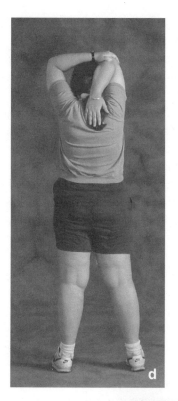

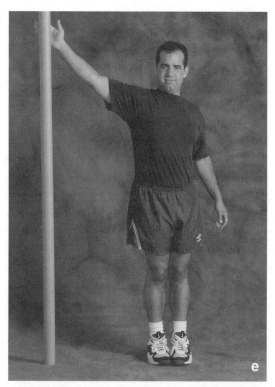

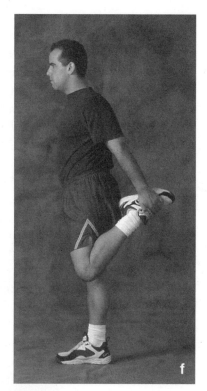

Figure 9.5 continued

d. Triceps stretch

e. Pectoral stretch

f. Quadriceps stretch

g. Low-back stretch

Weekly Aerobic Exercise Record

Week of _____

	Activity	Duration	Intensity	Notes
Monday				
Tuesday				
Wednesday				
Thursday				
Friday				
Saturday				
Sunday				

Figure 9.6
A sample of a weekly aerobic exercise record.

Figures 9.6 and 9.7 are examples of simple forms a client can use to keep a record of their aerobic and strength-training workouts. You may wish to create individualized forms for each client, as some will be more inclined to keep detailed records than others.

Rate of Change in Body Weight

There are a myriad of factors that influence an individual's rate of weight loss or change in body-fat percentage. Therefore, there is no simple way to give a client an exact estimate for how fast they will lose weight or improve their body-fat percentage.

Clearly, the greater the number of calories an individual burns each week through exercise, the more likely a greater negative energy balance will be established. The number of calories consumed, however, also is a significant factor in achieving long-term weight management.

It is important not to use the rate of weight loss as a measure of the effectiveness of a weight-management program. For example, as lean tissue is developed through the strength-training program, changes in body weight will not accurately reflect the potential decrease in body fat. It is better to focus the client's attention on such benefits as enhanced body image, the ability to complete a specific exercise, nutritional and behavior goals. Establishing realistic body-weight goals is a key factor in long-term success (Foreyt, 1994; Kosich, 1995). In most cases, the maximum, effective long-term rate of weight loss is between 1 and 1½ pounds per week (Foreyt, 1994).

Medications and Stimulants

There are many agents, from prescribed and over-the-counter medications to alcohol and nicotine, that can have a dramatic effect on a client's acute response to exercise. In many cases, the use of such agents will be discovered at the clients assessment and screening (see Chapter 6).

Prescription Medications

If a client is taking any type of prescription medications, you must make certain that their physician is aware of the exercise program design. Some

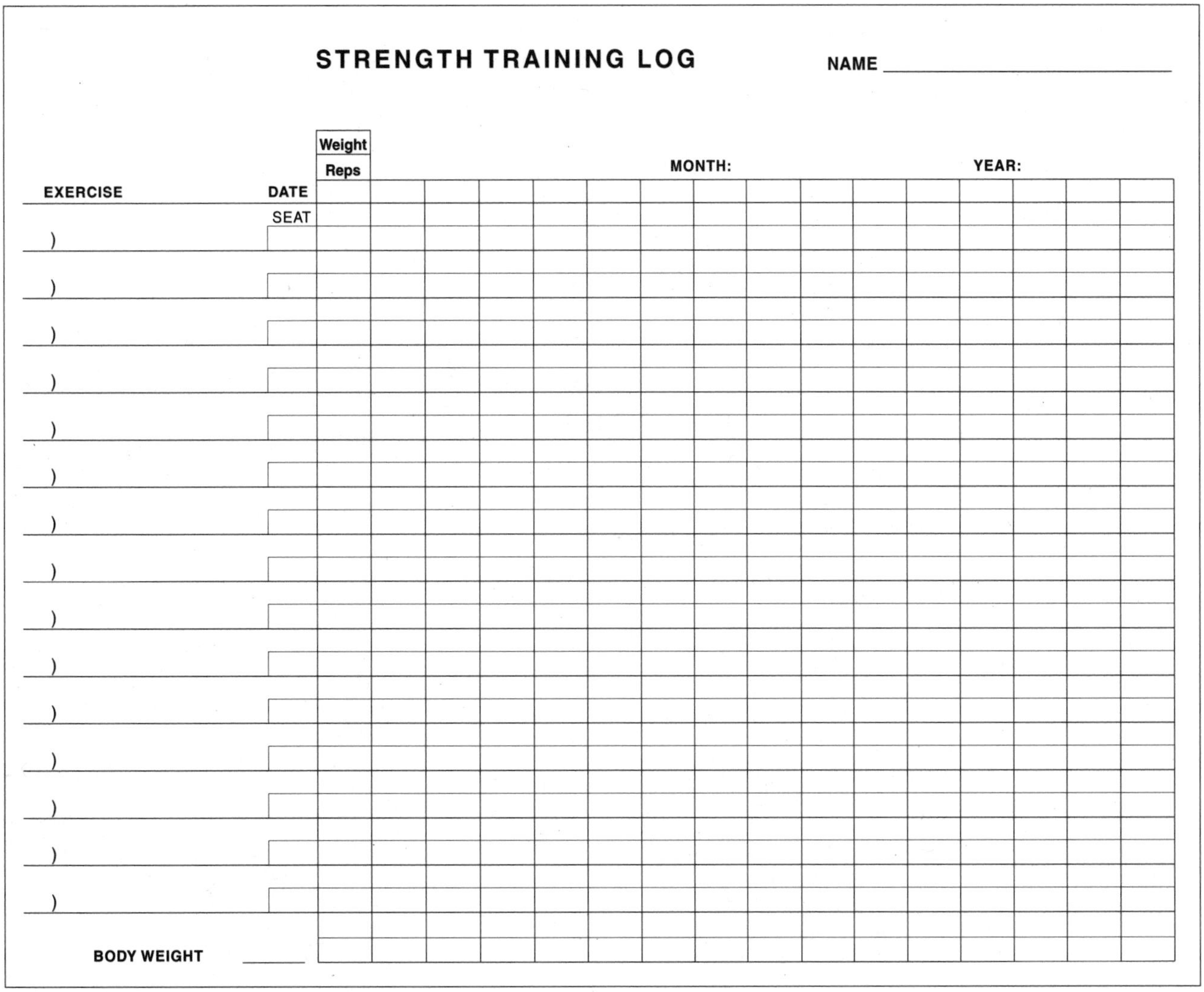

STRENGTH TRAINING LOG

NAME _____

EXERCISE	DATE	Weight / Reps	MONTH:	YEAR:
)	SEAT			
)				
)				
)				
)				
)				
)				
)				
)				
)				
)				
)				
)				
)				
)				

BODY WEIGHT _____

medications, such as **beta blockers**, which are frequently used for treating heart problems and **hypertension,** may make it impossible for an individual to reach their predicted training heart rate. This is because drugs such as beta blockers can have an attenuating, or lowering, effect on both heart rate and blood pressure response. It is important to receive a recommendation from a client's physician regarding appropriate exercise heart rate and/or RPE, as well as any other limitations.

Diuretic medications may reduce the body's ability to regulate internal temperature, as well as possibly cause electrolyte imbalances. As with beta blockers, a client taking diuretics should receive guidelines from the prescribing physician for exercise intensity, fluid intake and electrolyte replacement.

Over-the-counter (OTC) Medications

Two of the most common over-the-counter medications are diet pills and cold remedies. These medications stimulate the activity of the **sympathetic nervous system**, increasing both heart rate and blood pressure. While generally less dramatic than the **sympathomimetic effect** (simulating the effect of catecholamines such as epinephrine) or prescription amphetamines (Costill, 1994), both diet pills and certain cold medications may cause a client to reach their training heart rate at a lower-than-normal intensity. You must carefully

Figure 9.7
Strength training log.

Table 9.4
National Nutrition Guidelines

The USDA Dietary Guidelines for Americans

✔ Balance the food you eat with physical activity—maintain or improve your weight.
✔ Choose a diet with plenty of grain products, vegetables and fruits.
✔ Choose a diet low in fat, saturated fat and cholesterol.
✔ Eat a variety of foods.
✔ Choose a diet moderate in salt and sodium.
✔ Choose a diet moderate in sugars.
✔ If you drink alcoholic beverages, do so in moderation.

The American Heart Association

✔ Dietary fat intake should be less than 30% of total calories.
✔ Dietary carbohydrate intake should be 50-60% of total calories.
✔ Dietary protein intake should be 10-20% of total calories.
✔ Cholesterol intake should be less than 300 mg/day.
✔ Sodium intake should be less than 3,000 mg/day.
✔ AHA recommendations are also made for saturated, polyunsaturated and monounsaturated fats:
  ✔ Saturated fats should be less than 10% of total calories.
  ✔ Polyunsaturated fats should be up to 10% of total calories.
  ✔ Monounsaturated fats should be 10-15% of total calories.

The National Cancer Institute

In addition to supporting the US Dietary Guidelines for Americans the National Cancer Institute makes the following statements (NIH Pub # 87-2878):

✔ Americans should eat between 20-30 grams of fiber per day. For those who wish to consume more fiber, NCI recommends that individuals not exceed 35 grams daily.

✔ Fiber rich foods, not fiber supplements, are the sources of fiber to choose unless your doctor advises you otherwise.

✔ Americans should consume a diet in which no more than 30% of calories come from fat.

✔ Choose vegetables which are dark green leafy and other green vegetables, the red, yellow and orange vegetables and fruits, the citrus fruits and juices made from any of these.

✔ Other good vegetable choices include the cabbage family (cruciferous vegetables) which include bok choy, broccoli, Brussels sprouts, cabbage, cauliflower, collards, kale, kohlrabi, mustard greens, rutabagas, and turnips and their greens.

✔ Eat a variety of vitamin-rich foods, rather than relying on vitamin and mineral supplements to help protect yourself from cancer.

The Food Guide Pyramid (see Chapter 8)

monitor your client's relative aerobic intensity in these types of situations (Haskell, 1995).

Caffeine

Caffeine may influence exercise capacity (Costill, 1994) through a glycogen-sparing effect and enhanced catecholamine response (stimulation of the sympathetic nervous system). However, it may also lead to potentially negative consequences such as nervousness and **insomnia**. Caffeine's **diuretic** effect,

which can impair thermoregulation, is of particular importance to the beginning exerciser.

Nicotine

Some athletes use nicotine as a stimulant while others report that it has a calming effect. Regardless, the well-documented health risks of nicotine use far outweigh any potential performance benefit. Whether from cigarettes or smokeless tobacco, nicotine increases heart rate, blood pressure, peripheral resistance and blood lipid levels.

If that isn't enough, cigarette smoking has the added disadvantage of decreasing oxygen binding with hemoglobin because of its greater affinity for binding with carbon monoxide. This makes it more difficult for oxygen to get to the exercising muscles.

The fact that those who quit smoking tend to gain some weight should not be used as an excuse to continue smoking. For those who have recently quit, the key to effective weight management is to control the factors that influence energy balance. Eating a sensible diet and increasing caloric expenditure through exercise is the most appropriate course of action in most cases.

Alcohol

While some use alcohol as a stimulant, it does, in fact, act on the central nervous system (CNS) as a depressant. Most studies report that, because of its depressive effects, alcohol ingestion prior to exercise impairs performance, causing earlier fatigue, less total work output, etc., (Costill, 1994).

Because alcohol is a concentrated source of calories, providing 7 kcal/gram, or nearly 200 calories per ounce, it is easy to add a lot of calories to one's daily intake through alcohol consumption. In addition, alcohol acts as a diuretic, potentially inhibiting the body's ability to regulate internal temperature during exercise because of increased water loss.

Implementing the Nutrition Program

A myriad of cultural, biological and emotional factors influence people's food selections. These choices, which include the types and amounts of foods consumed, affect a person's state of health and risk of developing **chronic**

disease. Your task is to help your client match their dietary choices as closely as possible with national guidelines.

As a lifestyle and weight management consultant, you should be familiar with four sets of dietary recommendations (Table 9.4):

✔ the USDA Dietary Guidelines for Americans
✔ the Guidelines of the American Heart Association
✔ the Guidelines of the National Cancer Institute
✔ the **Food Guide Pyramid** (see Chapter 8)

Using these guidelines as tools will help you to guide your clients' dietary patterns to healthy, delicious food choices.

The Nutrition Interview

In order to help your clients make appropriate nutritional changes, you need to understand their current dietary patterns. For example, it would not be wise to advise someone to lower the fat content of their diet if they are already eating only 15 percent to 20 percent of their calories as fat. Similarly, it would not be wise to advise a client to drink wine to lower their risk of cardiovascular disease if they have a past history of alcoholism.

In order to obtain accurate information about your client's dietary habits, ask unbiased questions. An example of a biased question is: "What do you usually have for breakfast?" or "You don't drink alcoholic beverages, do you?" Research has shown that individuals will change their responses to biased questions to suit what they perceive to be the interviewer's expectations and judgments.

Examples of other biased interview questions:

How many alcoholic beverages do you drink?

What vegetables do you eat for dinner?

So, you didn't eat anything else, right?

What did you have for a snack?

You just had one piece of that, right?

Unbiased interview questions encourage honest, objective answers because they don't lead the individual to believe that there is a correct answer. Examples of unbiased interviewing questions:

What is the first thing you eat or drink after you get up in the morning?

Do you drink alcoholic beverages?

Do you use butter or margarine?

Do you eat fruit?

Did you have any other foods, beverages or snacks after that meal?

Did you have any foods or beverages in the afternoon, perhaps as a snack?

If the participant reports that they do eat a certain food (e.g., orange juice):

How often do you drink orange juice?

When you drink orange juice, how much (what volume) do you consume?

If the participant reports that they ate an unspecified quantity of something (e.g., cake):

You said that you had some cake, but you weren't sure how much. Did you eat the whole cake or half the cake?

Understanding Your Client's Current Dietary Habits

Reserve some time during the initial interview with your client to talk about their eating habits. There are several methods of information gathering that can help you understand your client's dietary habits. These include interviewing, record keeping and administering questionnaires.

Interviewing

This is probably the most common and misused method of information gathering. When done correctly, the data you obtain can be a powerful tool in helping your client reach their goals; if conducted inappropriately, however, such as with a judgmental bias, the interview could harm your relationship with the client. As noted in Chapter 2, listen actively when conducting a nutrition interview so that you hear everything the client is saying, both verbally and non-verbally. Pose your questions carefully to yield accurate information, but remember that all the information you gather will be subject to the client's memory of eating, awareness of foods in general and willingness to disclose information. The three main types of nutritional intake interviews are:

✔ Typical Pattern
✔ Past 24 hours
✔ Food Frequency

The Typical Pattern interview involves asking the client about the foods they usually consume on weekdays and weekends. It is important to draw a distinction between work days and days off, since many people eat differently on days when they, or their family members, have more leisure time. Ask about the foods and beverages they consume from the time they wake up until they go to sleep. Probe for additional items traditionally included in a meal (such as bread at a sit-down restaurant) that the client may not immediately think of. If they are vague about quantities, it may be helpful to suggest a quantity that is far higher than you would expect the client to reasonably consume. The following interchange, as well as the cake example above, illustrate this point.

LWMC: *You told me that you drink a lot of soda pop in the afternoon. How much do you regularly drink?*

CLIENT: *Oh, I don't know. Some. I mean, a few. You know, a few cans.*

LWMC: *A few? Like 20 cans?*

CLIENT: *Oh goodness no! Maybe six, not 20! Who could drink 20 cans of soda?*

You may feel that 20 cans of soda is an unreasonable quantity, however, a less-skilled interviewer might have asked, "a few, do you mean three?" and the client would agree, even if they had consumed more. The caloric difference between three and six cans of regular soda pop is about 450 calories, or greater than the typical caloric deficit from food required for most moderate weight-loss clients. Of course, another alternative is that your client may drink 10 cans of soda, which might far exceed your expectations, but they are more likely to answer truthfully when compared to a standard of 20 rather than a standard of three. If you do much nutritional interviewing you may come across a client who does consume atypical amounts of certain foods. They may not feel comfortable disclosing that information unless they feel that they are not "abnormal." Over-exaggeration is a way to make this client feel more at ease.

The Past 24 Hours interview involves asking the client about the foods eaten during the past 24-hour period or the previous day. You can use the same interviewing skills described above, but it is important to ask if these habits represent the typical eating patterns of the client. Because the past 24 hours may have been atypical (the client may not have been feeling well, celebrating a birthday, unusual work circumstances, etc.), this method is less popular with nutrition professionals.

The Food Frequency interview asks the client about the diet they typically follow rather than investigating the intake of a specific day. You can use the Food Guide Pyramid to help with this type of interview. Start at the bottom of the pyramid and work your way up. See the Food Guide Pyramid, which lists the typical foods in each category in Chapter 8. Questions to ask when utilizing this method include:

Do you eat foods from this food group? (show picture, list or name foods)

If yes, how many times during the day, week, month or year do you eat those foods? (For example, "I drink orange juice twice a week.")

How much (quantity) do you consume of this food?

Or you can ask:

Assuming a standard portion size is (use your **food model**), how much of this food do you usually consume?

Using a Food Frequency interview in this way can help you quickly ascertain your client's typical eating pattern and will illustrate if their food pyramid is out of balance or upside down.

Food Journals and Records

Food journals or records are widely used by health professionals and commercial weight-loss programs. The purpose of keeping a food record is to heighten an individual's awareness of eating behaviors so that they can use their nutrition knowledge to make appropriate food choices, as opposed to eating as an automatic behavior. Although many individuals will find this self-monitoring strategy a helpful tool for making lifestyle changes, others find it intrusive. You should not expect or request that every client keep a continual record over extended periods of time (many months or years) as this will make some clients feel frustrated and destined to fail. Other clients will benefit from a short-term food journal that includes "spot checks" on behavior, such as keeping a record for one or two days per week, or just during problem times. The goal of self-monitoring is to help the individual develop an internal awareness of what they are eating to help replace their old habits.

While they are generally helpful, there are potential areas of concern about food records that you should be aware of. In some cases, clients may

Figure 9.8
Sample food
frequency
questionnaire.

How Does Your Diet Measure Up?

Check the answer which best describes the way you have been eating recently.

1. How much meat/protein do you usually eat each day?
   1 ☐ I mainly eat beans, grains and vegetables to meet my protein needs.
   2 ☐ I eat four to six ounces of seafood, poultry or lean red meats per day.
   3 ☐ I eat six to 10 ounces of meat, poultry or seafood per day.
   4 ☐ I eat 10 or more ounces of meat, poultry or seafood per day.

2. In general, what type of cheese do you eat?
   1 ☐ I eat only nonfat, low fat and part skim milk cheeses.
   2 ☐ I eat a mixture of cheeses including non-fat, low fat and whole-milk cheeses.
   3 ☐ I eat mainly whole-milk cheese (such as Cheddar, Swiss, Monterey Jack, Munster and cream cheese).

3. In general, how much cheese do you eat?
   1 ☐ I eat cheese three times per week or less.
   2 ☐ I eat cheese four to seven times per week.
   3 ☐ I eat more than one serving of cheese a day.

4. What type of milk/yogurt do you use?
   1 ☐ I use only ½% or 1% milk, nonfat or low fat yogurt.
   2 ☐ I use skim milk but regular yogurt.
   3 ☐ I use 2% milk, whole milk and whole milk yogurt or I avoid dairy products altogether.

5. How many egg yolks do you use per week?
   1 ☐ I eat two egg yolks or less per week.
   2 ☐ I eat three to five egg yolks per week.
   3 ☐ I eat five or more egg yolks per week.

6. How often do you usually eat regular bologna, hot dogs, corned beef, spareribs, sausage, bacon, deli tuna or chicken salad?
   1 ☐ I do not eat any of these meats or meat salads or I select nonfat/very low fat versions of them.
   2 ☐ I eat them about once or twice per week.
   3 ☐ I eat them about three to five times per week.
   4 ☐ I eat more than five servings per week.

7. How many regular (not nonfat) baked goods and how much regular (not nonfat) ice cream do you usually eat? Examples: cake, cookies, coffee cakes, sweet rolls, doughnuts, etc.
   1 ☐ I avoid regular commercial baked goods and ice cream.
   2 ☐ I eat commercial baked goods and ice cream once a week.
   3 ☐ I eat commercial baked goods or ice cream two to four times per week.
   4 ☐ I eat commercial baked goods or ice cream more than four times per week.

8. How often do you eat fat-free or very low fat cookies, cakes, brownies, ice cream or frozen yogurt, etc.?
   1 ☐ I avoid these products or have them less than twice a week.
   2 ☐ I eat these products several times a week.
   3 ☐ I eat more than one serving of these products a day.

9. What is the main type of fat you use in cooking?
   1 ☐ I use a cooking spray or I do not use added fat.
   2 ☐ I use olive oil, canola oil, sesame oil, peanut oil or avocado oil.
   2 ☐ I use safflower, sunflower, or soybean oil or soft margarine.
   3 ☐ I use shortening, fatback, butter, stick margarine or bacon drippings.

10. What spread do you usually use on bread, vegetables, etc.?
    1 ☐ I don't use any spread or I use a non-fat/fat-free spread
    2 ☐ I use diet margarine or other reduced-fat and calorie products/spreads.
    3 ☐ I use a soft, tub or squeezable liquid margarine.
    4 ☐ I use stick margarine or butter or regular mayonnaise.

11. How often do you eat fresh or frozen fruits and vegetables?
    1 ☐ Daily I eat five or more servings of both fruits and vegetables.
    2 ☐ Daily I eat two to four servings of both fruits and vegetables.
    3 ☐ Weekly I eat about five servings of both fruits and vegetables.
    4 ☐ Weekly I eat less than four servings of both fruits and vegetables.

12. How many servings of complex carbohydrates (starches) do you eat each day?
    Examples: pasta, rice, beans, corn, bread, cereal, potatoes, etc.
    1 ☐ I eat at least six to 11 servings a day.
    2 ☐ I eat three to five servings a day.
    3 ☐ I eat two or less servings a day.

13. How often do you eat foods like regular chips, fries or party crackers?
    1 ☐ I avoid these foods or choose the non-fat or low-fat ones.
    2 ☐ I eat one or less servings of these products per week.
    3 ☐ I eat these foods two to four times per week.
    4 ☐ I eat these foods more than five times per week.

14. How often do you take a calcium supplement?
    1 ☐ Daily I consume an adequate amount of calcium through foods in my diet according to the Optimal Calcium Intake Chart below and take no supplements.
    2 ☐ Daily I take a calcium supplement providing the amounts in the Optimal Calcium Intake Chart below.
    3 ☐ Occasionally I take a calcium supplement because I am not sure if I am getting enough calcium.
    4 ☐ Daily I take a calcium supplement providing more than 2000 mg/day.

Optimal Calcium Intake. NIH Consensus Statement 1994, June 6-8. 12 (4):1-31.

Men, ages 25-65	1000 mg/day
Men, over age 65	1500 mg/day
Women, ages 25-50	1000 mg/day
Women, over 50 (postmenopausal)	
on estrogen	1000 mg/day
not on estrogen	1500 mg/day
Women, over age 65	1500 mg/day
Women, pregnant and nursing	1200-1500 mg/day

Your total score _____

How to interpret your score:

Less than 20:
You probably have a balanced low fat diet which has many healthful attributes. Keep up the good work!

21-29:
You are making some good food choices, but still have some room for improvement. Your meal pattern may not be quite balanced by being too high in fat or inadequate in fruits, vegetables, grains and/or calcium.

Above 30:
Your diet is fairly high in fat and/or nutritionally inadequate. This may be increasing your diet-related health risk. With a few changes, you can dramatically improve your diet and reduce your risk of diet-related chronic disease.

make statements such as, "I can only eat right if I am writing down everything I eat," or "If I don't record my eating, I can't remember what I ate." In the first case the client is using food records to police their behaviors, and in the second the food record may be acting as a barrier to helping the client become aware of their own eating. Remind your clients that food recording helps them focus and learn about their eating style. It is not meant to make them feel guilty.

While some people may purchase and prepare healthy food at home, eating out may be a different story. Many view restaurants as a time to eat whatever they want. Therefore, it is important that you understand all aspects of your client's dietary habits.

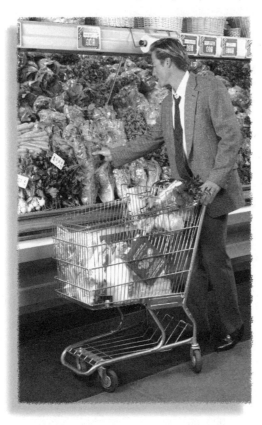

Another type of food journal is the specific nutrient journal, most commonly used to track fat gram intake. It is often used to target one or two areas of concern, such as high-fiber or high-calcium foods, as opposed to keeping track of all foods consumed. This type of record is often easier for participants to keep and may be more useful in helping them make prudent dietary choices.

You may find it helpful to have a client record behaviors, thoughts, feelings or emotions associated with eating. This type of record does not typically focus on the nutrient quality of the diet, but rather the reasons behind eating. It can help participants understand the ABCs (**antecedent**, **behavior**, **consequences**, see Chapter 2) of their eating, and be a potent tool for lifestyle change. If you suggest this type of tool to your client, it becomes your responsibility to examine the record for signs that warrant referral to an appropriate healthcare provider. Such signs include symptoms of depression or disturbing thoughts around food and eating that cause you to suspect disordered eating.

Food Frequency Questionnaires

There are several types of food frequency questionnaires; some are sophisticated, computer-scored tools often used for research, while others are more simple tools that quickly characterize typical intake patterns. This latter type will probably be most helpful to you. One type of quick food frequency questionnaire is the "How Does Your Diet Measure Up" questionnaire (Figure 9.8). Its use is similar to the Food Frequency interview, but it is a written, self-administered instrument.

Food Models and Portion Estimates

Research has shown that people, dieters in particular, don't know exactly how much food they eat. They may misunderstand and misreport their food consumption by as much as 50 percent of their total caloric intake. This is due to two reasons: unawareness of eating habits and unfamiliarity with portion sizes.

To help your clients have a better understanding of the quantities that represent a portion, it is a good idea for you to have access to a set of food models or visual portion estimates. Food models are plastic replicas that demonstrate one serving of a food from the Food Guide Pyramid. Visual portion estimates depict the same thing but are life-size photos rather than three-dimensional models. Either type can be a helpful aid to your client as they describe their dietary intake. They also are helpful tools when teaching clients the amounts of foods that make up a serving or "exchange" for portion control, calorie control or monitoring of fat-gram intake.

Choosing Your Tool

It is important to recognize that not every tool will work with every client. You may find that you are comfortable with one or two tools that you will use most frequently; you might also choose to modify or adapt a tool to suit the specific population you serve. It is not advisable to develop your own nutrition materials. Refer to nutrition resources from recognized organizations, such as the American Dietetics Association, the U.S. Department of Health and Human Services, the U.S. Department of Agriculture, the American Heart Association and the National Cancer Institute, for well-developed and tested nutrition education and screening tools. If you modify a tool be careful to avoid inserting your personal bias.

Addressing Your Client's Needs

The first step in addressing your client's nutritional needs is to compare their current food intake to the national guidelines. The second step is to help your client develop an active plan to move toward achieving those guidelines.

Your client may have many nutritional needs that can adequately be addressed by you. If you notice that whole categories of foods from the pyramid are missing from their diet, or that it does not follow the Dietary Guidelines for Americans, the guidelines of the American Heart Association or the National Cancer Institute, then use those guidelines to make concrete suggestions to help improve the quality of their diet. Work with your client to develop a plan. But remember, it is not within your **scope of practice** to prescribe a diet for your client. If they are in need of special dietary counseling or have food allergies, severe disease or disease risk, or refuse to include whole categories of food in their diet, refer them to a registered dietitian.

Your strongest tools will be the set of four national guidelines and some educational material on dietary fat. Since dietary fat is related to **obesity,** heart disease, some cancers and gall bladder disease, among others, and since obesity is related to many serious medical conditions, eating a moderate amount of dietary fat will be an important message to convey to most of your clients, especially if their goal is weight management.

Nutritional Program Planning for the Weight Loss Client

It is likely that many of your clients will have a weight-loss goal so it is important to reinforce healthy behaviors rather than encourage changes in numbers on the scale. Some clients will find slow weight loss frustrating and will not understand the value of the improvements in their total health. It is your job to help them appreciate the positive gains they are making as well as to monitor them for potential hazards.

It is estimated that the average middle-aged woman who is 5'4" tall, weighs between 120 and 140 pounds (54.5-88.4 kg) and exercises for about 30 minutes

Table 9.5

Examples of Food Servings Which Make up Healthy Caloric Intake Levels for Long-term Health and Weight Management.

Number of Calories	Starches and Breads	Fruits	Vegetables	Dairy Foods	Protein Foods	Fat Grams	Calories from Fat
1400	6	3	4	2	4	38	24%
1600	7	3	4	2	4	50	28%
1800	8	3	4	2	5	60	30%
2200	10	4	5	2	6	73	30%
2400	12	4	4	2	6	80	30%

Example servings from each Food Guide Pyramid group given for a 30% fat diet (except for 1,400 calorie level). These examples are given to illustrate the amounts of food which can be eaten in a healthy diet and are not meant to be used as a nutrition prescription.

three times per week can maintain her weight on 1,800 to 2,200 calories per day. The estimates for men are between 2,000 and 2,600 calories per day. Regardless of excess body weight, it is inappropriate for caloric intake in adults to fall much below these levels, and certainly not below 1,400 calories per day for anyone who is moderately active, at least 5 feet tall and weighs within a healthy body-weight range. You must discourage your clients from following starvation, **very-low-calorie** (less than 800 calories) and low-calorie (800 to 1,200 calorie) **diets,** as they can be dangerous and actually impede weight loss. A healthy caloric deficiency for achieving weight loss is about 300 calories a day from food, combined with 200 calories burned per day with physical activity, programmed (planned) or otherwise (incidental). More than this does not promote healthy weight loss. There is a maximum rate at which the body can safely lose weight. It is currently thought to be around 1 percent of body weight per week, which has also been estimated as between one-half to 2 pounds per week.

Estimating Caloric Needs

Although it is not within your scope of practice to prescribe a specific calorie level to a client, you can explain that fast weight loss and low-calorie diets are not recommended for long-term weight loss or its maintenance. A healthy person requires approximately 10 calories per pound of body weight to meet the needs of their resting metabolic rate. Energy for general movement or exercise requires additional calories. A middle-aged, 200-pound client who is 60 pounds overweight needs about 2,000 calories, plus more for energy for physical movement, to maintain their weight. If they were at an "ideal" weight of 140 pounds, they would require 1,400 calories to maintain their resting metabolic rate, plus more for physical movement. This client should successfully be able to lose weight while consuming between 1,800 and 2,400 calories per day. Their weight loss may be slower than if they followed a 1,200 calorie per day diet, but their overall progress is likely to be much faster in terms of health and fitness gains and the ability to make lifestyle changes that will last. They will lose weight by making gradual changes to their eating habits that they will maintain for the rest of their lives. That is the ultimate goal of nutrition management and counseling for the weight-loss

The Food Guide Pyramid Nutrition Screening and Education Tool

Do you eat fried foods?

Do you consume alcoholic beverages?

Do you drink regular soda or sweetened beverages?

Do you eat snack foods such as chips or snack crackers? Are they fat-reduced or fat free?

Do you eat sweets like doughnuts, cookies, cake, ice cream, pies?

Are they fat-reduced or fat free?

Do you eat butter, margarine, oil, salad dressings, or other fats/spreads?

Are they fat-reduced or fat free?

Do you consume dairy products such as milk, yogurt or cheese What is the percent fat?

Do you eat animal products such as beef, pork, poultry, seafood or eggs? Are they standard or fat/calorie reduced? Do you eat beans or nuts? How are these foods prepared?

Do you eat vegetables? What kind? How are these foods prepared?

Do you eat fruit, dried fruit or fruit juices? What kinds?

Do you eat rice? Do you eat pastas?

Do you eat breads? Whole grain or milled?

Do you eat cereals or other grains? What kind?

Do you eat snack foods such as pretzels, popcorn, rice cakes, etc.?

How are these foods prepared? Are they standard or fat-reduced?

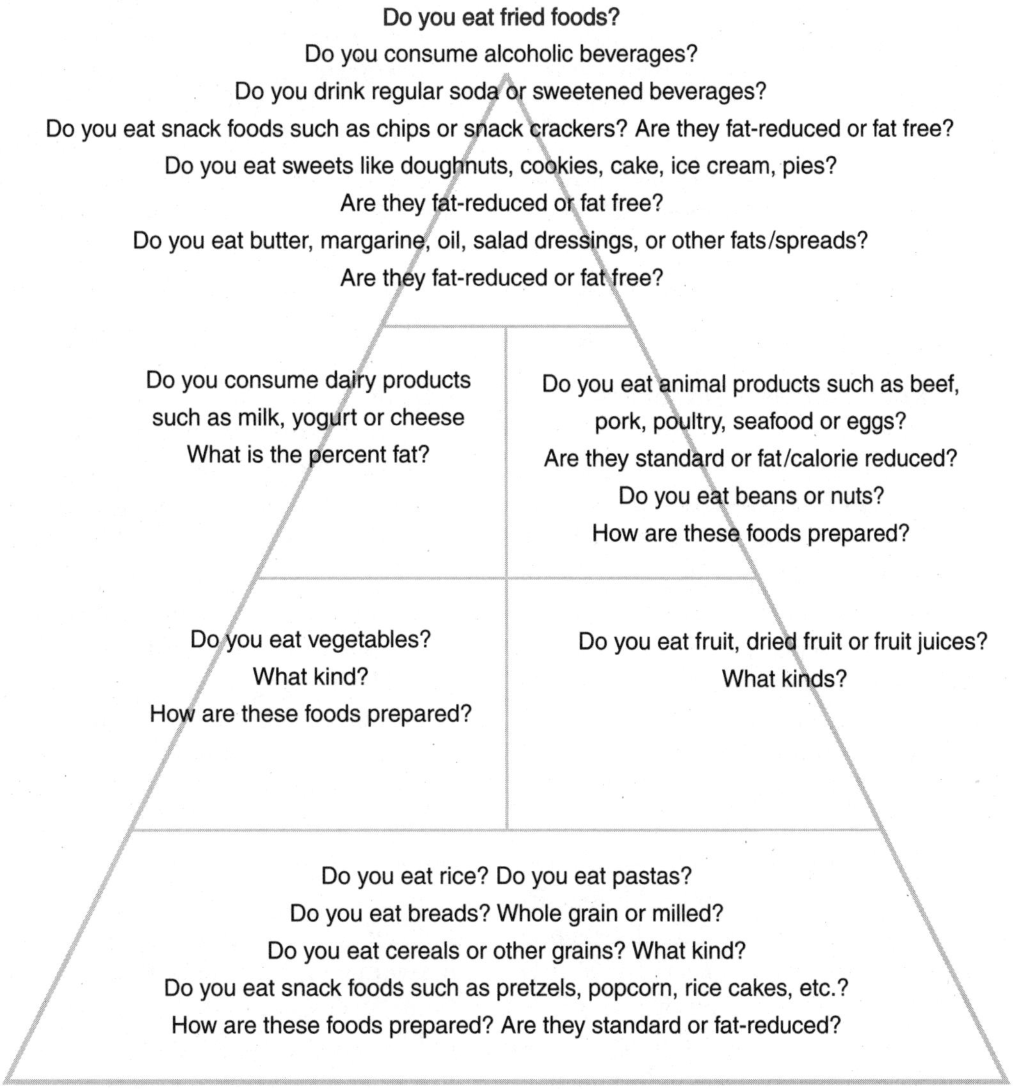

If client states yes to any question, ask portion size and how often (daily, weekly, monthly, yearly).

If whole groups of foods are missing due to food intolerance or preference, refer client to registered dietitian.

Setting Nutrition Goals

	My Current Eating Pattern	My Eating Goals
Bread / Starches Group		6 to 11+ servings/day
Vegetables Group		3 to 5+ servings/day
Fruits Group		2 to 4+ servings/day
Dairy Group		2 to 3 servings/day
Proteins Group		4 to 8 ounces/day
Fats, Sweets, Alcohol Group		40 to 60 fat grams/day

Source: Plaisted & Molloy, 1996.

Figure 9.9
The Food Guide Pyramid Nutrition Screening and Education Tool can be used to show clients how their current diets measure up to the guidelines.

client. Table 9.5 illustrates appropriate servings from the Food Guide Pyramid for several levels of energy intake.

Use this formula to estimate caloric needs:

Body Weight x 10 Calories per pound + additional energy for activity

Advise your clients to never eat less than a calorie level of:

Healthy Body Weight x 10 calories per pound

When working toward a healthy nutritional intake you may find it helpful to use the Food Guide Pyramid. Figure 9.9 illustrates the Food Guide Pyramid Nutrition Screening and Education Tool, a combined screening and teaching tool that you can use to show your client how their current diet measures up to the guidelines, and exactly how they can begin to make healthier choices. Use the goal-setting section at the bottom of the page to set goals together and chart progress. Give the client a copy of this sheet and keep one in their file. This exercise can easily be repeated at follow-up intervals to estimate the nutritional changes the client has made. Remember, it is not appropriate for you to set calorie levels, prescribe a diet or recommend supplements of any kind under any circumstance. However, recent research from the Diabetes Case Control Trial demonstrated that individuals following guidelines for a heart-healthy diet with nutrition-wise food choices made stronger health improvements than did those following more complicated and structured guidelines. The general guidelines that you provide should be easy to follow and are likely to translate into long-term changes in behavior and health.

You can use the Food Guide Pyramid Nutrition Screening and Education Tool to point out sources of calories in your client's diet that do not provide many nutrients. These often appear as concentrated fats, sugars and alcohol. Concentrated fats, such as mayonnaise or cream cheese, can often be replaced with reduced-fat or fat-free alternatives, and do not necessarily need to be excluded from the diet. Concentrated sweets, particularly in the form of soft drinks, provide calories and virtually nothing else. Again, many diet, sugar-free, or calorie-reduced versions of these drinks are available. Other concentrated sweets come in the form of fat-free dessert items, such as cookies and candies. There is room for these types of foods within the context of a healthy diet, but individuals must be cautious of the amounts they eat. People will often eat more of a dessert food item than they normally would because it is fat free. What they don't realize is that the number of calories in fat-free desserts are the same, or close to, their non-modified counterparts.

Alcohol is calorie-dense while being nutrient poor. It is not advisable for any individual to drink more than two alcoholic beverages per day, or for alcohol to be regularly included in an individual's diet if they desire weight loss. A serving of alcohol is defined as one jigger (1-¼ ounce) of liquor, 4 to 6 ounces of wine or one can of beer. Alcohol lowers the blood sugar and affects the judgment center of the brain, making it likely that the individual will fall into old eating patterns or disregard the health goals they are working on.

Weight History/ History of Dieting

It is unusual for a weight-loss client to have no prior experience with dieting. Many of your clients will have long dieting histories and will report their failures. This is your opportunity to emphasize to your client that people do not fail at diets, but that diets fail people. They are all too often unrealistic and misrepresent healthy ways of eating. You should explain that healthy eating can be pleasurable, tolerable and promote weight loss.

Most people who have long histories of dieting have learned myths about food, body weight and nutrition that you will have to counteract. Some of the more common myths you are likely to encounter include: "starchy foods make you fat," "you must eat a citrus fruit before every meal," "some foods are good foods and some foods are bad foods," or "I can only lose weight if I eat less than 1,200 calories." You might want to make a list of the myths you hear and the facts that dispel them.

There are no magic bullets when it comes to health, and nowhere is this more true than in the field of nutrition. There are no individual foods that are "good" or "bad." There is room for all foods, in moderation, within the context of a healthy diet; it all depends on how the diet is balanced. Help your clients understand that the purpose of eating is to nourish the body and that it can be pleasurable, but it is not an issue of moral judgment. Be aware of clients who report that they are "bad when they eat bad foods." Many individuals with previous dieting experience have been trained to feel this way when they eat foods not listed on their meal plan or those that fall into a category of "bad foods." Often you can correct these misconceptions with the explanation that no foods are good or bad, and that there is room for all foods within a healthy diet. If your client continues to struggle with self-esteem issues and feelings of guilt related to eating, it is reasonable to point out this observation and refer the client to a registered dietitian specializing in eating disorders, or a psychologist.

It is likely that individuals with a lifelong history of dieting will have complex issues with their eating and body weight, and will believe more concrete myths about food. You also may find that these individuals have found some tools or techniques that have helped them in the past, such as working from a healthy set of recipes at home, joining a support group or fitness center, or counting fat grams. If a technique worked for a client in the past to promote their health, then support its use now. However, some methods are cumbersome, unrealistic or support disordered thinking about food and eating, and it is not wise to support these thoughts, behaviors or tools. Examples of these dieting methods could include avoiding all social functions, excluding entire categories of foods from the diet or skipping meals in an attempt to lose weight.

Setting Healthy Weight Goals

It is appropriate for you to help your client set a healthy weight-loss goal. As with any other area of health, the goal depends on where your client is starting from. You probably would not recommend that a sedentary individual sign up for a marathon event in the next couple of months. Similarly, do not set "marathon" weight-loss goals for your client. The actual goal should be based on all of the following:

✔ age
✔ amount of weight to lose
✔ physical activity level
✔ lowest adult weight
✔ medical concerns*
✔ history of dieting
✔ emotional state (mild depression, compulsive or disordered eating)*

Figure 9.10
Example of pertinent information for the health record.

Date	Action Taken	Progress Note	Follow-up Plan
1/19/95	Health and Nutrition Screening conducted	Client determined to be low nutritional risk level	Set meeting for 2/2/95 to develop nutrition education plan
2/2/95	Nutrition Education Plan developed - used Food Guide Pyramid to set food goals (see attached)	Client reports 3 pound weight loss with beginning of exercise program; wants to keep weekly weight log	Suggested to review progress on exercise and eating goals each week after evening workout
4/14/95	Asks about fat grams in foods	Gave client name of recommended nutrition book with fat gram information	Ask next week how book helped
5/2/95	Shows fat gram record of past week - excited about averaging 35 fat grams or less each day	Gave feedback that fat gram intake far too low for an active adult, suggested approximately 60 fat grams/day as a "low fat" intake for active men desiring moderate weight loss	Plan to monitor weight to assure that rate of weight loss does not exceed 2 pounds/week
7/8/95	Asked about recent dizzy spells after workouts	Referred client to primary care doctor to evaluate symptoms; asked to not exercise until cleared to do so	Ask client to report back on outcome of doctor evaluation - left note at front desk to ask him for doctor's clearance before exercising again
8/3/95	Client reports having glucose intolerance per physician's diagnosis, asks about nutrition plan to manage problem	Referred client to RD specializing in diabetes (works in local diabetes education program)	Asked client to notify LWMC of RD's recommendations in order to provide appropriate support
10/8/95	Client attended healthy dining out seminar at club	N/A	N/A

Source: Molloy, 1996.

If you are working with these clients, it should only be with the express approval and continued supervision of their primary healthcare provider (physician, psychiatrist, psychologist).

In general, a weight-loss goal should be no more than 5 percent to 10 percent of initial body weight. It is better to set realistic and achievable goals than to set insurmountable ones. Periodically re-assess these goals with your client, providing feedback and continued support throughout their progress. Under no circumstances should a weight-loss goal be set at lower than ideal body weight.

For many individuals it is unrealistic that they will ever be able to reach their "ideal" body weight. In these cases, promote a healthy weight goal that can be achieved in small steps. For those who have a considerable amount of weight to lose, suggest a weight goal equal to the lowest weight they were able to maintain for a reasonable amount of time in the last 10 years (Goodrick, 1994).

Record Keeping

It is crucial that you record pertinent information in the client's health record. Include the date of activity, the action taken, a progress note and the follow-up plan for each specific action. See Figure 9.10 for a demonstration of clear record keeping.

Working with Eating Behaviors

We already know that people's food selections are influenced by a myriad of cultural, biological and emotional factors. Therefore, it is important that you make recommendations for each client based on the context of their lifestyle.

There are several eating behaviors for which you may be able to provide beneficial assistance. Remember that people often eat without being aware of their actions. This may be in front of the television, while driving a car, while working at a desk or on a computer or while grocery shopping. It is not that these are unhealthy behaviors, but that they are unmindful behaviors. For many adults, making lifestyle nutrition changes becomes easier when they recognize such automatic habits. When they are able to focus on the meal or snack that they are eating they feel more satisfied and take pleasure in the food. This is particularly important when the client has cut back on the amounts or types of foods that they consume.

Some clients will find it easier to focus on the experience if they eat in specific places, such as at a table. However, the place is not as important as "being in the present moment" or being mind-

10	Stuffed/Food coma
	Illness
9	Nauseous
8	Pain
	Lethargic
7	Distended
6	Uncomfortable
	Full
5	Satisfied
4	Hungry
	Strong hunger pangs
3	Irritable
	Light headed and dizzy
2	Nauseous
1	Starvation

Figure 9.11
The hunger rating scale.

ful of the experience. Be cautious to not make eating a "ritual," where the client feels they must sit at a certain place, use specific utensils or chew their food a certain number of times. Ritualizing an eating behavior implies that there is magic to eating a healthy diet and reinforces disordered thoughts about eating and body weight. You can counteract tendencies toward such disordered thoughts by helping your client learn how their body communicates with them about hunger and satisfaction. When they are focused on the experience of eating, they become aware of satisfaction and fullness, rather then when they have cleaned their plate. You may find the hunger rating scale (Figure 9.11) helpful in teaching your clients to be aware of their body signals.

You also will have clients who eat only one or two meals a day, or do not eat at all during the day, but "graze" for several hours in the evening. Recommend that these individuals eat at regular times. There is no magic to eating three times per day, and for some it is

Figure 9.12
Food guide pyramid
nutrition plan.

Nutrition Plan

For _____ Date _____

Goals _____

_____

_____

_____

Barriers/Obstacles _____

_____

_____

Food Guide Pyramid Goals _____

_____

_____

Next Visit _____

_____   _____
Client Signature   LWMC Signature

---

better to eat four, five or six small meals or meals with snacks. In general it is not advisable to eat all of one's food in one or two sittings, and it is good to recommend three or more meals during the day. If your client chooses to have meals and snacks, they must be careful to not eat more calories and food as they eat more frequently. Again, you can use the Food Guide Pyramid to plan healthy quantities of foods to eat as well as sound snack choices.

Follow-up Support

Regular follow-up sessions help reinforce the changes your client has already made and will help them to solve upcoming obstacles. The frequency of follow-up sessions will depend on your client's understanding of the plan, time commitments, finances and unanticipated events. Initially, you should meet with your client every one to two

weeks, eventually extending this to monthly visits. Because obesity is a chronic condition, frequent follow-up may need to be continued indefinitely, either with you or another support person or group. Care must be taken to determine the appropriate course for each individual; some people may not need, or be interested in, ongoing support that will internalize lifestyle changes. Figure 9.12 is an example of a form that can be used at each counseling session to determine the plan that your client will follow until the next session.

Contraindications for Weight Loss

There are certain circumstances when it is absolutely contraindicated for you to help a client lose weight. One obvious condition is pregnancy. Although a woman may be significantly

Table 9.6
Solutions to Common Obstacles

Obstacle	Possible Solution
Existing medical condition	Working with a physician, devise a program. Many conditions — diabetes, arthritis, hypertension — may improve with regular exercise.
Previous attempts resulted in injury	Start slowly, progressively increase intensity, duration and/or frequency.
Lack of time	Sleeping for 8 hours and working for 9 hours leaves 7 hours. 30-60 minutes for activity is a good health investment.
Too exhausted	Done correctly and with progression, regular exercise usually increases one's energy level.
Lack of motivational support	Find a friend or companion with a similar fitness level to exercise with.

overweight when she becomes pregnant, the American College of Obstetrics and Gynecology (ACOG) states that weight loss during pregnancy is contraindicated. Overweight women who are pregnant should be closely followed by their physician since their weight-gain requirements may be less than the 20 to 25 pounds recommended for most women. Registered dietitians are trained to design specific eating plans for pregnant women, and you may work in a supportive role with them or a physician.

Lactating (breast feeding) women also should follow a diet that does not promote weight loss. They actually need slightly more calories than pregnant women, so while many women want to lose weight immediately following delivery, you should discourage any attempt to reduce calories below the needs of lactation.

People of normal weight also may come to you for assistance with weight loss. If their desired weight places them below normal weight recommendations (according to accepted standards), they, too, must be discouraged from cutting calories. Use the Food Guide Pyramid and your exercise knowledge and skills to help them follow an exercise and nutrition program that will enable them to be more fit and nutritionally healthy without losing weight. Individuals with a recognized eating disorder, or a history of one, should be referred to an appropriate healthcare professional, and physician approval must be obtained before proceeding further. Finally, you may come across some clients who want to lose weight for the wrong reasons. They may feel that weight loss will make their life better, that they will be more accepted or attractive to other people. Help them realize that the benefits they expect from weight loss may not occur once the weight comes off. It may be appropriate to refer them for counseling before they begin a weight-loss program.

Overcoming Obstacles

Many people have, at one time or another, set weight-management goals, and most have also been side-tracked on their path to achieving them. Obstacles are a reality that will continually confront you as a lifestyle and weight management consultant. It is important to openly acknowledge and discuss with your client how even the "best laid plans" are continually subject to the real-life situations that will distract them from achieving pre-established, healthy lifestyle and weight management goals. Reflecting on the client's history will, in many cases, reinforce this fact. Some of the most common obstacles to program adherence are (Foreyt, 1994; Kosich, 1995):

✔ existing medical problems
✔ lack of time
✔ injury
✔ too exhausted to exercise
✔ lack of motivational support

There are certainly many other individual obstacles, and you will play a critical role in continually assisting clients in overcoming them. Table 9.6 suggests possible solutions to these common obstacles to regular exercise.

Summary

Your challenge as a lifestyle and weight management consultant is to help your clients realize that the most effective long-term weight-management program is one that encourages a sensible, but not rigidly structured, diet of adequate calories, combined with a lifestyle of regular, moderate- to vigorous-intensity exercise. These components must be blended with self-acceptance to ensure the greatest prospect for long-term success.

References and Suggested Reading

Alter, M.J. (1988). *The Science of Stretching.* Champaign: Human Kinetics.

American College of Sports Medicine. (1995). *Guidelines for Exercise Testing and Prescription,* (5th ed). Philadelphia: Lea & Febiger.

American College of Sports Medicine. (1990). The recommended quantity and quality of exercise for developing and maintaining cardiorespiratory and muscular fitness in healthy adults. *Medicine and Science in Sports and Exercise,* 22, 265-274.

American Council on Exercise. (1996). *Personal Trainer Manual.* San Diego.

Brownell, K. (1989). *The LEARN Program for Weight Control.* Dallas: American Health Publishing.

Costill, D. & Wilmore, J. (1994). *Physiology of Sport & Exercise.* Champaign: Human Kinetics.

Ellison, D. (1995). Beyond the Sit-up. *IDEA Today.* September, 33.

Ferguson, J. (1988). *Habits, Not Diets—The Secret to Lifetime Weight Control.* Palo Alto: Bull Publishing.

Foreyt, J. & Goodrick, G. (1994). *Living Without Dieting.* Houston: Warner Books, Harrison Publishing.

Goodrick, G., et al. (1994). Exercise adherence in the obese: self-regulated intensity. *Medicine, Exercise, Nutrition and Health.* 3, 335-338.

Haskell, W. (1995). More vs. Less. *IDEA Today,* 13, 9, 40-47.

Howley, E. & Franks, B. (1992). *Healthy Fitness Instructor's Handbook,* (2nd ed.) Champaign: Human Kinetics.

Kern, P., Ong, J., Saffari, B. & Carty, J. (1990). The effects of weight loss on the activity and expression of adipose-tissue lipoprotein lipase in very obese humans. *New England Journal of Medicine,* 322, 105.

Katch, F. & McArdle, W. (1991). *Nutrition, Weight Control and Exercise* (3rd ed). Philadelphia: Lea & Febiger.

Kosich, D. (1995) *GET REAL: A Personal Guide to Real-Life Weight Management.* San Diego: IDEA Press.

LaForge, R. & Kosich, D. (1995). Fat Burning: Just the Facts. *IDEA Today.* January, 65-70.

LaForge, R. & Kosich, D. (1994). Interval Exercise. *IDEA Personal Trainer.* November/ December, 18-24.

McArdle, W., Katch, F. & Katch, V. (1991). *Exercise physiology: Energy, nutrition and human performance* (3rd ed). Philadelphia: Lea & Febiger.

National Academy of Sciences. (1995). *Weighing the Options: Criteria for Evaluating Weight-Management Programs.* Washington, D.C.: National Academy Press.

National Task Force on the Prevention and Treatment of Obesity. (1994). Weight cycling. *Journal of the American Medical Association,* 272, 15, 1196-1202.

Pi-Sunyer, F. (1993). Medical Hazards of obesity. *Annals of Internal Medicine,* 119, 7 (part2), 655-660.

Sharkey, B. (1990). *Physiology of Fitness (3rd ed).* Champaign: Human Kinetics.

Westcott, W. (1993). *Be Strong: Strength Training for Muscular Fitness for Men and Women.* Dubuque: Brown & Benchmark.

Westcott, W. (1995). *Strength Fitness* (4th ed). Dubuque: Brown & Benchmark.

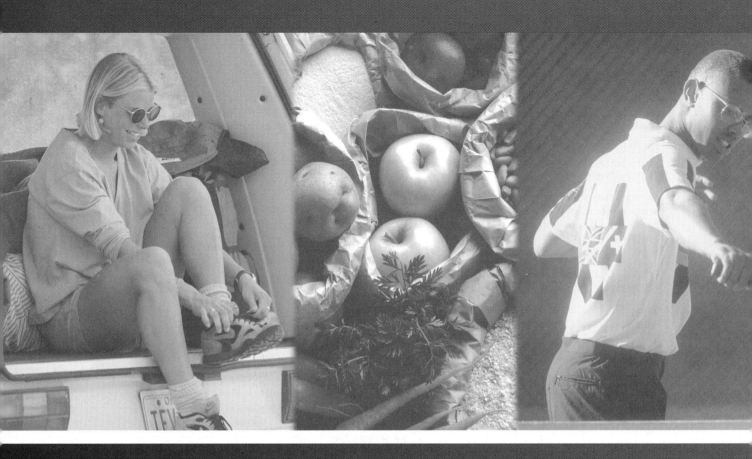

CHAPTER TEN

IN THIS CHAPTER:

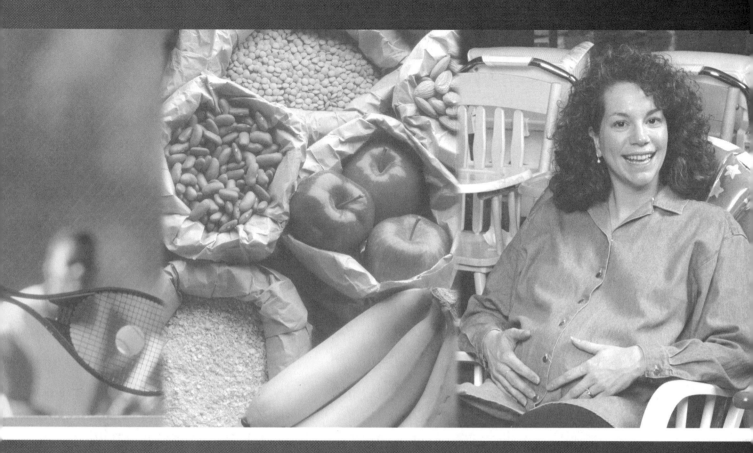

SPECIAL Populations

Lawrence J. Cheskin

*Lawrence J. Cheskin, M.D., F.A.C.P., is director of the Johns
Hopkins Weight Management Center in Baltimore, Maryland.
He is associate professor of medicine at the Johns Hopkins
University School of Medicine and holds a joint appointment
in International Health (Human Nutrition) at the Johns
Hopkins School of Hygiene and Public Health.*

Introduction

There are a number of medical conditions and special needs that require specific approaches to weight loss that are prescribed by a physician or specialist. As a lifestyle and weight management consultant, you will be working closely with the physicians, exercise physiologists and dietitians of clients who have these clinical concerns and needs. Clients with cardiovascular disease, diabetes, arthritis and other conditions must adhere to well-planned nutrition and physical activity programs if they are to effectively lose weight. Members of special populations such as pregnant women and the elderly have unique requirements as well. Your role with these clients will not be to develop exercise and nutrition regimens, but to provide the support and reinforcement that will make the programs prescribed by professionals successful. You will need to know as much as you can about the symptoms, effects and treatment of these conditions in order to aid your clients in their weight-loss efforts. This chapter will familiarize you with the modifications to lifestyle and weight management prescriptions that coincide with these conditions and needs.

Addressing Special Needs

Clients with special needs include those who report having health conditions that might affect their weight management plan and/or increase the risks of engaging in physical activities or dieting. These conditions include cardiovascular disease, diabetes mellitus and arthritis, as well as behavioral or psychiatric conditions such as eating disorders and depression.

It is important to have a sense of what is, and what is not, appropriate for you as a certified lifestyle and weight management consultant to do, particularly with respect to the care of clients from special populations and with special needs. Your job is to enable the client with special needs to carry out a plan for weight control that has been devised by other professionals with specific training, expertise and licensing in the disciplines of medicine, nutrition and psychology. Though it is not appropriate for you to give medical advice or devise a treatment plan for clients with special needs, you should carefully review the client's medical history through history taking or physical observation. You will have to rely on the client to report medical diagnoses to you, but you also can consult with their medical or other professional caregivers. It is appropriate to recommend that a client seek the advice of a qualified professional if they report symptoms that may be caused by a medical or psychiatric condition for which they are not currently receiving professional care. It is recommended that you insist that the client who you believe needs professional attention seek it before you proceed with implementing a lifestyle or weight management plan.

Since weight control plans usually require what may be difficult lifestyle changes for a client, your role as an implementor and source of encouragement is critical. Many well-made plans have failed to succeed without someone like yourself to guide and encourage the client toward permanent improvements in their lifestyle. Perhaps there is no other job more important or satisfying than helping a client with special needs, or one who falls into one of the special populations described in this chapter.

The purpose of this chapter is to give you an overview of several important special-needs health conditions and special populations; describe the benefits of weight management for each group; give examples of medical, dietary, exercise and behavioral treatments often prescribed for each group; and point out some of the risks of improper weight management plans for such individuals.

Cardiovascular Disease

Cardiovascular diseases are still the number one killer of adults in developed nations like the United States. The prevalence of asymptomatic cardiovascular disease is even higher than that of people who exhibit symptoms of the condition. Common symptoms include chest discomfort upon exertion (**angina pectoris**), shortness of breath on slight exertion (dyspnea on exertion), shortness of breath when lying flat (a sign of congestive heart failure), and **palpitations.**

You should be comfortable with the terminology commonly used in discussing cardiovascular diseases as these terms are often misapplied by clients (Table 10.1).

Table 10.1
Cardiovascular Disease Terminology

Cardiovascular Disease (CVD)	Range of diseases affecting the heart and blood vessels
Atherosclerotic Cardiovascular Disease (ASCVD)	Caused by accumulation of plaques containing cholesterol in the heart, coronary vessels or other vessels
Coronary Artery Disease (CAD)	Partial or complete occlusion of one or more coronary arteries which supply blood to the heart muscle; a major cause of exertional chest pain (angina pectoris) and "heart attacks" or myocardial infarctions (MI)
Arrhythmia	Abnormal heart rhythm
Bradycardia	Abnormally slow resting heart rate (fewer than 60 beats per minute)
Tachycardia	Abnormally fast resting heart rate (more than 100 beats per minute)
Congestive Heart Failure (CHF)	Inadequate heart function, which leads to fluid accumulation and heart enlargement
Myocardial Infarction	Sudden insufficient blood flow through a coronary artery which causes permanent damage to a portion of the heart
Peripheral Vascular Disease	Disease of the arteries or veins of the limbs, usually the legs

The odds of developing cardiovascular disease are increased if one or more risk factors are present (Table 10.2).

Obesity is a strong risk factor for cardiovascular disease as are increased blood pressure, high blood lipids and diabetes (Table 10.2).

While risk factors are important in identifying clients with a greater chance of having or developing problems, the absence of risk factors by no means guarantees the absence of cardiovascular disease, nor does it mean they have no risk of developing it. It is important to recognize that many people with atherosclerotic cardiovascular disease are asymptomatic. Others have mild symptoms that have not led them to seek medical attention, and still others may develop symptoms while under your supervision.

Why is it important to be aware of whether a client has cardiovascular disease or is at risk of developing it?

First, there are safety considerations. Clients with cardiovascular disease have an increased risk of developing sudden disturbances in their heart rhythm, which in severe instances can lead to sudden death or myocardial infarction. While arrhythmias and myocardial infarction can occur at any time, physical or emotional stress is often a precipitating event. Safety requires that you be aware of the signs of possible trouble as well as the kinds of restrictions that are sometimes placed by physicians or other professionals on the physical activity of individuals with cardiovascular disease.

Signs of danger include chest pain, arm pain, shortness of breath, nausea, palpitations, lightheadedness or fainting, profuse sweating and cold, clammy skin. Physical activity should stop immediately if any symptoms develop and the client should lay down. The emergency medical system should be activated, especially if you can't feel the client's pulse, they are unresponsive or not breathing. In such cases begin cardiopulmonary resuscitation while waiting for the ambulance to arrive.

A second reason you should be aware of cardiovascular disease in your clients is that their physician or other professional responsible for prescribing a diet and exercise plan may place certain restrictions on their individual plan. Physical activity restrictions are usually based on the amount of limitation the cardiovascular disease places on the client's tolerance of exercise, or the degree of exertion that may precipitate a cardiovascular symptom.

The degree of restriction is typically based on the level of activity that induces shortness of breath. Individuals with severe cardiovascular disease may be affected after taking only a few steps. For others, only activity of high intensity causes symptoms. You must adhere to the restrictions dictated by the client's plan, and the timing of any relaxation of exercise restriction should be left to the medical care provider. With time and training, a client with cardiovascular disease will often improve in exercise tolerance.

Finally, it is important for you to be aware of your client's history of cardiovascular disease because they may often benefit from lifestyle modification involving safe and effective physical activity and specific dietary restrictions.

Hypertension

Commonly known as high blood pressure, **hypertension** is a silent killer. People who have it can't feel its effects as it rarely causes symptoms. Hypertension is the most common form of cardiovascular disease, and is a major risk factor for heart disease and stroke.

Table 10.2
Risk Factors for Cardiovascular Disease

✔ Advanced Age

✔ Physical Inactivity

✔ Male Gender

✔ Hypertension

✔ Family History of Heart Disease

✔ Diabetes Mellitus

✔ High Blood Lipids/Cholesterol

✔ Cigarette Smoking

✔ Obesity

It is particularly common among African-American males.

Hypertension is detected by taking a blood pressure reading. A consistent systolic blood pressure (the higher number) of more than 140 mmHg, and/or a diastolic blood pressure (the lower number) of 90 mmHg or greater is considered too high. (A normal reading would be 120 mmHg/80 mmHg.)

Blood pressure readings should be taken while the client is at rest since their blood pressure may be higher during or shortly after physical exertion or any form of stress. If a client is hypertensive, refer them to a physician for treatment before beginning an exercise or weight-loss program.

Hypertension may be caused by a high-salt diet, kidney disease, atherosclerosis or a positive family history. The cause, however, is often unknown. Even so, hypertension can be treated and controlled to prevent the complications of prolonged hypertension: heart attack, stroke and kidney failure.

Treatment for hypertension, which is usually completed in stages, depends on the severity of the disease. The first stage of treatment includes changes in diet (specifically, restricting salt or sodium intake), and increased physical activity. For severe hypertension, especially if associated with symptoms such as headaches or transient ischemic

CHAPTER TEN

SPECIAL
POPULATIONS

attacks (mini-strokes), pharmacologic treatment (second stage treatment) is begun at the same time as dietary changes. Exercise generally does not begin until the hypertension has been brought under reasonable control by drug treatment. Drugs used for treatment include **diuretics**, **beta blockers**, angiotensin-converting enzyme inhibitors and **vasodilators.**

You can be instrumental in helping your clients control their hypertension. If your hypertensive client is already receiving medication, diet and exercise

Hypertension is particularly common among African-American men, placing them at increased risk for heart disease and stroke.

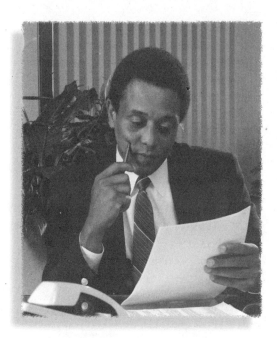

can be even more helpful. In many cases, it is possible for the physician to reduce or even stop medication as a result of improvements in diet and/ or fitness. It is essential that you obtain the approval of the physician who has prescribed medications for the treatment of hypertension before embarking on an exercise and weight-control-program. The physician can make you aware of possible situations you may encounter. For example, patients on beta blockers will not show the usual heart-rate increase that follows exertion. They will thus tire easily and not be able to achieve their target heart

rate. Ratings of perceived exertion, such as the Borg Scale, should be used to regulate exercise intensity in such individuals.

In general, aerobic exercise should be emphasized for the client with hypertension, as this has been shown to lower blood pressure in many people. This decrease is not seen initially, nor during acute exercise, but is often apparent over a period of months involving regular aerobic activity. Clients with hypertension should exercise at low to moderate intensity (50 percent to 70 percent of maximum heart rate) with periodic monitoring of blood pressure. Begin at low intensity and, with physician approval, slowly increase the intensity over a period of months as tolerated.

During acute exercise a rise in blood pressure is expected, both in hypertensive and non-hypertensive clients. If, however, systolic blood pressure rises above 250 mmHg, or diastolic blood pressure rises above 110 mmHg, exercise should be stopped immediately and you should recheck the blood pressure. If it is not decreasing, medical attention should be sought, especially if there are related symptoms such as lightheadedness, confusion or headache. Clients also should stop exercising if their blood pressure or pulse rate falls below pre-exercise levels.

Strength-training exercises should generally be avoided, or at least modified, since they tend to aggravate hypertension.

Diabetes

Diabetes mellitus is a chronic metabolic condition characterized by a decreased ability to utilize glucose, the body's main source of fuel. This results in **hyperglycemia,** excessive levels of glucose in the bloodstream. Over the long term, uncontrolled diabetes can lead to cardiovascular, cerebrovascular and peripheral vascular disease, kidney disease and vision loss. The short-term effects include excessive thirst and urination. Control of hyperglycemia symptoms through weight loss, exercise and/or medications is believed to reduce the risks of long-term effects of diabetes.

There are two forms of diabetes: type I, or insulin dependent diabetes mellitus (IDDM), and type II, or non-insulin dependent diabetes mellitus (NIDDM). Type I is characterized by a deficiency of insulin, a hormone necessary for the absorption of glucose into cells, and is often a more severe illness than type II. Regular injections of insulin are required to control the symptoms of patients with type I diabetes. Children and young adults with diabetes usually suffer from this relatively rare type.

Type II diabetes is characterized by normal or high levels of insulin production, accompanied by an insensitivity to its actions (also called insulin resistance). Most patients with type II diabetes are middle-aged or older and obese. Obesity is the number one risk factor in developing type II diabetes. Fortunately, weight loss (and exercise) are beneficial in reducing insulin resistance and the risk of type II diabetes. Many patients with this type of the disease do not require injections of insulin. Their hyperglycemia can be controlled by diet manipulations (primarily weight control through restriction of total caloric intake) or orally administered medications that lower glucose levels.

Exercise can help both type I and type II diabetics. Moderate exercise tends to lower blood glucose levels by promoting the entry of glucose into cells. However, prolonged or severe exercise may lower blood glucose levels too much. This is called **hypoglycemia**, and may be accompanied by lightheadedness, fatigue, nausea, headache,

trembling, sweating, or even seizures or total loss of consciousness.

Hypoglycemia can be precipitated in a diabetic by such things as not eating regularly, taking too much insulin, an infection or vomiting. Consuming a glass of juice or other sugary beverage will often correct an episode of hypoglycemia, but you should seek medical attention if any symptoms occur when working with a diabetic client of either type. You may want to encourage your clients with diabetes to consume a snack of complex carbohydrates one hour before exercising to help avoid a hypoglycemic episode.

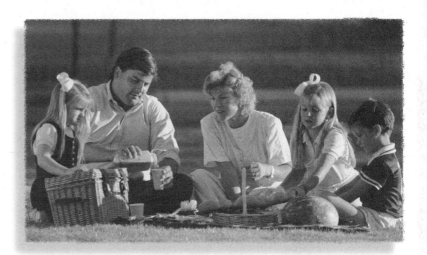

Since diabetes can mask or hide the presence of concurrent cardiovascular disease, it is particularly important that the diabetic client undergo a physician's assessment, which should include an ECG-monitored exercise test prior to embarking on an exercise program.

The diet most often prescribed for diabetics emphasizes calorie control. In the past it was felt that it was important to restrict the consumption of simple carbohydrates, but this approach is falling out of favor. The role of the registered dietician is very important in devising a diet plan for both type I and type II diabetics — often a delicate balancing act is required to avoid both hypoglycemia and hyperglycemia.

Obesity is the number one risk factor in the development of type II diabetes. Fortunately, weight loss and exercise are effective in reducing insulin resistance and may reduce the need for medications to control this disease.

Some specific suggestions for working with a diabetic client include emphasizing aerobic activity and stressing the importance of regular exercise and a stable diet to minimize swings in blood glucose levels.

In addition, for diabetics with poor peripheral circulation and/or peripheral **neuropathy**, attention to foot care is important. There may be a decreased ability to sense discomfort in the extremities, especially the feet. Any change in foot color, or signs of trauma, skin breakdown or ulceration should receive proper medical attention.

Morbid Obesity

Morbid obesity is defined as more than 100 pounds over, or twice "ideal" body weight, or as having a body-mass index (weight in kg/square of height in meters) of 40 or greater. For example, a 5'6" person weighing 250 pounds or more would be considered morbidly obese.

Morbid obesity is seen in only about one in 20 persons who are obese. People who were obese children are more likely to fit into this category than those with adult-onset obesity. Morbid obesity produces both medical and psychological consequences. Virtually every part of the body can be adversely affected. There is an increased risk of heart disease, hypertension and type II diabetes mellitus, which rises with the degree of obesity, as well as a number of other conditions such as joint disease, skin breakdown and endocrine disorders. Psychologically, morbidly obese people have a greater risk of depression, largely a consequence of the social stigma of obesity.

The constellation of problems associated with morbid obesity can often be improved with weight loss. Although it was thought that a morbidly obese person should reduce their weight to a near normal level in order to achieve substantial medical benefits, it is now clear that as little as a 10 percent reduction in initial body weight can result in significant medical benefits. Blood pressure may improve, high cholesterol and **triglyceride** levels will come down, insulin resistance will diminish and the overall fitness and outlook of the person may improve. It is, therefore, usually best to set modest initial weight-loss goals as they are more likely to be achieved and sustained than aggressive goals, and often yield substantial medical benefits.

The method of weight reduction prescribed for a person with morbid obesity will vary according to the desires and characteristics of the client. The two major categories of diet are low-calorie diets (LCD), and very-low-calorie diets (VLCD). A diet that provides 800 or more calories per day is a low-calorie diet, while one of fewer than 800 calories is a very-low-calorie diet. VLCDs have fallen out of favor in recent years because they pose a greater risk of diet-associated complications than LCDs. They are still useful in some patients with severe obesity, but a similar degree of weight loss can often be achieved with a somewhat less restrictive diet.

There is a tendency among clients desiring weight loss to seek aggressive dieting methods. While this is not necessarily the best long-term approach, there is some rationale for prescribing moderately aggressive diets in the morbidly obese. First, a client is encouraged by fairly rapid weight reduction. Second, few people are able to adhere to a calorie-restricted diet for an extended length of time. It is often impractical for a morbidly obese person to follow a diet that delivers 500 fewer calories per day than their estimated needs (3,000 instead of 3,500 total calories per day), because it will take at least one year of continuous dieting to lose about 50 pounds. On the other hand, any diet, aggressive or not, will likely fail if emphasis is not placed on helping the client make permanent changes in types and portions of foods chosen, eating behaviors and amount of physical activity.

Psychological and emotional support is important, both in facilitating the success of weight loss and in dealing with the consequences of success or the lack of it. Assistance can be provided through support groups, individual counseling by a qualified therapist or a social support network. You should be aware of this need for support in sustaining change. As a consultant you can provide a ready ear as well as encourage the client to seek support from other sources.

The exercise and fitness program may, of necessity, be initially limited for the morbidly obese client. Even in the absence of medical complications, the client's fitness level may be so poor that a moderate walking program could be too strenuous. An aggressive exercise program also may increase the risk of injuries. It is usually worthwhile, however, to include modest fitness goals in a comprehensive weight management approach. In addition to the medical and lifestyle benefits, it also has been shown that weight maintenance after weight loss is better in those individuals who maintain physical activity than in those who do not.

Eating Disorders

While the term eating disorder is sometimes used to describe the condition of obesity, it is generally reserved for specific psychiatric diagnoses such as anorexia nervosa, bulimia nervosa and binge-eating disorder. It is important that you understand the nature of these conditions and are aware of the need to refer a client to an appropriate professional if you suspect that

they suffer from one of these disabling conditions.

Anorexia nervosa is seen chiefly in young, white, middle-to-upper class women. The condition is characterized by extreme thinness, lack of appetite and an altered body image in which the person believes herself to be overweight even though she may be severely underweight. Anorexia nervosa is sometimes accompanied by a compulsive adherence to an increasingly intensive exercise regimen. If you have a client who wishes to lose weight but seems thin, you should encourage them to seek the advice of a physician or therapist. It is inappropriate to help such a client lose more weight.

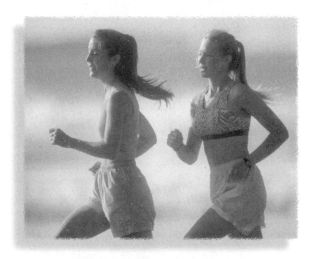

Bulimia nervosa is characterized by frequent binge eating, followed by purging, usually by self-induced vomiting or the use of potent diuretics or laxatives. The person suffering from bulimia nervosa is often able to maintain a normal body weight despite excessive caloric intake by purging. The possibility that a client has bulimia nervosa may be apparent at the initial meeting. In other cases it may manifest itself later in the course of your work with the client.

As with anorexia nervosa, referral to a professional skilled in the diagnosis and treatment of eating disorders is necessary.

Anorexia nervosa is sometimes accompanied by a compulsive need to exercise. If you suspect that a client suffers from this or any other eating disorder, you must refer them to an appropriate professional for diagnosis and treatment.

Depression is the most
common psychiatric
condition in the U.S.
If you notice a client
exhibits signs of depres-
sion such as prolonged
sadness, mood swings
and changes in appetite
and sleep patterns, it is
essential that you refer
them to a qualified pro-
fessional.

Binge-eating disorder (BED) is a recently recognized disorder that is similar to bulimia nervosa. An individual
with BED engages in frequent binge
eating but does not purge. Binge eating,
however, is not enough to define BED.
Binges must consist of abnormally
large amounts of food, consumed at
an unusually rapid pace at one sitting,
while alone. The person may feel out
of control and unable to stop eating,
followed by guilt or depression after
the episode. In addition, the frequency
of binges must average two times or
more per week to meet the criteria for
binge-eating disorder.

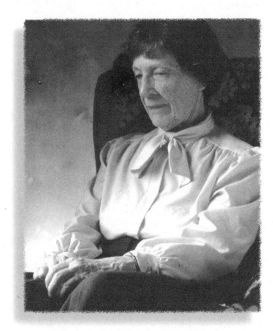

Clients with this disorder are often
overweight because they don't purge
the large amounts of food they consume. The first aim of treatment, however, is to control the binge eating
rather than to achieve weight loss. Referral to a skilled professional is again
recommended. Clients with BED are
often quite good at adhering to a strict
diet and exercise program, and this
may halt their bingeing. It is common,
though, for bingeing to resume or increase once the diet is over or "broken."
Thus, it is safest to wait to begin a diet

with a client whom you suspect may
have BED until they have sought the
help of an eating disorders specialist.

Depression

Depression is arguably the most common psychiatric condition in the United
States, and is prominent among people
with eating disorders. The signs and
symptoms of depression include prolonged sadness, mood swings and
changes in appetite and sleep patterns.

While signs of depression are seen in
many people on occasion, you should
be aware of persistent symptoms. There
are some people who are depressed who
do not exhibit obvious signs or symptoms. Anger, for example, can sometimes mask an under-lying depression.

If you feel that a client you are working with shows evidence of depression —
particularly if you feel that they may do
harm to themselves — you must see that
they get professional attention. In some
cases, a client suffering from depression
may be very compliant with a diet or
exercise program, and insist that losing
weight is all that they need to improve
their condition. This is not usually true.
Try to point out that there are a number of successful treatments for depression that can alleviate suffering. Among
the treatments available are various
medications and psychotherapy. Weight
loss and exercise can begin or resume
once the client has begun treatment
and gained the approval of a qualified
professional.

Anxiety Disorders

Anxiety disorders are a response to
stressful circumstances and are accompanied by exaggerated behavior.

Although it may seem that what an
anxiety disorder is obvious, some explanation is warranted. The symptoms of
an anxiety disorder are often sporadic,
but may last many days or months. Symptoms include a sense of impending

doom; jitteryness; autonomic symptoms such as cold, sweaty palms and dry throat; as well as shallow, rapid breathing; rapid heart rate; lightheadedness and trembling. In general, women are more likely then men to suffer from panic attacks and other anxiety disorders.

When episodes of extreme anxiety occur without obvious precipitants, and last minutes to hours, they are called panic attacks. Panic attacks are a subset of anxiety disorders and people who experience them may respond to treatment with anti-depressants. This may be because people with anxiety disorders often have a history of depression.

Weight management is unlikely to have a direct effect on the reduction of anxiety symptoms in clients with this disorder, so no special diet or exercise components are needed to work with them effectively. It may be worthwhile, however, to find out what kinds of situations have led to anxiety or panic attacks in a client's past. Precipitating situations can thus be avoided.

For example, if the client suffers from anxiety when physically challenged, a less-aggressive exercise program would clearly be necessary. If a client becomes anxious while you are with them, stop whatever activity is occurring. Allow the client to sit down and try to relax, and speak reassuringly, slowly and softly. Try to maintain a calm manner. It is best to avoid making physical contact with the person.

Referral to a qualified health professional who can provide treatment, such as a psychologist, is recommended. Treatment for anxiety disorders includes medications such as the benzodiazepines and anti-depressants, as well as psychotherapy. Anti-anxiety medications may have a sedating effect, and it is advised that they not be taken when driving or operating machinery. You should discuss whether modifications in the client's exercise program should be made with health provider. These may include avoiding the use of exercise equipment, which might be dangerous if the client becomes sedated from the medication.

Special Populations

Children

The benefits of weight management in children are numerous. They are subject to many of the same medical problems as adults, including hypertension, heart disease and obesity. Since such medical problems are less common in children than adults, the medical conditions are less likely to be manifest initially. Establishing good eating behavior and exercise habits early in life can aid in the prevention of these medical conditions.

The prevalence of obesity among children is rising even faster than among adults. Although only about 20 percent of obese adults were obese children, about 80 percent of obese children go on to become obese adults.

Characteristics of childhood-onset obesity are worth noting. First, there are a number of rare, inherited conditions and diseases of the neuroendocrine system which can lead to childhood obesity. These conditions usually appear early in life, and typically result not only in obesity but in growth retardation. Thus, children who are tall for their age as well as obese are unlikely to have one of these conditions.

Second, there is a great deal of stigmatization of obese children in the United States. A study in which young children were shown pictures of obese and non-obese children and asked to describe them demonstrated that prejudice begins as early as age six. The obese children in the pictures were typically described as less intelligent, less attractive and more lazy than the non-obese children pictured. Social stigmatization extends to economics as well. Most obese children are poor.

Third, there is some evidence that obese adults who were obese children are less responsive to treatment. This may be in part physiologic, but it is more likely that any behavioral contributors to obesity are easier to control in children than they are in adults. This is because the habits of children have been established for less time. In addition, the environment of a child can be controlled more readily than that of an adult who has greater freedom and financial independence.

Fourth, it is important to recognize that obesity runs in families. An obese child is likely to have at least one obese parent, so it is important to involve parents in the implementation of a weight management plan for their child. Ideally, they will implement similar changes in their own lives.

Since obese children will be exposed to the medical risks associated with obesity for a longer time than those who become obese as an adult, they are more likely to suffer medical problems in the long run. Weight management is likely to reduce the risks of many of the medical complications of obesity.

In implementing a lifestyle and weight management plan for a child, it is important to take some precautions. Since obese children are still growing, it is usually best to allow their growth to catch up with their weight (unless morbidly obese), rather than attempt substantial weight loss. This is because growth may be impeded by an aggressive weight-loss plan. Regarding exercises for obese children, it is best to avoid high-impact sports and any activity that entails an increased risk of injury.

As noted, it is important to involve parents or other family members in the planning and implementation of

a program. Children benefit from a supportive environment and lots of encouragement even more so than adults. It is always best to focus on positive behavior change. Do not emphasize or encourage the child to dwell on the scale.

Children can be very rewarding to work with. Patience and encouragement go a long way toward improving the life of a child suffering from the consequences of a weight problem.

Older Adults

While there are a variety of age-associated changes in bodily function that affect almost every organ system, the magnitude of the change is quite variable. It is widely believed that maintaining physical fitness and reasonable body weight can lessen the deleterious effects of aging. This is particularly beneficial to the cardiovascular system, as heart disease is the chief source of mortality in older adults. The risk of falls and frailty also is reduced in physically fit older adults.

Though many medical problems may be well advanced in older adults, it is certainly worthwhile for each older adult to consider the benefits of lifestyle change to enhance physical fitness and achieve and maintain a reasonable body weight. As a consultant, you can be of great help to older adults in achieving these lifestyle goals. An awareness of the special situations that aging imposes on weight management and fitness planning is essential.

One of the most important effects of aging worth noting is that body weight and composition tends to change as the body grows older. Even among healthy older adults, there is, on average, a gradual increase in body weight (perhaps one half to one pound a year) and a decrease in muscle mass. This latter phenomenon tends to depress a person's resting energy expenditure as metabolically active muscle is replaced by fat, and body-fat percentage increases. These changes in body composition are often accompanied by decreases in physical activity levels as well as a caloric intake that does not decline proportionately. The result is gradual weight gain. This scenario suggests that increasing physical activity and/or decreasing caloric intake can be beneficial in preventing weight gain in older adults.

Increasing fitness can both help control weight gain and help prevent the frailty and consequent injuries that so negatively affect the quality of life of many older adults.

Aging also affects the cardiovascular system so that heart rate, maximum heart rate, stroke volume and cardiac output all decline. Maximum oxygen consumption declines 9 percent each decade after age 30, so the typical older adult tires more easily and walks more slowly than their younger counterparts. Despite the decrease in cardiac output, blood pressure tends to increase with advancing age as arteriosclerosis narrows the diameter of blood vessels and increases vascular resistance. Systolic blood pressure is usually increased more than diastolic.

Aging adversely affects the skeletal system as well, particularly in older women. Osteoporosis is very common as bone mass and strength decline. These changes, along with reduced elasticity, mobility, and flexibility of joints, tendons and muscles, and slowed reflexes, result in a high risk of falls and fractures. Levels of physical fitness fall further with the decreased mobility imposed by injury, and recovery of functional capacity becomes more difficult. Fractures, particularly of the hip, can seriously affect the quality of life and the ability to live independently, and can even lead to death in many older adults.

Regular physical activity, especially progressive resistance and weight-bearing exercises, can help to maintain bone mass. Maintaining an adequate intake of calcium and vitamin D is also a useful intervention method that does not require a prescription. Physicians may prescribe estrogen replacement therapy for post-menopausal women.

These adverse consequences of aging can be avoided by maintaining physical fitness and a reasonable body weight throughout the life cycle. Your role as a consultant in helping the older adult is 1) to recommend that the client obtain physician clearance and advice before

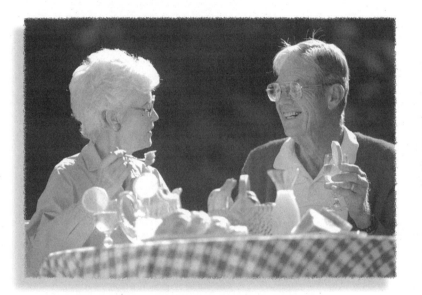

embarking on any exercise or weight loss regimen; and 2) to ensure that the older adult carries out the prescribed exercise and weight management plan in a safe and effective manner.

Some specific recommendations follow:

✔ Regarding diet, it is important that caloric intake not be too severely restricted. Gradual weight loss of about one pound per week is safest. There is seldom a need to lose weight more rapidly than this. Rapid weight loss may not be well tolerated in older adults, particularly if they have cardiovascular conditions requiring anti-hypertensive medications and diuretics. It also is important that a

It is widely believed that maintaining physical fitness and reasonable body weight can lessen the deleterious effects of aging, such as increased risk of disease and disability.

Table 10.3

American College of Gynecologists and Obstetricians' Recommendations for Exercise in Pregnancy

The following recommendations are for women who do not have any additional risk factors for a complicated pregnancy:

1. Women can continue to derive health benefits from physical activity performed at least three times per week.

2. Women should avoid exercise in the supine position after the first trimester, and prolonged periods of motionless standing should also be avoided.

3. Pregnant women should modify exercise intensity according to how they feel. They should stop exercising when fatigued and not exercise to exhaustion. Some women may be able to continue doing weight-bearing exercises at intensities similar to those prior to pregnancy. Non-weight-bearing exercise such as cycling and swimming generally may be continued throughout pregnancy.

4. Exercise that might result in a loss of balance or trauma to the abdominal area should be avoided.

5. Women who exercise must be sure to consume enough calories to compensate for the added calorie cost of both physical activity and pregnancy.

6. Pregnant women who exercise must be careful to maintain proper hydration and wear appropriate clothing to augment heat dissipation.

Source: ACOG, 1994

calorie-restricted diet contain adequate protein, calcium and other minerals, and vitamins. Single ingredient diets and fad diets should be avoided.

✔ Regarding the fitness program, it may be helpful to organize recommendations around the FITT mnemonic.

F Frequency of exercise can often be as high as it is for younger adults, as long as rest days are included at least once weekly. Be sure to warm up and perform flexibility exercises slowly.

I Intensity requires modification in older adults. Start slowly, and progress gradually through all exercises. Target heart rates should begin at 40 percent of maximum reserve, and go no higher than 70 percent with training. You must closely monitor the client for signs of distress such as shortness of breath, chest pain, lightheadedness or tiring. Recall that medication may mask signs of distress or prevent rises in heart rate with exertion. Use a perceived exertion scale in addition to monitoring heart rate and blood pressure.

T Time of each training session should begin at 10 to 15 minutes, and advance slowly to no longer than 60 minutes, depending on the client's tolerance.

T Type of exercise also should be altered for older adults. All types of aerobic activity can be appropriate, but the client's individual fitness level and concurrent medical conditions may make some activities more suitable than others. Low-impact activities are safest, especially for individuals with arthritic or orthopedic problems. The obese client may do best with water aerobics and swimming. Walking is often an ideal exercise and requires no special equipment or facilities. Weight training can be beneficial in building strength and bone mass, but must be approached cautiously, particularly for those with arthritis or orthopedic conditions. Light resistance is best, such as that provided by 1- to 3-pound hand weights. Be aware that balance may be impaired in some older adults.

Working with older adults requires

an understanding of the relevant physiologic changes of aging, and alertness to the increased risks of injuries and complications of diet and exercise programs. Keeping these special considerations in mind can enhance your ability to safely accomplish meaningful improvements in the older client's quality of life.

Pregnant Women

Pregnant women have different physiologic needs and responses to diet and exercise compared to non-pregnant women. You will have to be aware of the relevant physiologic alterations caused by pregnancy and work within the limitations imposed by them. As with other special conditions and populations, urging the pregnant client to seek the advice of her physician and adhering to the guidelines of professional organizations are important.

In general, dieting for weight loss is discouraged, even if the pregnant woman is obese, while exercise is permitted and encouraged. However, the American College of Obstetricians and Gynecologists (ACOG) recommends that women who have the following conditions should not exercise during or immediately following pregnancy:

✔ cardiac disease
✔ vaginal bleeding or placenta previa
✔ incompetent cervix
✔ ruptured membranes
✔ history of three or more
  spontaneous miscarriages

Even in the absence of one of these conditions, if there are other medical problems present, or if the client is extremely obese or underweight, it is advisable to seek the input of the pregnant client's obstetrician. ACOG guidelines for exercise during pregnancy are shown in Table 10.3.

The nutritional requirements of pregnant women are increased both in total calories needed and in specific nutrients, vitamins and minerals. It is important that prescribed vitamins and minerals, including iron, be taken faithfully. Pre-natal visits with the client's obstetrician or mid-wife should include dietary recommendations. For the woman who was obese prior to pregnancy, weight gain is often more than average during pregnancy, and more weight tends to be retained one year after delivery than for the non-obese pregnant woman. This is not desirable. Rather than encourage weight reduction during pregnancy (which can be injurious

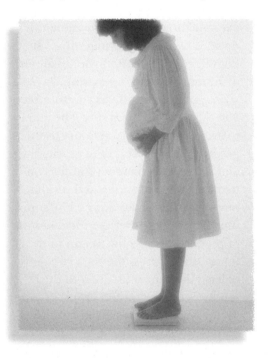

Dieting for weight loss during pregnancy is discouraged, even if the pregnant woman is obese. Exercise, however, is generally permitted and encouraged.

to fetal growth and development), it is usually recommended that the woman's diet be regulated so that pregnancy-related weight gain is reduced. This may be accomplished through a combination of exercise (when not contraindicated), portion control and a reduction in fat intake.

The physiologic changes of pregnancy also affect the exercise regimen. For example, ACOG's recommendation that maternal core temperature not be allowed to exceed 38 degrees C

(100.4 degrees F) stems from the fact that a pregnant woman has a higher basal body temperature and metabolic rate than when not pregnant, and may overheat sooner. Thus, special caution should be taken to avoid exercising in warm or humid conditions, or when the pregnant client has a fever. Overheating in an air-conditioned environment is quite possible as well. Exercise intensity should be reduced, and recovery time increased for the pregnant client.

Another physiologic factor of pregnancy that affects exercise tolerance is related to the energy requirements of the fetus. Fatigue and hypoglycemia may easily set in with even moderate levels of exercise intensity. Hypoglycemia can be delayed or avoided by ingesting a snack high in complex carbohydrates about 30 minutes prior to exercising.

Pregnancy also affects comfortable and safe exercise positions. The aim is to avoid back strain and injury as the pregnant client's center of gravity shifts and hormonal changes produce connective tissue relaxation and resultant joint instability. Exercising while supine must be avoided after the third month of pregnancy since the weight of the fetus can compress the vena cava, impairing the return of blood to the mother's heart, and the supply of blood to her brain. This results in lightheadedness and rapid fatigue.

The decision to exercise should be made in conjunction with a woman's physician. There is currently no evidence to indicate that pregnant women must limit the intensity of their exercise or lower their target heart rates due to potential adverse effects. Instead, perceived exertion should be used to monitor exercise intensity as it is often a more reliable measure than heart rate. Fatigue and breathlessness should always be avoided. Immediately stop the exercise session and call for medical attention if the pregnant client experiences vaginal bleeding, fainting, severe nausea, clear fluid emerging from the vagina, neurologic signs such as disorientation, blurring of vision, severe or persistent headache or if she feels either very hot or cold and clammy.

In the second and third trimesters of pregnancy, recommend aerobic activities that minimize joint stress (water aerobics, swimming and walking). Straining and holding the breath during exertion (known as the Valsalva maneuver) should be avoided, and only light resistance strength training with higher repetitions should be performed. Lamaze and **Kegel exercises** may replace the exercises done earlier in pregnancy.

Exercise may resume four to six weeks after delivery, but if a cesarean section was performed, only with the obstetrician's permission. Reduce exercise intensity when breast feeding to prevent lactic acid concentration in the breast milk. Because there has been a period of time without exercise prior to and after delivery, an exercise program should be resumed at a slow and steady pace.

Summary

As the benefits of lifestyle modification become more widely appreciated, the prevalence of obesity continues to rise and the American population ages, the need for certified lifestyle and weight management consultants is expected to rise dramatically. An increasing proportion of clients will fall into the special conditions and special population categories. Both the risks and benefits of lifestyle modifications are often greater in such clients. Knowledge of the physiology and special requirements of special populations and clients with special conditions will enable you to achieve successful results with the greatest degree of safety.

References

Brownell, K.D. & Fairburn, C.G. (eds). (1995). *Eating Disorders and Obesity: A Comprehensive Handbook.* New York: Guildford.

Cheskin, L.J. (1994). *Obesity.* In Bayless, T.M. (ed). *Current Therapy in Gastroenterology* (4th ed.). St. Louis: Mosby.

Epstein, L.H., Valoski, A., Wing, R.R. & McCurley, J. (1990). Ten-year follow-up of behavioral, family-based treatment for obese children. *Journal of the American Medical Association,* 264, 2519-2523.

Folsom, A.R., Prineas, R.J., Kaye, S.A., et al. (1989). Body fat distribution and self-reported prevalence of hypertension, heart attack and other heart disease in older women. *International Journal of Epidemiology,* 18: 361-367.

Hubert, H.B., Feinleibm, McNamara, P.M. & Castelli, W.P. (1983). Obesity as an independent risk factor for CFD. *Circulation,* 67: 968-77.

Wadden, T.A. & Van itallie, T. (eds). (1992). *Treatment of the Seriously Obese Patient.* New York: Guilford.

Zieve, P.D. (1995). *Handbook of Ambulatory Medicine.* Baltimore: Williams & Wilkins.

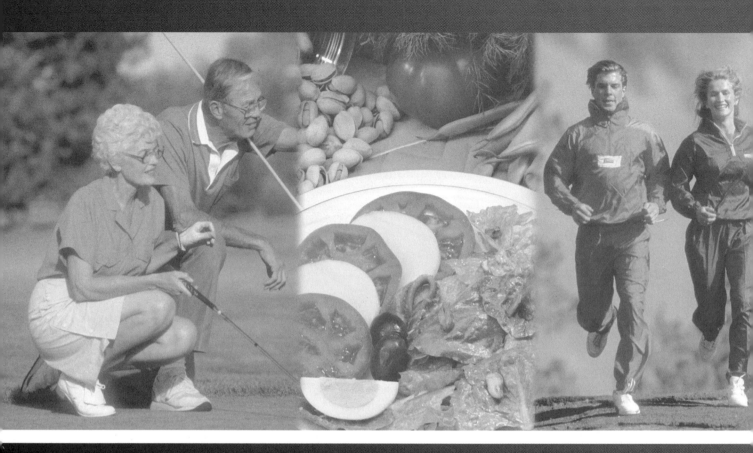

CHAPTER ELEVEN

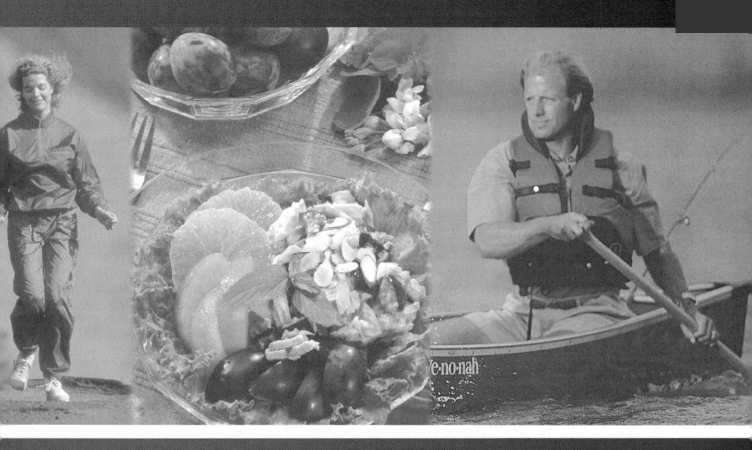

Responsibilities

LEGAL, PROFESSIONAL AND ETHICAL

by David L. Herbert

with the assistance of

Kimberly A. Johnson

David L. Herbert, Esq., is a senior partner at Herbert, Benson & Scott, a law firm in Canton, Ohio. He is also the co-editor of The Exercise Standards & Malpractice Reporter.

Introduction

As a lifestyle and weight management consultant you need a basic understanding of the legal system and the operation of various laws and legal principles that may have an impact upon your ability to serve your clients. The following information will help you understand the broad legal implications of your position; however, individualized legal assistance should be obtained before embarking upon the delivery of service to consumers.

The legal system is divided into three branches — federal, state and local. Most of the legal principles discussed in this chapter will be based upon state law concepts. However, a variety of federal and local laws also may affect you.

The Legal System

The legal system may differ from state to state. Consequently, only general legal principles will be discussed, interspersed with examples of specific state statutes and case law, where applicable. Principles related to **contract law**, **tort law**, **criminal law** and state statutory regulation of defined professionals and activities are provided.

Contract Law

Relationships between those providing products or services and their clients are, for the most part, governed by contract law. Contracts may be either in written or oral form; however, when dealing in this defined service area, contracts should be in written form and adequately define and delineate the duties and responsibilities of the consultant and the client. Specific services, service delivery methods and service frequency, along with payment amounts and terms should all be specified within such contracts.

Contracts are based upon the exchange of mutual promises supported by something of value, referred to in law as "consideration," such as products, services or money bargained for and given in exchange for some other consideration. In this setting, contracts will form the basis of your, the consultant's, relationship with your clients.

Minors and those who otherwise lack the requisite capacity to contract, such as those who are not mentally competent, cannot lawfully contract with you as a provider. Consequently, contractual relationships with such individuals must be avoided.

Releases, waivers and **informed consent documents** (which are discussed later in this chapter) are forms of contracts. In many jurisdictions, these contractual documents are valid and binding. In some states, however, their use may be unlawful. In other situations, their use may be prohibited in certain settings. In many states, moreover, releases executed by one party (a husband, for example) may not be binding upon another person who is not a party to the release documents (a wife).

The services you are to provide to your clients should be defined and specified in written form. The amount to be paid for service delivery should be explicitly stated and contained within any contract.

Tort Law

Tort law is a system of **jurisprudence** that governs the management and disposition of personal injury and wrongful death lawsuits. "Torts," or wrongs, are determined within this system. Such wrongs are founded upon the alleged breach of certain duties that one person owes to another, generally referred to in law as "negligence" or in the professional healthcare setting as "malpractice." The breach of such duties that subsequently results in harm and damage to another is redressable through this system by an award of damages to the injured party.

Personal injury claims and wrongful death actions make up a large part of the cases filed each year in virtually every jurisdiction. Those in healthcare, sports, sports administration or the fitness industry are involved in many of these cases. Often, in the course of such litigation, standards derived from respected authorities and/or professional associations are utilized to assist in establishing the so-called legal "**standard of care.**" Such standards are used to evaluate conduct to determine if the care rendered by a provider to a client or patient was appropriately provided. Expert witnesses are frequently used in these cases to provide opinion testimony as to whether there was a breach of care or standard that is deemed damaging in nature.

Criminal Law

Criminal law also is part of the judicial system. Through a variety of statutory enactments, certain defined conduct is statutorily prohibited or proscribed under threat of criminal prosecution of those violating such laws. Violation of criminal laws are categorized into three classifications: capital crimes for murder cases; felonies for other serious crimes; and misdemeanors generally punishable by less than one year imprisonment.

Criminal laws exist in virtually every jurisdiction, prohibiting, among other matters, the unauthorized practice of medicine and other allied healthcare professional practices. As a consultant, you must be aware of these laws and refer to them in order to govern your activities and provision of services.

The Standard of Care

Those engaged in the delivery of service to consumers have a duty to render that service in accordance with the so-called "standard of care." Deviation from that standard, as previously stated, can be actionable if substandard care causes harm and damage to the client.

In the fitness and wellness industry, a variety of written standards exist that establish benchmarks of expected behavior for those providing service. Standards from the American Council on Exercise (ACE), the American College of Sports Medicine (ACSM), the Aerobic and Fitness Association of America (AFAA), the International Health, Racquet and Sportsclub Association (IHRSA), the National Strength and Conditioning Association (NSCA) and the Young Men's Christian Association (YMCA), among others, all provide

written statements of expected behavior that could be utilized in legal proceedings to establish expected parameters of care. These standards provide information and direction in the areas of client screening, assessment, recommendations for activity, supervision, emergency response and documentation.

In this regard, you should be aware that you have an obligation, prior to recommending activity, to obtain sufficient information from a client to determine if that client can, upon assessment of that information, safely carry on recommended activity. The standards of the ACSM specify that a **health history questionnaire** or a **Par-Q**-type form must be obtained and analyzed before activity is recommended to a consumer by a wellness/fitness professional. If such a screening device indicates that a **medical clearance** is necessary before a client begins activity, then such a clearance must be obtained prior to recommending activity. Should the client neglect or refuse to obtain clearance, the ACSM standards specify that no activity recommendations should be provided.

Deviation from such written standards would be actionable if a client is injured or suffers an untoward event as a subsequent result. Consequently, it is important for you as a consultant to ensure that you comply with the published standards, not only for screening and assessing clients, but for recommending and supervising activity, and providing emergency response if needed.

You should be aware of the fact that the standard of care for service delivery to clients is constantly changing. As new scientific or professional developments unfold in this practice area, changes to the standard of care will inevitably take place. As a consequence, you will need to stay abreast of and keep current as to developments in this field.

One of the most practical ways to

stay on top of professionally important changes to the standard of care is to participate in continuing education and similar programs. In addition, you clearly have an obligation to keep current with professional publications and resources that might have an impact on your ability to serve your clients. Consultants who neglect these continuing education and self-development requirements run the risk of providing service that does not meet the current standard of care.

State Regulation of Healthcare – Permitted and Unpermitted Activities

The provision of services to consumers in many professions is frequently the subject of local, state and/or federal regulation. Such regulations take many forms and cover a host of activities, from door-to-door sales solicitations, to the practice of medicine and other branches of healthcare. While federal and local regulations may affect a number of such services, state laws generally regulate healthcare professionals and the delivery of healthcare-related services.

The practice of medicine and nursing, dentistry, chiropractic and physical therapy are governed by state law in virtually all jurisdictions. Athletic training, various forms of therapy and the practice of dietetics/nutrition also is regulated in many jurisdictions. Some emerging professional services, such as clinical exercise physiology, are now receiving state attention through the enactment of licensing statutes.

State licensing statutes and enactments for various providers differ from state to state. While some state licensing statutes might be similar in nature, many are often very different between jurisdictions. Moreover, the defined

roles, responsibilities and obligations specified by law as to diverse, licensed providers may be overlapping, ill-defended or susceptible to more than one interpretation or analysis. As a result, a sometimes confusing patchwork of state laws is imposed upon healthcare providers and allied professionals that can even overlap into areas which are seemingly unregulated.

Pursuant to most state statutory frameworks, individuals who, for example, wish to practice medicine, must be licensed to do so by the state in which they intend to provide service. Those who are not licensed are prohibited by state civil and criminal statutes from engaging in the profession or in rendering such professional services. In addition, unlicensed individuals can be subject to injunction or other civil orders prohibiting them from engaging in unauthorized practices. However, when other healthcare statutes that define who can do what within a particular healthcare profession are examined and analyzed, the distinction between licensed healthcare provider enactments can become blurred. Moreover, certain other practices also can be subject to diverse interpretation as to whether activity is regulated or proscribed. This becomes particularly true for professionals who move out of and away from traditionally regulated areas, such as medicine or nursing, and into developing areas, such as clinical exercise physiology, lifestyle and weight management consulting or a host of others.

Despite the foregoing, individuals must ensure that they are entitled to provide specified services with or without **licensure**, **registration** or **certification** by that jurisdiction. To make that determination, individuals, including those involved in lifestyle and weight management consulting, must determine what they can and cannot do under

Table 11.1

Listing of State Laws Regulating Dietitians and Nutritionists

The following states currently have some form of law to regulate dietitians and nutritionists.
(Further information is available from The American Dietetic Association in Chicago, Illinois):

Alabama (1989)**
    licensing of dietitian/nutritionists

Arkansas (1989)
    licensing of dietitians

California (1982)
    registration* of dietitians

Connecticut (1994)
    certification of dietitians

Delaware (1994)
    certification of dietitians/nutritionists

District of Columbia (1986)
    licensing of dietitians and nutritionists

Florida (1988)
    licensing of dietitians, nutritionists
    and nutrition counselors

Georgia (1994)**
    licensing of dietitians

Idaho (1994)
    licensing of dietitians

Illinois (1991)
    licensing of dietitians and nutrition counselors

Indiana (1994)
    certification of dietitians

Iowa (1985)
    licensing of dietitians

Kansas (1989)**
    licensing of dietitians

Kentucky (1994)**
    licensing of dietitians and
    certification of nutritionists

Louisiana (1987)**
    licensing of dietitians/nutritionists

Maine (1995)**
    licensing of dietitians and dietetic technicians

Maryland (1994)**
    licensing of dietitians and nutritionists

Minnesota (1994)
    licensing of dietitians and nutritionists

Mississippi (1994)
    licensing of dietitians and
    nutritionist title protection

Montana (1987)**
    licensing of nutritionists and
    dietitian title protection

Nebraska (1995)**
    licensing of medical nutrition therapists

Nevada (1995)*
    certification of dietitians

New Mexico (1989)
    licensing of dietitians, nutritionists
    and nutrition associates

New York (1991)
    certification of dietitians and nutritionists

North Carolina (1991)
    licensing of dietitians and nutritionists

North Dakota (1989)**
    licensing of dietitians and
    certification of nutritionists

Ohio (1986)
    licensing of dietitians

Oklahoma (1984)
    licensing of dietitians

Oregon (1989)
    certification # of dietitians

Puerto Rico (1974)**
    licensing of dietitians and nutritionists

Rhode island (1991)**
    licensing of dietitians and nutritionists

Tennessee (1987)
    licensing of dietitians/nutritionists

Texas (1993)**
    certification # of dietitians

Utah (1986)
    certification of dietitians

Vermont (1993)
    certification of dietitians

Virginia (1995)*
    certification of dietitians and nutritionists

Washington (1988)
    certification of dietitians and nutritionists

Wisconsin (1994)
    certification of dietitians

* This is an entitlement law, which protects the use of the title by individuals meeting state-mandated qualifications.

** This is the year amended and/or reauthorized.

\# These laws provide the certified practitioner with a license, and are termed "voluntary licensing" laws.

particular state laws and regulations in their delivery of specified services.

Licensure for some occupations and professions is allowed for individuals who meet specified **competencies** and requirements under state law. Typically, these providers must obtain a license before providing service. Registration

Case	Summary	Ruling
Foster vs. Georgia Board of Chiropractic Examiners, 359 S.E. 2d 877 (1987)	A chiropractor prescribed treatment for a patient which included ingestion of certain substances including free amino acids and organamim.	License to practice chiropractic was suspended, since the chiropractor did prescribe such items for treatment of a patient's ailments.
State of Ohio vs. Winterich, 157 Ohio St. 414 (1952)	Foods were recommended to a patient, but were not given to respond to or treat any disease.	Trial court's conviction of the chiropractor for unauthorized practice of medicine was reversed. The reversal was based, in large part, on the fact that the foods that were recommended to the chiropractor's patient were not given to treat any disease.
Stetina vs. State of Ohio Medical Licensing Board, 513 N.E. 2d 1234 (Ind. App. 2 Dist., 1987)	Nutritionist determined a patient had certain problems that could be remedied by an enema, mineral water, kelp, amelade, projestine and raw food.	The nutritionist was not prevented from lecturing or educating the public, nor from selling products, as long as he did not examine, diagnose, treat or sell products (or prescribe or offer such advice) based upon an assessment of an individual's specific needs or problems.
Ohio Board of Dietetics vs. Brown, 83 Ohio App. 3d 342 (Ct. of Appeals, Cuy. Cty. 1993)	Defendant admittedly gave nutritional counseling to "patients" without a license.	The court determined that until he obtained a license, he was properly barred from engaging in nutritional counseling or assessments, or any other activity prohibited by the Code.
Strandwitz vs. Ohio Board of Dietetics, 83 Ohio App. 3d 183 (Ct. Appeals, Franklin Cty., 1992)	Two clinical nutritionists brought a declaratory judgment action, seeking a court ruling that they were exempt from state licensing requirements.	The court ruled that any person, regardless of their title, who engages in nutritional assessment, nutritional counseling, nutritional education or any of the activities governed by the statute, must adhere to the regulations of the law and be licensed.

Figure 11.1
Overview of case law related to the unauthorized practice of medicine or other allied healthcare.

is a state-imposed process by which those who have met established requirements register with a state agency prior to delivering service. State-imposed certification, on the other hand (not to be confused with professional association certification), generally prohibits the use of certain titles by those who do not meet state-established criteria to practice a given occupation or profession.

A few "rules" will assist you in determining whether there is a need to seek state licensure/registration/certification prior to providing services. It is important to consult with an attorney and/or a state regulating agency regarding state regulatory statutes in your jurisdiction. If the service area is subject to state control, compliance must first be obtained before offering some services. If there is a lack of statutory guidance as to whether services are controlled by law, declaratory judgment proceedings or similar actions may be available to obtain court guidance.

Be careful not to overstep your bounds of practice if you live in a state where regulation does not prohibit delivery of service. You should always be aware of the fact that service provided to "treat," "alleviate," "cure," "rehabilitate" or even in some jurisdictions to "prevent" disease, illness, infirmity, condition or injury may be deemed to be the practice of medicine or some other allied healthcare profession. In these circumstances, delivery of such services is prohibited except when it is provided by a licensed practitioner and, then, only within the permissible scope of service delivery (Table 11.1).

Avoid using titles that are limited for use by physicians or other licensed and/or regulated healthcare providers. As a consultant, you should not use any of the following terms: nutritionist, registered nutritionist, doctor of nutrition, doctor of dietetics, or any healthcare specific acronym such as "M.D.," "Dr.," "D.C." or "R.D." unless you lawfully possess such a title or designation.

Never refer to your clients as "patients." Using this term while delivering services might convey the wrong connotation and raise questions as to whether or not you are required to be licensed as a healthcare provider. Terms such as "customer" or "client" are preferable to the term "patient," in order to avoid the appearance of rendering healthcare-related services.

Always inform your clients that you are not a healthcare practitioner or, if so licensed, that the licensure is in a defined area. These statements should be made orally and in writing. If, in the course of delivering services, you feel that a client should be referred to a licensed practitioner, that recommen-

dation should be made to the client and documented in your records.

There is a growing body of case law on the unauthorized practice of medicine or other allied healthcare (Figure 11.1). Decisions in these cases are generally not favorable to those who provide advice and consultation that can be interpreted or perceived as the practicing of medicine or a field of allied healthcare without a license. The consequences of such illegal activities have ranged from suspensions to injunctions to being barred from engaging in counseling and assessment.

In addition, practices that may be lawful in one state may be unlawful in another state. Non-licensed providers must take care to ensure that the requirements of their state law are met when rendering services. State laws must be considered, analyzed and addressed by legal counsel prior to providing services.

Finally, medical terminology should be avoided when delivering services. Terms such as "diagnosis," "diagnostic testing," "prescription," "treatment" or "cure" should be avoided.

Legal and Professional Duties and Responsibilities

As previously mentioned, lifestyle and weight management consultants have defined duties and responsibilities toward their clients. These duties include those established by practice standards as determined and applied to actual case scenarios. Key duties and responsibilities associated with delivering services include client screening and assessment, referral to a healthcare provider when deemed necessary based on the screening assessment, appropriate recommendations for activity, proper supervision of activity, keeping client information confidential and the provision of emergency response in the event of an untoward event.

While issues related to screening and assessment have been discussed, you must realize that this duty is one that the profession has imposed upon itself, and one that the judicial system would probably sanction in the course of resolving individual claims and litigation.

Deficiencies related to recommendations for activity or in the supervision of that activity also have been the subject of frequent claim and suit, as have deficiencies or defects related to exercise devices/machinery and free weights.

In addition, deficiencies related to the provision of appropriate emergency response have been the subject of numerous claims and suits. You must be able to respond to a client's emergency needs for first aid and CPR, as well as have access to an emergency response system. Case law, supported by applicable industry standards, particularly those from the American College of Sports Medicine, impose specific obligations upon professionals to have emergency response plans in place to deal with foreseeable client emergencies. Such plans must be in writing, and must be rehearsed and readily accessible to all personnel responding to such events. Working communication systems also must be in place to summon off-premises emergency response personnel.

Industry standards provide that a consent form must be obtained from a client prior to performing a fitness assessment. Consent documents for such procedures are utilized to ensure that the client properly understands the procedure they are about to undergo, and that you obtain the client's "informed" decision and consent to administer the procedure. While not always required by law in some jurisdictions, especially during non-surgical procedures, obtaining a consent also is related to your

compliance with professional standards. Examples of various consent forms for fitness testing of apparently healthy adults are included in Appendix C.

While confidentiality requirements are not generally imposed upon you by state statute, as is often the case with physicians and some other healthcare professionals, data that is obtained from clients and contains personally identifiable and sensitive client information must be protected from unauthorized disclosure, since this can lead to a variety of claims. These claims can center upon allegations of: 1) violation of privacy rights; 2) intentional or negligent infliction of emotional distress; and 3) breach of contract. Because your clients will expect and demand that information about them be kept confidential, you should develop and follow established policies to ensure that such information is protected. Remember that violations of such policies can lead to substantial claims and litigation.

You also should be aware of the fact that professional associations may choose to impose ethical and even contractual obligations upon its members as a condition of obtaining or retaining membership and/or certification provided by such groups. If obligations are imposed upon association members, it is your duty to adhere to them.

The American Council on Exercise (ACE), for example, has developed a set of Professional Practices and Disciplinary Procedures that authorize them to revoke or take action with respect to those who seek or maintain ACE certifications. While these procedures establish a disciplinary process for specified violations of ACE certification standards, you should be aware of the fact that the practice statement and disciplinary process require additional professional responsibilities and accountability for violations of specified certification practices.

Records, Record Keeping and Communication

Most lawyers who practice negligence law will tell professionals engaging in record development, record keeping and client communications that, "If it's not recorded, it didn't happen!" Regardless of whether that statement is absolutely true, it does provide strong impetus for all professionals to thoroughly document client records and communications to assist, not only in providing better client services, but also in helping to establish the proper and appropriate delivery of service.

Client records should be maintained in separate client files and should contain the original of any signed form or document, including the consultant/client contract, any **informed consent forms** and any prospective release or **assumption of risk** documents, together with authorizations to release information and the client's developing record. Such records should be kept in a safe and secure storage facility under lock and key. Records should be kept and maintained for a period of time to coincide with the relevant statutory period (statute of limitations) within which a suit could be brought by the client against you, or indefinitely as determined by your legal counsel.

All significant and other professionally or legally important communications between you and your clients should be in writing. Never trust yourself to remember what was said or agreed upon, particularly for any length of time.

Defenses to Claims and Suits

Even though the judicial system is available to redress a variety of alleged wrongs, not all actions are ultimately successful. Defenses to some client actions may be predicated upon issues related to your adherence to the standard of care, while many others may relate to the client's knowing assumption of the risks associated with particular activities, or their provision of prospectively executed releases or **waivers** related to the activity.

Properly worded assumption of risk forms, releases or waivers can often be of significant benefit in defending against claims and suits. However, these documents must be: 1) lawful; 2) properly written; 3) understood by the client; and 4) duly executed by the client. Examples of such documents are contained in Appendix C. Individualized legal assistance is necessary, however, to develop any legally effective forms for you to use with clients in particular jurisdictions.

In some states, the negligence of the client, referred to in law as "**contributory negligence**," may also act as a bar to a successful suit. In such circumstances, the defense must be affirmatively stated and established to bar any civil suit. In other states, a system of "**comparative negligence**" is used to apportion fault between an injured party and any defendant. Pursuant to this system, any negligence of the plaintiff will not generally bar relief, but will be used to reduce the amount they can recover in terms of damages.

Copyright Law Compliance

In the course of structuring programs or in carrying out activities within programs, information that is copyrighted by another may not be adapted to your program unless: 1) your use of materials is exempt from copyright laws; 2) the use is permissible under laws by reason of a statutory allowance; or 3) express consent is obtained for use from copyright holders. Where copyrighted materials, such as musical routines, are to be adapted for commercial use by the consultant in the course of providing service to clients, royalty payments to copyright holders through licensing groups may be required.

Insurance

You need to secure and maintain adequate professional and general liability insurance prior to the delivery of relevant client services. Such policies may be available through professional associations or insurance brokers. However, policies that are available for such purposes must be carefully read and interpreted to ensure that coverage is afforded in all activity areas provided by you to your clients. Particular attention should be given to any policy exclusions for which insurance may not be afforded as to the provision of specific services.

Professional Ethics

You also should be aware that organizations such as ACE, ACSM, IHRSA and others have developed **codes of ethics** to govern professional conduct. These codes are supplementary to other professional standards of practice, as well as any other requirements imposed by the legal system. Nonetheless, adherence to such requirements may be necessary to maintain professional standing or certification. Moreover, violations of such established codes potentially can be cited in the event of claim and suit as additional grounds for legal redress.

Conclusion

A variety of legal principles and requirements are imposed upon a diverse body of professionals providing services to consumers, including lifestyle and weight management consultants. As such, you must appreciate these legal principles and requirements if you are planning to deliver services within this area. However, this discussion is not a replacement for individualized legal assistance from competent legal practitioners specializing in this area.

References

American College of Sports Medicine. (1992). Sol, N. & Foster, C. (Eds.) *ACSM's Health/Fitness Facility Standards and Guidelines.* Champaign: Human Kinetics.

American Council on Exercise. (1995). *Code of Ethics.* San Diego.

American Council on Exercise. (1996). Cotton, R.T. (ed.) *Personal Trainer Manual.* (2nd ed.) San Diego: American Council on Exercise.

American Council on Exercise. (1995). *Professional Practices and Disciplinary Procedures.* San Diego.

Herbert, D.L. & Herbert, W. G. (1993). *Legal Aspects of Preventive, Rehabilitative and Recreational Exercise Programs.* (3rd ed.) Canton: Professional Reports Corporation.

IRSA. (1993). *Standards Facilitation Guide.* Boston: IRSA

Koeberle, B. (1990). *Legal Aspects of Personal Fitness Training.* Canton: Professional Reports Corporation.

APPENDIX A

Code of Ethics

Code of Ethics

ACE-certified Professionals are guided by the following principles of conduct as they interact with clients, the public and other health and fitness professionals.

ACE-certified Professionals will endeavor to:

✔ Provide safe and effective instruction.

✔ Provide equal and fair treatment to all clients.

✔ Maintain an understanding of the latest health and physical activity research and its applications.

✔ Maintain current CPR certification and knowledge of first-aid services.

✔ Comply with all applicable business, employment and copyright laws.

✔ Uphold and enhance public appreciation and trust for the health and fitness industries.

✔ Maintain the confidentiality of all client information.

✔ Refer clients to more qualified fitness, medical or health professionals when appropriate.

APPENDIX B

Certification Exam Content Outline

Certification Exam Content Outline

Purpose

In September 1994, the American Council on Exercise® (ACE®) and Columbia Assessment Services, Inc. conducted a role delineation study to identify primary tasks performed by lifestyle and weight management consultants. The purpose of this study was to establish and validate appropriate content areas for the ACE Lifestyle & Weight Management Consultant Certification Examination. The results of this process include this exam content outline, which sets forth the tasks, knowledge and skills necessary for a lifestyle and weight management consultant to perform job responsibilities at a minimum professional level. It is the position of ACE that the recommendations outlined here are not exhaustive to the qualifications of a lifestyle and weight management consultant but represent a minimum level of proficiency and theoretical knowledge.

Please note that not all knowledge and skill statements listed in the exam content outline will be addressed on each exam administration.

Description

ACE-certified Lifestyle & Weight Management Consultants will be competent to analyze a client's health habits, providing basic education and support to facilitate healthy weight management and lifestyle changes. Clients and employers working with a certified consultant will be assured that the consultant has a broad background of knowledge and skills needed to facilitate healthy lifestyle changes. These knowledge and skills include those that are necessary to develop an integrated and comprehensive approach to weight management, such as basic exercise programming, basic nutrition education and facilitating change skills.

The ACE Lifestyle & Weight Management Consultant Certification is available to those who meet the following prerequisites: being at least 18 years of age, obtaining current adult CPR certification and passing an entry-level written examination measuring ACE-identified competencies. The certification will be valid for a two-year period at which time it may be renewed. Requirement for renewal will be 1.5 continuing education credits (CECs) and applicable fee.

These recommendations apply only to those individuals working with apparently healthy individuals who have no special medical or psychological needs. It is not the intent of ACE to provide recommendations for consultants to deliver specialized programs outside of their scope of practice, such as those requiring a clinical exercise physiologist, registered dietitian or psychotherapist.

Percentages indicate how much of the exam is devoted to each area and the number of questions on the examination are shown in parentheses.

I. Client Assessment
28% (50 questions)
- A. Interview and communication methods
- B. Client screening for program development and referral
- C. Determination of client profile
- D. Recognition of conditions and/or behaviors that necessitate referral

II. Development of Client Plan
22% (38 questions)
- A. Utilization of assessment data
- B. Long- and short-term goal establishment
- C. Creation of client plan

III. Implementation and Facilitation of Client Plan
32% (56 questions)
- A. Establishing a constructive professional relationship
- B. Client instruction utilizing a variety of techniques and materials
- C. Client monitoring

IV. Professional Responsibility
18% (31 questions)
- A. Communication of the scope and limitations of the professional relationship
- B. Applicable laws, regulations and scope of practice
- C. Documentation of client-related data, communications and progress
- D. Assurance of continuing competence and professional growth
- E. Initiation of emergency procedures
- F. Adherence to the American Council on Exercise Code of Ethics
- G. Insurance needs of the lifestyle and weight management consultant

---

Attention Exam Candidates!

When preparing for an ACE certification exam, be aware that the material presented in this manual, or any text, may become outdated due to the evolving nature of the fitness industry, as well as new developments in current and ongoing research. These exams are based on an in-depth job analysis and an industry-wide validation survey. By design, these exams assess a candidate's knowledge and application of the most current scientifically based professional standards and guidelines. The dynamic nature of this field requires that ACE certification exams be regularly updated to ensure they reflect the latest industry findings and research. Therefore, the knowledge and skills required to pass these exams are not solely represented in this or any industry text.

In addition to learning the material presented in this manual, ACE strongly encourages all exam candidates and fitness professionals to keep abreast of new developments, guidelines and standards from a variety of valid industry resources.

Domain I: Client Assessment

A. Establish an environment that is conducive to communication utilizing effective interview and communication methods in order to establish rapport and obtain accurate and comprehensive information.

Knowledge of:

1. Communication techniques (e.g., active listening, appropriate eye contact, reflecting and other attending behaviors).
2. Effective interviewing techniques (e.g., open-ended questioning, clarifying, paraphrasing, probing, informing, summarizing).
3. Factors that build and enhance rapport (e.g., empathy, genuineness, nonjudgmental responses).
4. Cultural, ethnic and personal differences as they affect communications, lifestyle, dietary habits and personal and interpersonal behavior.
5. Environmental factors that affect communication (e.g., location, noise, temperature, distractions, sense of privacy).
6. Body language, other nonverbal behaviors and the incongruities between verbal and nonverbal behaviors.
7. The factors that influence an individual's self-image and their impact on the communication process.
8. Common assumptions with regard to client's body size, eating habits, exercise habits and the impact of such assumptions on the client.
9. The complexity of issues related to obesity, body size, eating disorders and related lifestyle factors.
10. Governmental regulations and acceptable procedures as they apply to the confidentiality of client information.

Skill in:

1. Applying interviewing and communication techniques.
2. Interpreting body language and recognizing incongruities between verbal and nonverbal behaviors.
3. Selecting an appropriate environment for consultation sessions.
4. Building rapport.
5. Modifying interaction style and content appropriate to client's personal characteristics (e.g., gender, age, cultural/ethnic background) and individual behavioral style.
6. Avoiding prejudicial statements, negative body language, and/or unproductive assumptions with regard to client's body size, eating habits, exercise habits, past success/failures with weight management, etc.

B. Initially screen the client by reviewing health history in order to determine suitability for services and/or the need for referral.

Knowledge of:

1. Components of a client screening and health history form that document the client's physical and psychological health status, such as age, gender, body weight, blood pressure, personal health risk factors, mental health treatment history, symptoms of common psychological disorders (e.g., anxiety, depression, stress), family health history, biomechanical injuries/limitations, medications, weight loss history, physical activity patterns, nutrition profile, etc.
2. Physical and psychological conditions which may require referral to appropriate allied health

professionals (e.g., cardiovascular disease, diabetes, anorexia, bulimia, chronic dieting, compulsive over-eating, morbid obesity, hypertension, elevated lipids, pregnancy, HIV/AIDS, being underweight, asthma, COPD, stroke, arthritis, anxiety disorder, depression).

3. Effects and appropriate precautions to take with respect to prescription and non-prescription drugs (e.g., beta blockers, diuretics, antihistamines, tranquilizers, antidepressants, antianxiety, thyroid medications, alcohol, diet pills, cold medications, caffeine, nicotine).

4. Primary and secondary cardiovascular risk factors and their significance relative to referral and appropriate application of assessment tools.

5. Patterns of use of alcohol and other drugs and related health guidelines that determine abuse.

6. Applicable guidelines and position statements published by accepted organizations (e.g., American College of Sports Medicine [ACSM], American College of Obstetricians and Gynecologists [ACOG], American Heart Association [AHA], American Diabetes Association [ADA], Institute of Medicine [IOM], National Cholesterol Education Program [NCEP], U.S. Department of Agriculture [USDA]) and their implications for referral and weight management program participation.

7. Characteristics of appropriate allied health professionals (e.g., credibility, reliability, convenience, cost effectiveness, certification/ licensure) and resources to use for referrals.

8. Appropriate allied health professionals to use as referrals (e.g., physicians, psychotherapists, registered dietitians, certified fitness professionals).

9. Appropriate referral procedures/ methods for making referrals to allied health professionals.

10. Significance and limitations of measurement data obtained from assessment screening and testing.

Skill in:

1. Recognizing the characteristics of physical and psychological conditions that may indicate the need for referral.

2. Processing the client's health history and interview and observation data relative to accepted guidelines, and making safe and effective decisions regarding continuance and/ or referral.

3. Identifying and taking appropriate precautions with respect to prescription and non-prescription drugs.

4. Conferring with allied health professionals to interpret health data/ conditions.

5. Identifying appropriate allied health professionals to include in a referral program.

6. Recognizing alcohol and drug abuse and consulting with medical/mental health professionals.

C. **Determine client profile that includes current and past health conditions, risks, experience with health and fitness lifestyle change and goals by collecting and assessing all appropriate information in order to establish a baseline and understand the client's needs and expectations.**

Knowledge of:

1. The components of a comprehensive client profile including current and past health conditions, client's readiness to change, health risks, experience with health and fitness lifestyle change and personal weight

management goals.

2. Components of a client screening and health history form that adequately document the client's physical and psychological health status (e.g., age, gender, body weight, blood pressure, personal health risk factors, family health history, biomechanical injuries/limitations, medications, weight loss history, physical activity patterns, nutrition profile, client's readiness to change).

3. The factors that indicate a client's readiness to change (e.g., intrinsic and extrinsic motivators, past success with lifestyle change and weight management, goal setting experiences).

4. Genetic, psychological and physiological factors related to obesity and how they affect approaches to weight management.

5. Methods used to identify client goals.

6. Methods used to identify the methods and impact of a client's previous attempts at weight management.

7. Methods used to identify a client's perceived and unperceived needs and expectations for change.

8. Cognitive, affective, and psychomotor factors and learning styles that influence progress and goal attainment.

9. Knowledge of field test techniques used to determine aerobic, flexibility and strength fitness (e.g., walking tests, step tests, trial and error).

10. Warning signs and symptoms that require intervention during fitness tests.

11. Common aerobic fitness tests and protocols, and the purpose and value of testing.

12. The steps used to estimate percent body fat using circumference measurements (e.g., McArdle 3-site circumference test).

13. Body composition tests and protocols (e.g., hydrostatic weighing, skinfold calipers, bioimpedence).

14. The benefits and deficiencies of body composition testing and the appropriateness of applying this testing with respect to a given client's personal characteristics, needs and desires.

15. When to focus on healthy habits in lieu of a body weight/composition emphasis.

16. The relevance of assessment data in establishing client profile and short- and long-term goals.

17. Physiological effects and appropriate precautions to take with respect to beta blockers, diuretics, antihistamines, tranquilizers, alcohol, diet pills, cold medications, caffeine and nicotine.

18. The motivational/demotivational implications of fitness testing.

19. The applicability of assessment data to the development of the client profile.

20. Simple assessment tools to evaluate the client's preferences, probability of success, locus of control, rewards and support needs.

21. The relationship of body mass index (BMI) and waist-to-hip ratio (WHR) to body weight and the determination of appropriate body weight.

Skill in:

1. Assessing client screening, health history and field test data in the formulation of client profile.

2. Formulating a comprehensive client profile, including current and past health conditions, health risks, experience with health and fitness lifestyle change, readiness to change and personal weight management goals.

3. Conducting a thorough needs an

alysis in order to accurately recognize client's motivations/needs.

4. Recognizing the cognitive, affective, and psychomotor factors and learning styles that may warrant modifications in approach and possible consultation with an expert.

5. Evaluating the appropriateness, implications and application of past experiences with weight management relative to identified goals and expectations.

6. Determining aerobic, flexibility, strength fitness, and body composition utilizing accepted field tests and/or trial and error.

7. Recognizing warning signs and symptoms that require intervention during fitness tests.

D. Recognize conditions and/or behaviors on an ongoing basis using observation and assessment in order to identify the need for referral.

Knowledge of:

1. The significance of psychological and physical changes that may warrant referral (e.g., irregular eating patterns, injury, pregnancy, chest pain, dizziness, angina).

2. Appropriate allied health professionals to use as referrals (e.g., physicians, psychotherapists, registered dieticians, certified fitness professionals).

Skill in:

1. Identifying and determining the significance of psychological and physical changes and special needs that may warrant referral.

Domain II: Development of Client Plan

A. Utilize the assessment data by comparing it with accepted standards and guidelines in order to formulate recommendations for the client plan.

Knowledge of:

1. Applicable standards, guidelines, and position statements published by accepted organizations (e.g., ACSM, ACOG, ADA, AHA, IOM, NCEP, USDA, YMCA) to use in the formulation of recommendations.

2. Methods of interpreting the client profile as it relates to established guidelines.

Skill in:

1. Conferring with allied health professionals to interpret health data/conditions.

2. Applying acceptable standards and guidelines to use in the formulation of recommendations.

B. Collaboratively establish the client's specific long- and short-term goals by discussing recommendations and the client's needs, expectations and potential obstacles in order to formulate an achievable, realistic and measurable plan.

Knowledge of:

1. Principles of goal setting.

2. Qualities of a well-stated goal (i.e., specific, measurable, action-oriented, realistic, timed).

3. Safe and effective rates of change in physical fitness and body weight with respect to the development of weight management program recommendations.

4. Genetic, psychological and physiological factors related to obesity.

5. Typical obstacles that may interfere with the attainment of goals. (e.g., time restraints, weather changes, family obligations, financial issues).

6. Facilitating change as it applies to

the role of the weight management consultant (e.g., goal setting, support, motivation).

7. Adult learning fundamentals (e.g., basic assessment, learning and teaching styles, motivation).

8. Communication skills to ensure collaborative goal setting.

9. The six categories of nutrients and their functions.

10. The current Dietary Guidelines for Americans published by the USDA.

11. Nutrient and caloric content and fat/carbohydrate composition of common foods.

12. Cholesterol, lipoproteins and triglycerides as they apply to cardiovascular risk and dietary choices.

13. Safe and effective weight-loss methods.

14. The amount of safe and effective weight loss per week recommended for an unsupervised client.

15. The concepts of energy balance including factors that determine basal metabolic rate (BMR).

16. Energy requirements of common physical activities.

17. Unsafe or inappropriate approaches to weight loss (e.g., fasting, spot reducing, diet pills, drugs, fad diets).

18. Health, psychological and performance benefits of participation in physical activity programs.

19. The components of a physical fitness program.

20. The relationship of physical activity and exercise to health, physical fitness and weight management with respect to the mode, intensity, frequency and duration of activity.

21. Methods used to facilitate client's acceptance, responsibility and accountability for program goals.

Skill in:

1. Collaboratively setting goals that are specific, measurable, realistic,

action-oriented and time-bound.

2. Applying principles and knowledge of exercise, nutrition and weight management to the establishment of short- and long-term goals.

3. Using behavior change principles in goal-setting.

4. Using adult learning techniques with respect to the setting and prioritization of goals.

5. Delineating a client's responsibilities and accountability.

6. Applying safe and effective weight-loss methods.

7. Estimating the timeline for weight-loss goal attainment.

8. Communicating the benefits of weight management and participation in physical activity programs.

9. Determining special needs based on personal characteristics (e.g., age, gender, cultural influence).

C. Create a client plan incorporating safe, effective and alternative strategies that take into account client obstacles and methods for evaluating progress in order to achieve the client's goals.

Knowledge of:

1. Obstacles that may interfere with weight management program success (e.g., environmental, personal, financial, emotional, religious, ethnic/cultural factors).

2. Problem-solving strategies to overcome obstacles.

3. Methods for evaluating progress.

4. Modifications necessary for clients with special needs, including those who have been cleared by their physician to take part in a community-based/nonclinical weight management program.

5. Resources that provide acceptable standards and guidelines to use in the formulation of recommendations

(e.g., ACSM, YMCA, ACOG, USDA, ADA).

6. Different approaches to weight management and/or body composition change and the associated efficacy of each.

7. Self-monitoring techniques.

8. Food guide pyramid (number of servings per section), macronutrients and micronutrients.

9. Common nutritional supplements, weight loss products (e.g., chromium picolinate, herbs, isolated amino acids) and their effectiveness in weight management.

10. Caloric content of fats, proteins and carbohydrates.

11. The definition of kilocalories as applied to caloric intake and expenditure.

12. Basic exercise science with respect to aerobic vs. anaerobic activity, muscle mass changes and exercise program development.

13. Components of an activity program (i.e. aerobic, strength, flexibility).

14. Basic exercise programming with respect to frequency, intensity, duration and progression as applied to weight management.

15. Appropriate modes of physical activity (e.g., swimming, walking, biking, strength training) and their integration into a weight management exercise program.

16. Appropriate facilities, activities and organizations to refer clients to based on their activity needs.

17. Safe and effective fitness programs and products.

18. Dietary deficiencies and related health risks.

19. The characteristics (i.e., balance, variety, moderation) of a healthy eating plan.

Skill in:

1. Identifying obstacles to weight management program success and developing strategies to overcome them.

2. Reviewing goals, assessing progress and re-establishing goals based on findings.

3. Applying resources that provide acceptable standards and guidelines to use in the formulation of recommendations. (i.e., ACSM, YMCA, ACOG, USDA, ADA).

4. Safely and effectively applying different approaches to fat weight loss and/or body composition change.

5. Setting up self-monitoring systems for client's use.

6. Approximating caloric intake and expenditure.

7. Basic exercise programming, utilizing all of the components of an activity program (i.e. aerobic, strength, flexibility).

8. Applying the basic exercise programming principles (frequency, intensity, duration, progression).

9. The selection of appropriate physical activities for a weight management program.

10. Integrating safe and effective fitness programs and products into a weight management program.

Domain III: Implementation and Facilitation of Client Plan

A. **Establish a constructive professional relationship by employing effective interpersonal skills in order to support the client's efforts toward achieving goals.**

Knowledge of:

1. Communications techniques (e.g., active listening, appropriate eye contact, reflecting and other attending behaviors).

2. Factors that build and enhance rapport (e.g., empathy, genuineness, nonjudgmental responses).

3. Age, gender, cultural, ethnic and personal differences as they affect communications, lifestyle, dietary habits, and personal and interpersonal behavior.

4. Body language, other nonverbal behaviors and the incongruities between verbal and nonverbal behaviors.

5. The factors that influence an individual's self-image and their impact on the communication process.

6. The importance and application of feedback, re-enforcement, acknowledgment and encouragement.

7. Common assumptions with regard to client's body size, eating habits and exercise habits and the impact such assumptions have on the client.

8. Group dynamics and group stage development with their accompanying strategies as they affect the behavior of group members.

9. Types of groups (support vs. therapy) and their purposes and functions.

10. Group leader roles and styles.

11. Consultant's limitations concerning types of groups, group facilitation and the selection and referral of group members.

12. Impact of such factors as group size and frequency of meetings on group effectiveness.

Skill in:

1. Applying effective communication techniques.

2. Interpreting body language and recognizing incongruities between verbal and nonverbal behaviors.

3. Applying techniques that build rapport between consultant and client.

4. Modifying interaction style and content appropriate to client's personal

characteristics (e.g., gender, age, cultural/ethnic background) and individual behavioral style.

5. Observing and supporting client's efforts toward program goals.

B. Instruct the client by utilizing a variety of techniques and materials in order to develop the knowledge and/or skills required to promote adoption and adherence to the client's plan.

Knowledge of:

1. Adult learning fundamentals (e.g., basic assessment, learning and teaching styles, motivation).

2. Cognitive, affective, and psychomotor factors and learning styles in order to select appropriate educational techniques and materials.

3. Educational materials (safe, effective and client-appropriate).

4. The role and effect of social support in behavior change.

5. Relapse-prevention principles and maintenance strategies.

6. The relationship of exercise and nutrition to weight management.

7. Basic guidelines for preparing healthy foods.

8. High-fat and low-fat cooking methods.

9. Low-fat substitutions for traditionally high-fat foods.

10. Caloric density of foods as it relates to fat content and nutritional value, especially with respect to calorically dense, low/nonfat foods.

11. Food Guide Pyramid, including serving sizes.

12. Methods used to determine appropriate calorie levels for weight loss and weight maintenance.

13. Basic menu planning (translating the Food Guide Pyramid into daily food choices).

14. Food selection techniques when shopping or eating away from home.
15. Interpretation of current federally mandated food labeling.
16. Guidelines regarding the percent of calories from macronutrients (i.e. carbohydrates, fat, protein).
17. The six categories of nutrients and their functions.
18. The current Dietary Guidelines for Americans published by the USDA.
19. Nutritional misinformation and misconceptions.
20. Cholesterol, lipoproteins and triglycerides as they apply to cardiovascular risk and dietary choices.
21. Supplements and weight loss products (e.g., vitamins, minerals, chromium picolinate, herbs, isolated amino acids).
22. Risks associated with over-supplementation, liquid protein diets, diet pills and other commercially available weight management products.
23. The definition of kilocalories as applied to caloric intake and expenditure.
24. The concepts of energy balance.
25. Health risks associated with obesity.
26. Basic theories that address genetic and physiological causes of obesity (e.g., metabolic theories, "set point," fat cell distribution, size and number).
27. Risk factors and contributors that lead to obesity (e.g., culture, environment, heredity, inactivity, family history).
28. Commercially available, scientifically sound weight management programs and products.
29. Basic exercise science with respect to aerobic vs. anaerobic activity, muscle mass changes and exercise program development.
30. Components of an activity program (i.e. aerobic, strength, flexibility).
31. Basic exercise programming with

respect to frequency, intensity, duration and progression as applied to weight management.
32. Appropriate modes of physical activity (e.g., swimming, walking, biking, strength training) and their integration into a weight management exercise program.
33. Body composition and its relationship to obesity and weight management.
34. Appropriate application, safety and effectiveness of various weight management techniques (e.g., diet only, diet and exercise, exercise only, surgical interventions, pharmacological intervention, fasting, spot reducing).
35. Current myths and misconceptions related to nutrition, exercise and weight management.
36. Proper hydration during physical activity.
37. Environmental factors (e.g., heat, cold, pollution, elevation) related to physical activity.
38. Appropriate strategies to lead an effective group program through its developmental stages.
39. Methods for dealing with difficult clients in both the group setting and individual consulting.

Skill in:

1. Selection and application of appropriate educational techniques and materials.
2. Applying principles and knowledge of exercise, nutrition and weight management.
3. Assisting client in developing and/or enhancing social support systems.
4. Preparing client for lapses and plateaus and developing a plan of action to handle them.
5. Creating and facilitating group interaction.
6. Dealing with difficult clients in both

a group setting and individually.

7. Teaching clients to be good group members.

C. Monitor the client's participation in, and the effectiveness of, the plan through the use of direct observation, reassessments, client's self-reports and discussions in order to evaluate progress and update the client's plan, as necessary.

Knowledge of:

1. Timing, selection and procedures related to periodic reassessments.
2. Significance, limitations and incongruities of assessment data obtained through observation, client self report and direct measurement.
3. Barriers to program success (e.g., time management, self-image, self-efficacy, lifestyle, injury, personal characteristics, environment).
4. Relapse prevention principles and maintenance strategies.
5. Communication techniques (e.g., active listening, appropriate eye contact, reflecting and other attending behaviors).
6. Effective interviewing techniques (e.g., open-ended questioning, clarifying, paraphrasing, probing, informing, summarizing).
7. Safe and effective rates of change in physical fitness and body weight.
8. Knowledge of the complexity of issues related to obesity, body size, eating disorders and related lifestyle factors.

Skill in:

1. Application of reassessment techniques.
2. Evaluating reassessment data with respect to client plan.
3. Modifying client plan with respect to client progress and goals.

Domain IV: Professional Responsibility

A. Communicate and document, as necessary, the scope and limitations of the professional relationship between the consultant and client by delineating ethical and legal boundaries in order to protect the client and minimize liability.

Knowledge of:

1. Professional boundaries as they relate to the client/consultant relationship.
2. Consultant's responsibility in the clarification and documentation of roles in a professional relationship.
3. Lifestyle and weight management consultant's scope of practice as it relates to client's needs, consultant's knowledge and skills, and limitations to the scope of the service that a consultant can provide with respect to the fields of exercise, nutrition and behavior change.
4. Assumption of risk, including the use of waivers, warnings and informed consents.

B. Maintain professional standards by complying with all applicable laws and regulations and staying within the consultant's scope of practice and bounds of competence in order to make appropriate referrals, protect the client and minimize liability.

Knowledge of:

1. Copyright laws as they apply to print media, music and film.
2. Standard of care with respect to health screening, client referral and weight management program development and implementation.
3. Laws applicable to exercise programming, nutrition education and counseling.

4. Lifestyle and weight management consultant's scope of practice as it relates to client's needs, consultant's knowledge and skills, and limitations to the scope of the service that a consultant can provide with respect to the fields of exercise, nutrition and behavior change.

5. Personal issues and biases that may interfere with effectiveness.

C. Document client-related data, communications and progress by utilizing a record-keeping system that is confidential, accurate, current and retrievable in order to maintain continuity of care and minimize liability.

Knowledge of:

1. Significance of client data, communications and progress.
2. Effective and confidential record-keeping methods.

Skill in:

1. Assessing the significance of client data, communications and progress.
2. Effective record-keeping.

D. Assure continuing competence and professional growth by staying current with scientifically based research, theories and practice in order to provide the most effective services.

Knowledge of:

1. Available continuing education programs (e.g., conferences, college/ university courses, seminars, workshops, correspondence courses).
2. Appropriate and relevant publications (e.g., journals, consumer books, texts, videos, tapes).

E. Initiate emergency procedures by taking appropriate actions as defined in an emergency action plan to protect the client's safety.

Knowledge of:

1. CPR procedures.
2. Worksite emergency action plan.
3. Appropriate EMS system activation.

Skill in:

1. CPR
2. Utilizing the emergency action plan.
3. EMS system activation.

F. Adhere to the American Council of Exercise Code of Ethics by complying with this code in order to uphold professional standards.

Knowledge of:

1. ACE Code of Ethics.
2. Limitations to confidentiality (e.g., mandated reporting of abuse, court subpoena).
3. Process for reporting violations of the ACE Code of Ethics and the ACE Application and Certification Standards.

G. Obtain appropriate insurance in order to protect the client and minimize financial risk.

Knowledge of:

1. Professional liability insurance and its application to consultant's situation.

APPENDIX C

Sample Forms

Sample Forms

The following forms have been reprinted from *Legal Aspects of Preventive, Rehabilitative and Recreational Exercise Programs*, (3rd ed.), by D. L. Herbert and W. G. Herbert, with permission from P.R.C. Company, Canton, Ohio, and are offered for illustrative purposes only. A contract must adhere to the rules and regulations of the appropriate local governing entities and comply with the laws of the local jurisdictions in which they are executed. As with any contract, it is recommended that you seek professional legal assistance in developing its contents.

Informed Consent for Exercise Testing of Apparently Healthy Adults

(without known heart disease)

Name _____

1. Purpose and Explanation of Test

I hereby consent to voluntarily engage in an exercise test to determine my circulatory and respiratory fitness. I also consent to the taking of samples of my exhaled air during exercise to properly measure my oxygen consumption. I also consent, if necessary, to have a small blood sample drawn by needle from my arm for blood chemistry analysis, and to the performance of lung function and body fat (skin fold pinch) tests. It is my understanding that the information obtained will help me evaluate future physical activities and sports activities in which I may engage.

Before I undergo the test, I certify to the program that I am in good health and have had a physical examination conducted by a licensed medical physician within the last _____ months. Further, I hereby represent and inform the program that I have completed the pre-test history interview presented to me by the program staff and have provided correct responses to the questions as indicated on the history form or as supplied to the interviewer. It is my understanding that I will be interviewed by a physician or other person prior to my undergoing the test who will in the course of interviewing me determine if there are any reasons which would make it undesirable or unsafe for me to take the test. Consequently, I understand that it is important that I provide complete and accurate responses to the interviewer and recognize that my failure to do so could lead to possible unnecessary injury to myself during the test.

The test which I will undergo will be performed on a motor driven treadmill or bicycle ergometer with the amount of effort gradually increasing. As I understand it, this increase in effort will continue until I feel, and verbally report to the operator, any symptoms such as fatigue, shortness of breath or chest discomfort which may appear. It is my understanding, and I have been clearly advised, that it is my right to request that a test be stopped at any point if I feel unusual discomfort or fatigue. I have been advised that I should, immediately upon experiencing any such symptoms or if I so choose, inform the operator that I wish to stop the test at that or any other point. My wishes in this regard shall be absolutely carried out.

It is further my understanding that prior to beginning the test, I will be connected by electrodes and cables to an electrocardiographic recorder which will enable the program personnel to monitor my cardiac (heart) activity. During the test itself, it is my understanding that a trained observer will monitor my responses continuously and take frequent readings of blood pressure, the electrocardiogram, and my expressed feelings of effort. I realize that a true determination of my exercise capacity depends on progressing the test to the point of my fatigue. Once the test has been completed, but before I am released from the test area, I will be given special instructions about showering and recognition of certain symptoms which may appear within the first 24 hours after the test. I agree to follow these instructions and promptly contact the program personnel or medical providers if such symptoms develop.

2. Risks

It is my understanding, and I have been informed, that there exists the possibility of adverse changes during the actual test. I have been informed that these changes could include abnormal blood pressure, fainting, disorders of heart rhythm, stroke and very rare instances of heart attack or even death. Every effort, I have been told, will be made to minimize these occurrences by preliminary examination and by precautions and observations taken during the test. I have also been informed that emergency equipment and personnel are readily available to deal with these unusual situations should they occur. I understand that there is a risk of injury, heart attack, stroke or even death as a result of my performance of this test, but knowing those risks, it is my desire to proceed to take the test as herein indicated.

3. Benefits to be Expected and Alternatives Available to the Exercise Testing Procedure

The results of this test may or may not benefit me. Potential benefits relate mainly to my personal motives for taking the test, i.e., knowing my exercise capacity in relation to the general population, understanding my fitness for certain sports and recreational activities, planning my physical conditioning program or evaluating the effects of my recent physical activity habits. Although my fitness might also be evaluated by alternative means, e.g., a bench step test or an outdoor running test, such tests do not provide as accurate a fitness assessment as the treadmill or bike test nor do those options allow equally effective monitoring of my responses.

4. Confidentiality and Use of Information

I have been informed that the information which is obtained in this exercise test will be treated as privileged and confidential and will consequently not be released or revealed to any person without my express written consent. I do, however, agree to the use of any information for research or statistical purposes so long as same does not provide facts which could lead to the identification of my person. Any other information obtained, however, will be used only by the program staff to evaluate my exercise status or needs.

5. Inquiries and Freedom of Consent

I have been given an opportunity to ask questions as to the procedure. Generally these requests, which have been noted by the testing staff, and their responses are as follows:

_____

_____

_____

I further understand that there are also remote risks that may be associated with this procedure. Despite the fact that a complete accounting of all remote risks is not entirely possible, I am satisfied with the review of these risks, which was provided to me, and it is still my desire to proceed with the test.

I acknowledge that I have read this document in its entirety or that it has been read to me if I have been unable to read same.

I consent to the rendition of all services and procedures as explained herein by all program personnel.

_____   _____

Patient's Signature   Date

_____

Witness' Signature

_____

Test Supervisor's Signature

Alternative Form for Informed Consent for Exercise Testing Procedures of Apparently Healthy Adults

Name_____

1. Purpose and Explanation of Test

It is my understanding that I will undergo a test to be performed on a motor driven treadmill or bicycle ergometer with the amount of effort gradually increasing. As I understand it, this increase in effort will continue until I feel, and verbally report to the operator, any symptoms such as fatigue, shortness of breath or chest discomfort which may appear, or until the test is completed or otherwise terminated. It is my understanding, and I have been clearly advised, that it is my right to request that a test be stopped at any point if I feel unusual discomfort or fatigue. I have been advised that I should immediately upon experiencing any such symptoms, or if I so choose, inform the operator that I wish to stop the test at that or any other point. My stated wishes in this regard shall be carried out. **IF CORRECT, AND YOU AGREE AND UNDERSTAND, INITIAL HERE_____.**

It is further my understanding that prior to beginning the test, I will be connected by electrodes and cables to an electrocardiographic recorder which will enable the program personnel to monitor my cardiac (heart) activity. During the test itself, it is my understanding that a trained observer will monitor my responses continuously and take frequent readings of blood pressure, the electrocardiogram and my expressed feelings of effort. I realize that a true determination of my exercise capacity depends on progressing the test to the point of my fatigue. Once the test has been completed, but before I am released from the test area, I will be given special instructions about showering and recognition of certain symptoms which may appear within the first 24 hours after the test. I agree to follow these instructions and promptly contact the program personnel or medical providers if such symptoms develop. **IF CORRECT, AND YOU AGREE AND UNDERSTAND, INITIAL HERE_____.**

Before I undergo the test, I certify to the program that I am in good health and have had a physical examination conducted by a licensed medical physician within the last_____months. Further, I hereby represent and inform the program that I have accurately completed the pre-test history interview presented to me by the program staff and have provided correct responses to the questions as indicated on the history form or as supplied to the interviewer. It is my understanding that I will be interviewed by a physician or other person prior to my undergoing the test who will, in the course of interviewing me, determine if there are any reasons which would make it undesirable or unsafe for me to take the test. Consequently, I understand that it is important that I provide complete and accurate responses to the interviewer and recognize that my failure to do so could lead to possible unnecessary injury to myself during the test. **IF CORRECT, AND YOU AGREE, INITIAL HERE_____.**

2. Risks

It is my understanding, and I have been informed, that there exists the possibility of adverse changes during the actual test. I have been informed that these changes could include abnormal blood pressure, fainting, disorders of heart rhythm, stroke and very rare instances of heart attack or even death. I have also been informed that aside from the foregoing, other risks exist. These risks include, but are not necessarily limited to the possibility of stroke, or other cerebrovascular or cardiovascular incident or occurrence, mental, physiological, motor, visual or hearing injuries, deficiencies, difficulties or disturbances, partial or total paralysis, slips, falls, or other unintended loss of balance or bodily movement related to the exercise treadmill (or bicycle ergometer) which may cause muscular, neurological, orthopedic or other bodily injury as well as a variety of other possible occurrences, any one of which could conceivably, however remotely, cause bodily injury, impairment, disability or death. Any procedure such as this one carries with it some risk however unlikely or remote. THERE ARE ALSO OTHER RISKS OF INJURY, IMPAIRMENT, DISABILITY, DISFIGUREMENT, AND EVEN DEATH. I ACKNOWLEDGE AND AGREE TO ASSUME ALL RISKS. **IF YOU UNDERSTAND AND AGREE, INITIAL HERE_____.**

Every effort, I have been told, will be made to minimize these occurrences by preliminary examination and by precautions and observations taken during the test. I have also been informed that emergency equipment and personnel are readily available to deal with these unusual situations should they occur.

Knowing and understanding all risks, it is my desire to proceed to take the test as herein described. **IF CORRECT, AND YOU AGREE AND UNDERSTAND, INITIAL HERE_____.**

3. Benefits to be Expected and Alternatives Available to the Exercise Testing Procedure

I understand and have been told that the results of this test may or may not benefit me. Potential benefits relate mainly to my personal motives for taking the test. (i.e., knowing my exercise capacity in relation to the general population, understanding my fitness for certain sports and recreational activities, planning my physical conditioning program or evaluating the effects of my recent physical activity habits). Although my fitness might also be evaluated by alternative means, e.g., a bench step test or an outdoor running test, such tests do not provide as accurate a fitness assessment as the treadmill or bike test, nor do those options allow equally effective monitoring of my responses. **IF YOU UNDERSTAND, INITIAL HERE_____.**

4. Consent

I hereby consent to voluntarily engage in an exercise test to determine my circulatory and respiratory fitness. I also consent to the taking of samples of my exhaled air during exercise to properly measure my oxygen consumption. I also consent, if necessary, to have a small blood sample drawn by needle from my arm for blood chemistry analysis, and to the performance of lung function and body fat (skinfold pinch) tests. It is my understanding that the information obtained will help me evaluate future physical fitness and sports activities in which I may engage. **IF CORRECT, AND YOU AGREE, INITIAL HERE_____.**

5. Confidentiality and Use of Information

I have been informed that the information which is obtained in this exercise test will be treated as privileged and confidential and will consequently not be released or revealed to any person without my express written consent. I do, however, agree to the use of any information for research or statistical purposes, so long as same does not provide facts which could lead to the identification of my person. Any other information obtained, however, will be used only by the program staff to evaluate my exercise status or needs. **IF YOU AGREE, INITIAL HERE_____.**

6. Inquiries and Freedom of Consent

I have been given an opportunity to ask questions as to the procedures. Generally these requests, which have been noted by the testing staff, and their responses are as follows:

_____

_____

IF THIS NOTATION IS COMPLETE AND CORRECT, INITIAL HERE_____.

I acknowledge that I have read this document in its entirety or that it has been read to me if I have been unable to read same.

I consent to the rendition of all services and procedures as explained herein by all program personnel.

_____
Date

_____   _____
Witness' Signature   Participant's Signature

_____   _____
Witness' Signature   Spouse's Consent

_____
Test Supervisor's Signature

Informed Consent for Participation in an
Exercise Program for Apparently Healthy Adults

(without known or suspected heart disease)

Name _____

1. Purpose and Explanation of Procedure

I hereby consent to voluntarily engage in an acceptable plan of exercise conditioning. I also give consent to be placed in program activities which are recommended to me for improvement of my general health and well-being. These may include dietary counseling, stress reduction, and health education activities. The levels of exercise which I will perform will be based upon my cardiorespiratory (heart and lungs) fitness as determined through my recent laboratory graded exercise evaluation. I will be given exact instructions regarding the amount and kind of exercise I should do. I agree to participate three times per week in the formal program sessions. Professionally trained personnel will provide leadership to direct my activities, monitor my performance, and otherwise evaluate my effort. Depending upon my health status, I may or may not be required to have my blood pressure and heart rate evaluated during these sessions to regulate my exercise within desired limits. I understand that I am expected to attend every session and to follow staff instructions with regard to exercise, diet, stress management, and smoking cessation. If I am taking prescribed medications, I have already so informed the program staff and further agree to so inform them promptly of any changes which my doctor or I have made with regard to use of these. I will be given the opportunity for periodic assessment with laboratory evaluations at 6 months after the start of my program. Should I remain in the program thereafter, additional evaluations will generally be given at 12 month intervals. The program may change the foregoing schedule of evaluations, if this is considered desirable for health reasons. I have been informed that during my participation in exercise, I will be asked to complete the physical activities unless symptoms such as fatigue, shortness of breath, chest discomfort or similar occurrences appear. At that point, I have been advised it is my complete right to decrease or stop exercise and that it is my obligation to inform the program personnel of my symptoms. I hereby state that I have been so advised and agree to inform the program personnel of my symptoms, should any develop.

I understand that during the performance of exercise, a trained observer will periodically monitor my performance and, perhaps measure my pulse, blood pressure or assess my feelings of effort for the purposes of monitoring my progress. I also understand that the observer may reduce or stop my exercise program when any of these findings so indicate that this should be done for my safety and benefit.

2. Risks

It is my understanding, and I have been informed, that there exists the remote possibility during exercise of adverse changes including abnormal blood pressure, fainting, disorders of heart rhythm, and very rare instances of heart attack, stroke or even death. Every effort, I have been told, will be made to minimize these occurrences by proper staff assessment of my condition before each exercise session, staff supervision during exercise and by my own careful control of exercise efforts. I have also been informed that emergency equipment and personnel are readily available to deal with unusual situations should these occur. I understand that there is a risk of injury, heart attack or even death as a result of my exercise, but knowing those risks, it is my desire to participate as herein indicated.

3. Benefits to be Expected and Alternatives Available to Exercise

I understand that this program may or may not benefit my physical fitness or general health. I recognize that involvement in the exercise sessions will allow me to learn proper ways to perform conditioning exercises, use fitness equipment and regulate physical effort. These experiences should benefit me by indicating how my physical limitations may affect my ability to perform various physical activities. I further understand that if I closely follow the program instructions, that I will likely improve my exercise capacity after a period of 3-6 months.

4. Confidentiality and Use of Information

I have been informed that the information which is obtained in this exercise program will be treated as privileged and confidential and will consequently not be released or revealed to any person without my express written consent. I do, however, agree to the use of any information which is not personally identifiable with me for research and statistical purposes, so long as same does not identify my person or provide facts which could lead to my identification. Any other information obtained, however, will be used only by the program staff in the course of prescribing exercise for me and evaluating my progress in the program.

5. Inquiries and Freedom of Consent

I have been given an opportunity to ask questions as to the procedures of this program. Generally these requests, which have been noted by the interviewing staff member, and his/her responses are as follows:

_____

_____

I further understand that there are also other remote risks that may be associated with this program. Despite the fact that a complete accounting of all these remote risks is not entirely possible, I am satisfied with the review of these risks which was provided to me and it is still my desire to participate.

I acknowledge that I have read this document in its entirety or that it has been read to me if I have been unable to read same.

I consent to the rendition of all services and procedures as explained herein by all program personnel.

_____   _____

Patient's Signature   Date

_____

Witness' Signature

_____

Test Supervisor's Signature

Alternative Clauses to be Considered for
Possible Addition to Informed Consent Forms or Pre-Participation Forms

1. Anxious Patient - Additional Spousal Consent

I have been informed by _____, that a full disclosure of all known risks associated with the procedure to be performed by my spouse has not been given to my spouse. This is because in the professional opinion and judgment of _____ such disclosure would have adverse consequences to my spouse and would expose my spouse to an increased risk while undergoing the procedure due to his/her anxiety and nervousness as to the procedure itself and the risks involved with treatment procedures. Consequently, I have been informed by _____ of the following risks which were not disclosed to my spouse:

_____

_____

_____

_____

It is my agreement and consent that despite these risks, and the lack of full communication of same to my spouse, the procedure be carried out as to my spouse inasmuch as _____ has explained to me that the following benefits may be derived from the procedure:

_____

_____

_____

I agree with the assessment of _____, that further explanation as to the details of the test would undoubtedly cause increased anxiety and stress in my spouse and as a consequence thereof, I believe that no further disclosure should be made to my spouse and that the test procedure should be performed as previously described.

2. Prospective Release Claims

In consideration of my admission to this program, I do hereby agree to assume all risks of injury or death to myself while using the program's facilities and equipment. I represent that I am completely aware of all risks and hazards inherent in my participation in the program. I agree that the program and personnel shall not be liable for any dangers arising from personal injury or death to myself even if such injuries or death shall be caused by the negligence of the program or any of its agents. I agree to and do hereby release the program and all of its personnel and agents, successors and assigns from any and all damages, demands, claims, causes of action, present or future, disclosed or undisclosed, anticipated or unanticipated, caused by or resulting from the negligence of the program, or any of its employees or agents or otherwise, and arising out of my use or attempted use of any of the program's facilities or equipment.

This agreement shall be binding upon the undersigned and my heirs, executors, and administrators.

3. Severability Clause for Use With Prospective Release Form Containing Exculpatory Language

In the event that any court should conclude that any portion of this document is unenforceable or void, such a determination shall not affect the remaining provisions of the document, which shall survive such a declaration.

4. Release of Information Clause

I agree to allow the program to take my photograph or photographs either while I am at rest, or while exercising or performing any activity with the program. I further agree to allow the program to use any of my photographs for publicity purposes to advertise the program. I also agree to the use of any likeness of myself in connection therewith and to the disclosure of my name, address, age and other personal information in connection therewith.

5. Additional Language for Informed Consents for Patients In Those Jurisdictions Where Children May Have a Separate Cause of Action for Loss of Parental Consortium

I (We), the undersigned participant (and spouse of the participant), do hereby agree to indemnify and hold the program and its personnel absolutely harmless from any and all claims, causes of actions, or damages which may be sought or assessed against the program or its personnel by reason of any claim or demand or suit brought by my estate or by my (our) heirs or children as a result of any claimed injuries to me (us), or as the result of any claimed interference with the relationship of parent and child. I (We) agree to indemnify the program and its personnel against all costs, fees, including attorney fees, damages and expenses of any kind by reason of any claims or suits brought or threatened as aforesaid.

Agreement and Release of Liability

1. In consideration of being allowed to participate in the activities and programs of _____ and to use its facilities, equipment and machinery in addition to the payment of any fee or charge, I do hereby waive, release and forever discharge _____ and its directors, officers, agents, employees, representatives, successors and assignees, administrators, executors, and all others from any and all responsibilities or liability from injuries or damages resulting from my participation in any activities or my use of equipment or machinery in the above mentioned activities. I do also hereby release all of those mentioned, and any others acting upon their behalf, from any responsibility or liability for any injury or damage to myself, including those caused by the negligent act or omission of any of those mentioned, or others acting on their behalf or in any way arising out of or connected with my participation in any activities of _____ or the use of any equipment at _____.
   IF YOU AGREE, PLEASE INITIAL _____.

2. I understand and am aware that strength, flexibility and aerobic exercise, including the use of equipment, is a potentially hazardous activity. I also understand that fitness activities involve the risk of injury and even death, and that I am voluntarily participating in these activities and using equipment and machinery with knowledge of the dangers involved. I hereby agree to expressly assume and accept any and all risks of injury or death.
   IF YOU AGREE, PLEASE INITIAL _____.

3. I do hereby further declare myself to be physically sound and suffering from no condition, impairment, disease, infirmity or other illness that would prevent my participation or use of equipment or machinery except as hereinafter stated. I do hereby acknowledge that I have been informed of the need for a physician's approval for my participation in an exercise/fitness activity or in the use of exercise equipment and machinery. I also acknowledge that it has been recommended that I have a yearly or more frequent physical examination and consultation with my physician as to physical activity, exercise and use of exercise and training equipment so that I might have his or her recommendations concerning these fitness activities and equipment use. I acknowledge that I have had a physical examination and have been given my physician's permission to participate, or that I have decided to participate in activity and use of equipment and machinery without the approval of my physician and do hereby assume all responsibility for my participation and activities, and utilization of equipment and machinery in my activities.
   IF YOU AGREE, PLEASE INITIAL _____.

_____   _____

Date   Signature

Medical Approval

_____ has medical approval to participate in fitness activities and exercise

programs and in the use of _____ equipment and machinery at

_____ .

The following restrictions apply (if none, so state):

_____

_____

_____

_____

Physician's Signature

_____

Physician's Name

_____

Address

_____

Date

Express Assumption of Risk For Participation In Specified Activity

I, the undersigned, hereby expressly and affirmatively state that I wish to participate in _____ .
I realize that my participation in this activity involves risk of injury, including, but not to limited to (list)

_____

_____

_____

and even the possibility of death. I also recognize that there are many other risks of injury including serious disabling injuries which may arise due to my participation in this activity and that it is not possible to specifically list each and every individual injury risk. However, knowing the material risks and appreciating, knowing and reasonably anticipating that other injuries and even death are a possibility, I hereby expressly assume all of the delineated risks of injury, all other possible risk of injury, and even death, which could occur by reason of my participation.

I have had an opportunity to ask questions. Any questions which I have asked have been answered to my complete satisfaction. I subjectively understand the risks of my participation in this activity and knowing and appreciating these risks I voluntarily choose to participate, assuming all risks of injury or even death due to my participation.

_____   _____
Witness   Participant

_____
Dated

NOTES OF QUESTIONS AND ANSWERS

_____

_____

_____

This is, as stated, a true and accurate record of what was asked and answered.

_____
Participant

TO BE CHECKED BY PROGRAM STAFF

CHECKED INITIALS

1. RISKS WERE ORALLY DISCUSSED. _____
2. QUESTIONS WERE ASKED AND THE PARTICIPANT INDICATED COMPLETE UNDERSTANDING OF THE RISKS. _____
3. QUESTIONS WERE NOT ASKED, BUT AN OPPORTUNITY TO QUESTION WAS PROVIDED AND THE PARTICIPANT INDICATED COMPLETE UNDERSTANDING OF THE RISKS. _____

_____   _____
Staff Member   Date

Alternative Form - Express Assumption of
Risk/Prospective Waiver of Liability and Release Agreement

I, the undersigned, hereby expressly and affirmatively state that I wish to participate in fitness assessments, activities and programs and in the use of exercise equipment at various sites, including home, club or worksite, that may be provided or recommended by _____ (hereinafter "Facility"). I realize that my participation in these activities or in the use of equipment involves various risks of injury including, but not limited to (list)

_____

_____

_____

and even the possibility of death. I also recognize that there are many other risks of injury, including serious disabling injuries, that may arise due to my participation in these activities or in the use of equipment, and that such risks, including remote ones, have been reviewed with me. I also understand that under some circumstances I may choose to engage in activity in a non-supervised setting under circumstances where there is no one to respond to any emergency that may arise as a result of my participation or use of equipment on an individual basis, in an unsupervised setting. Despite the fact that I have been duly cautioned as to such unsupervised and unattended activity or equipment use, and despite the fact that I have been advised against such activity and equipment use in an unsupervised and unattended setting, I, knowing the material risks and appreciating, knowing and reasonably anticipating that other injuries and even death are a possibility as a result of my participation in fitness assessments, activities or programs or in the use of equipment in supervised/attended and unsupervised/unattended settings (within which settings I acknowledge that the risks of injury or death may be greater than in other settings), hereby expressly assume all of the delineated risks of injury, all other possible risks of injury and even the risk of death which could occur by reason of my participation in any of the assessments, activities or programs or in the use of equipment in any or all settings.
IF YOU AGREE, PLEASE INITIAL _____.

I have had an opportunity to ask questions regarding my participation in various activities and in the use of exercise equipment. Any questions I have asked have been answered to my complete satisfaction. I subjectively understand the risks of my participation in various activities or in the use of equipment, and knowing and appreciating these risks, I voluntarily choose to participate, assuming all risks of injury and death which may arise due to my participation
IF YOU AGREE, PLEASE INITIAL _____.

I further acknowledge that my participation in the activities and use of equipment is completely voluntary and that it is my choice to participate and/or use equipment, or not to participate, as I see fit.
IF YOU AGREE, PLEASE INITIAL _____.

In consideration of being allowed to participate in the activities and programs provided through (Facility) and/or in the use of its facilities and equipment, I do hereby waive, release and forever discharge (Facility), and all of its directors, officers, agents, employees, representatives, successors and assigns, and all others from any and all responsibility or liability for injuries or damages resulting from my participation in any activities at (Facility) or elsewhere. I do also hereby release all of those mentioned, and any others acting upon their behalf, from any responsibility or liability for any injury or damage to myself, including those caused by the negligent act or omission of any of those mentioned or others acting on their behalf, or in any way arising out of or connected with my participation in any of the contemplated activities or in the use of equipment through (Facility) or otherwise.
IF YOU AGREE, PLEASE INITIAL _____.

I understand and am aware that strength, flexibility and aerobic exercise including the use of equipment is a potentially hazardous activity. I also understand that fitness activities involve a risk of injury and even death, and that I am voluntarily participating in these activities and using equipment with knowledge of the dangers involved.
IF YOU AGREE, PLEASE INITIAL _____.

I do further declare myself to be physically sound and suffering from no condition, impairment, disease, infirmity or other illness that would prevent my participation in any of the activities and programs provided through (Facility) or in the use of equipment and machinery except as hereinafter stated:

_____. I do hereby acknowledge that I have been informed of the need or desirability for a physician's approval for my participation in exercise/fitness activity or in the use of exercise equipment. I also acknowledge that it has been recommended that I have a yearly or more frequent physical examination and consultation with my physician as to physical activities, exercise and as to the use of exercise equipment, so that I might have recommendations concerning these physical activities and equipment use. I acknowledge that I have either had a physical examination and have been given my physicians' permission to participate, or that I have decided to participate in activity and/or use of equipment without the approval of my physician and do hereby assume all responsibility for my participation and activities or in the utilization of equipment without that approval.
IF YOU AGREE, PLEASE INITIAL _____.

I, the undersigned spouse of the participant, do hereby further acknowledge that my spouse/participant wishes to engage in certain activities and programs provided by (Facility) including the use of various facilities and equipment. In consideration of my spouse's/participant's voluntary decision to engage in such activities, and in consideration of the provision of such activities and equipment to spouse by (Facility), I the undersigned do hereby waive, release and forever discharge (Facility) and its directors, officers, agents, employees, representatives, successors and assignees and all other from any and all responsibility or liability for any injuries or damages resulting from my spouse's participation in any activities or in my spouse's use of equipment as a result of participation in any such activities or otherwise arising out of that participation. I do further release all of those above mentioned and any others acting upon their behalf from any responsibility or liability for any injury to or even death of my spouse, including those caused by the negligent act or omission of any of those mentioned or others acting upon their behalf or in any way arising out of or connected with my spouse's participation in any of the activities provided by (Facility) or in the use of any equipment at any location. I specifically acknowledge that my execution of this prospective Waiver and Release relinquishes any cause of action that I may have either directly, through my spouse or independently by way of a loss of consortium or other type of action of any kind or nature whatsoever and I do hereby further agree to my spouse's participation in the activities as above mentioned and in the use of any equipment at any location.

IF YOU AGREE, PLEASE INITIAL _____.

IN WITNESS WHEREOF, the participant and the participant's spouse, if any, have executed this Express Assumption of Risk/Prospective Waiver of Liability and Release Agreement this ____ day of _____, 19_____, which shall be binding upon each of them and their respective heirs, executors, administrators and assigns. Each does hereby further agree to indemnify and hold (Facility) and all those identified or named herein absolutely harmless in the event that anyone claiming any cause of action as a result of any injury and/or death to participant or spouse attempts at any time to institute any claim or suit against (Facility) arising out of any of the activities or programs herein or in the use of any equipment.

Signed in the presence of:

_____   _____
                                              Participant

_____   _____
                                              Participant's Spouse

RELEASE OF INFORMATION FORM

TO WHOM IT MAY CONCERN:

Please furnish to _____ (hereinafter "Facility") and/or all of its personnel, information, copies of any and all hospital and medical records or reports of any sort, charts, notes, x-rays, lab reports and prescription information, including the right to inspect and copy such records. Facility is to be furnished with any and all other information without limitation pertaining to any confinement, examination, treatment or condition of myself, including medical, dental, psychological or other treatment, examinations, or counseling for any condition, medical, dental or psychological.

This AUTHORIZATION shall be considered as continuing and you may rely upon it in all respects unless you have previously been advised by me in writing to the contrary. It is expressly understood by the undersigned and you are hereby authorized to accept a copy or photocopy of this medical authorization with the same validity as though an original had been presented to you.

Dated this _____ day of _____, 19_____.

Signature _____

Name _____

Address _____

Phone_____

PRINCIPLES FOR EMERGENCY RESPONSE SYSTEMS IN ADULT EXERCISE FACILITIES

Staff Competency & Certification

- Require current AHA certification (or equivalent) in CPR for all staff who routinely interact with clients
- At appropriate intervals, schedule and require staff to practice CPR skills in the context of mock emergencies
- In any facility that provides exercise services for patients with known or suspected cardiopulmonary or metabolic diseases, require the presence of a licensed physician or his/her legally authorized surrogate who has the necessary skills, certifications and equipment to quickly and effectively activate the early steps of ACLS care

Protocols & Documentation

- Develop emergency response plans, including Physician Standing Orders (if appropriate), through a team development process that includes the principal supervisory exercise professional in the facility and a licensed physician (or other responsible representative of the community EMS system) who utilizes ACLS skills with some regularity in medical practices.
- Write emergency plans that fully conform to the most current AHA Guidelines; cross reference important procedural elements in the written plan of the facility with the most relevant sections from the AHA publication.
- Apply the emergency planning concept in ACSM's RESOURCE MANUAL only after prudent consideration of the facility's service objectives (e.g., health improvement or recreation) and attendant risks of cardiovascular complications in exercise for the highest risk participants.

---

* Very recently, the AHA revised its "Guidelines for Cardiopulmonary Resuscitation and Emergency Cardiac Care," JAMA 268 (16): 2171 - 2302, 1992). This new AHA publication contains several important changes, e.g., priorities for activation of EMS system when CPR must be initiated and for rapid electrical defibrillation when ventricular fibrillation is confirmed. In particular, the ACLS algorhythms are quite detailed and require more clinical sophistication to execute than the previous set. Moreover, the new ACSM's RESOURCE MANUAL FOR GUIDELINES FOR EXERCISE TESTING AND PRESCRIPTION, (2nd ed.), Lea & Febiger, Philadelphia, PA, 1993, p. 367 - 377, suggests different levels of response readiness for different situations. Unfortunately, the minimum standard of emergency care for adult exercise facilities has been made more uncertain by these new publications. Therefore, we suggest the process outlined in the previous principles as a basis for developing or updating emergency response plans for specific exercise facilities.

APPENDIX D

**Performance Guidelines
One-rescuer CPR: Adult**

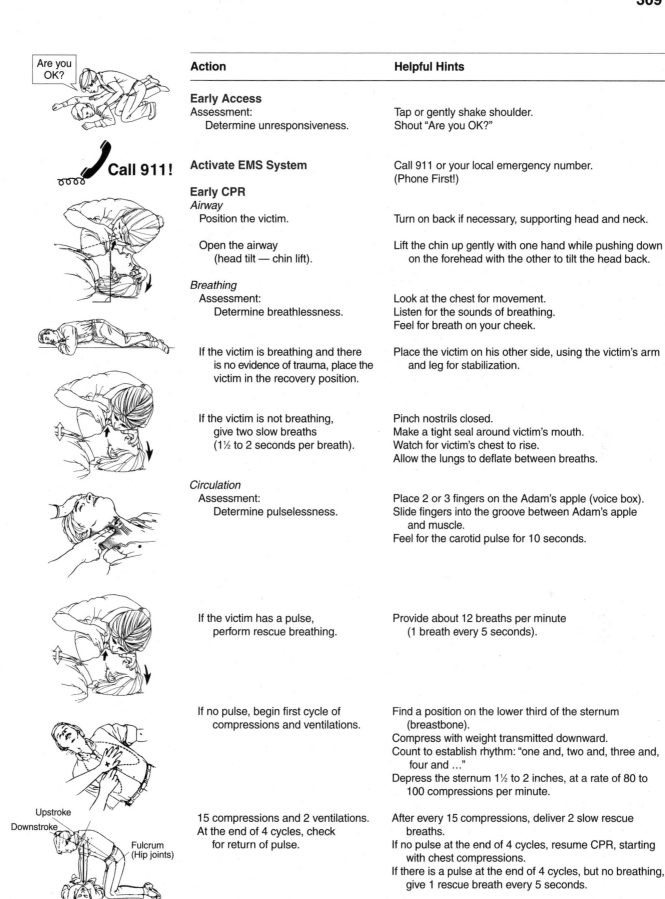

Action	Helpful Hints
Early Access Assessment: Determine unresponsiveness.	Tap or gently shake shoulder. Shout "Are you OK?"
Activate EMS System	Call 911 or your local emergency number. (Phone First!)
Early CPR *Airway* Position the victim.	Turn on back if necessary, supporting head and neck.

Open the airway
        (head tilt — chin lift).
	Lift the chin up gently with one hand while pushing down
	    on the forehead with the other to tilt the head back.

Breathing
    Assessment:
        Determine breathlessness.
	Look at the chest for movement.
	Listen for the sounds of breathing.
	Feel for breath on your cheek.

If the victim is breathing and there
      is no evidence of trauma, place the
      victim in the recovery position.
	Place the victim on his other side, using the victim's arm
	    and leg for stabilization.

If the victim is not breathing,
      give two slow breaths
      (1½ to 2 seconds per breath).
	Pinch nostrils closed.
	Make a tight seal around victim's mouth.
	Watch for victim's chest to rise.
	Allow the lungs to deflate between breaths.

Circulation
    Assessment:
        Determine pulselessness.
	Place 2 or 3 fingers on the Adam's apple (voice box).
	Slide fingers into the groove between Adam's apple
	    and muscle.
	Feel for the carotid pulse for 10 seconds.

If the victim has a pulse,
      perform rescue breathing.
	Provide about 12 breaths per minute
	    (1 breath every 5 seconds).

If no pulse, begin first cycle of
      compressions and ventilations.
	Find a position on the lower third of the sternum
	    (breastbone).
	Compress with weight transmitted downward.
	Count to establish rhythm: "one and, two and, three and,
	    four and …"
	Depress the sternum 1½ to 2 inches, at a rate of 80 to
	    100 compressions per minute.

15 compressions and 2 ventilations.
    At the end of 4 cycles, check
      for return of pulse.
	After every 15 compressions, deliver 2 slow rescue
	    breaths.
	If no pulse at the end of 4 cycles, resume CPR, starting
	    with chest compressions.
	If there is a pulse at the end of 4 cycles, but no breathing,
	    give 1 rescue breath every 5 seconds.

Source: *Basic Life Support Heartsaver Guide*, American Heart Association, 1993.

Glossary

Absorption   The uptake of substances into, or across tissues, e.g., skin, intestine and kidney tubules.

Adenosine Triphosphate (ATP)   The high-energy phosphate molecule that provides energy for cellular function.

Adipose tissue   Fatty tissue; connective tissue made up of fat cells.

Aerobic energy system   The metabolic pathway that, in the presence of oxygen, uses glucose for energy production. Also called aerobic glycolysis.

Amenorrhea   The absence of menstruation, usually in a premenopausal woman.

Amino acids   Nitrogen-containing compounds that are the building blocks of proteins.

Anaerobic creatine phosphate system   A metabolic pathway that resynthesizes ATP rapidly, and without oxygen, through the transfer of chemical energy from the high-energy compound creatine phosphate.

Anaerobic glucose system   The metabolic pathway that uses glucose for energy production without requiring oxygen, and produces lactic acid as a by-product.

Anaerobic threshold   The point during high-intensity activity when the body can no longer meet its demand for oxygen and anaerobic metabolism predominates. Also called lactate threshold.

Anemia   A reduction in the number of red blood cells and/or quantity of hemoglobin per volume of blood to below normal.

Angina pectoris   Chest pain caused by inadequate blood flow, and thus oxygen supply, to the heart. Often aggravated or induced by exercise or stress.

Anorexia nervosa   An eating disorder characterized by extreme thinness, distorted body image and a fear of becoming obese.

Antecedent   The stimuli that precedes a given behavior, sometimes referred to as a cue or a trigger.

Anthropometric   Pertaining to the measurement of the size, weight and proportions of the human body.

Antibodies   Immunoglobulin molecules that have a specific amino acid sequence and thereby interact only with the agent that induced its synthesis.

Arrhythmia   Abnormal heart rhythm or beat.

Assumption of risk   A legal defense used to show that a person has voluntarily participated in a specific activity after being made aware of its known dangers.

Asymptomatic   Without obvious symptoms.

Atherosclerosis   A condition in which yellowish plaques containing cholesterol and lipid material are formed within the inner lining of arteries.

Basal metabolic rate (BMR)   The minimal level of energy required to sustain the body's vital functions. BMR is measured immediately upon awakening, following a 12-hour fast and eight hours of sleep in a metabolic lab.

Behavior chain   A series of behaviors connected to each other in such a way that the resulting behavior will not occur if any links in the chain of behaviors are broken.

Behavioral contracts   See *Contingency contracts.*

Beta blockers (beta-adrenergic blocking agents)   Medications that block or limit sympathetic nervous system stimulation.

Binge-eating disorder (BED)   An eating disorder characterized by frequent binge eating (without purging) and feelings of being out of control when eating.

Bio-electric impedance analysis (BIA)   A noninvasive means of assessing body composition via an electrical current through the body. Impedence of the flow of electricity through the body is related to the level of body fat.

Bloating   Enlargement or distention of the abdomen due to gaseous production.

Body composition The makeup of the body in terms of the relative percentage of fat mass and fat-free mass.

Body mass index (BMI) A relative measure of body height to body weight used to determine the degree of obesity.

Bradycardia Slowness of the heartbeat, as evidenced by a pulse rate of less than 60 bpm.

Brown fat Metabolically active adipose tissue found primarily in animals who hibernate. Humans store very little brown fat.

Bulimia nervosa An eating disorder characterized by episodes of binge eating, followed by self-induced vomiting or the use of diuretics or laxatives.

Calorie The amount of heat required to raise the temperature of 1 kilogram of water 1 degree Celsius. Also called kilocalorie.

Carbohydrates An essential nutrient that provides energy to the body. Dietary sources include sugars (simple) and grains, rice, potatoes and beans (complex).

Catabolism Any destructive process by which complex substances are converted into more simple compounds by living cells.

Cell membrane The enveloping capsule of a cell composed of proteins, lipids and carbohydrates.

Certification The act of attesting that an individual or organization has met a specific set of standards.

Cholesterol A fat-like substance found in the blood and body tissues and in certain foods. Its accumulation in the arteries leads to a narrowing of the vessels (atherosclerosis).

Chronic disease Any disease state that persists over an extended period of time.

Codes of ethics Codes, supplementary to other professional standards of practice or legal requirements, developed by professional organizations to govern professional conduct.

Adherence to these codes is necessary to maintain professional standing or certification with such organizations.

Cognitions Current thoughts or feelings that can function as antecedents or consequences for overt behaviors.

Comparative negligence A system used in legal defenses to distribute fault between an injured party and any defendant.

Competencies Specific skills or knowledge that one must possess in order to have the capacity to function in a particular way (provide appropriate standard of care) for a specific job.

Complete proteins Foods that contain all 10 essential amino acids. Eggs and most meats and dairy products are considered complete protein foods.

Complex carbohydrates The starches or long chains of sugars (polysaccharides) that are found in whole grain breads and cereals, vegetables, fruits and beans.

Compulsive exercise A compelling urge to overexercise that is emotionally destructive, physically draining and may progress to anorexia nervosa and/or bulimia.

Concentric movement Contraction of a muscle in which the muscle shortens, or the proximal and distal attachments of the muscle come together.

Connective tissue The tissue that binds together and supports the various structures of the body. In a broad sense it includes collagenous, elastic, mucous, reticular, osseous and cartilaginous tissue.

Consequence The stimuli that follows a behavior. It may be positive, which increases the probability of the behavior recurring, or negative, which will have the opposite effect.

Contingency contracts Written agreements between client and consultant specifying target behavior, frequency of the behavior and a timeline. May identify rewards or consequences when the conditions are met or fail to be met.

Contract law A system of law governing relationships between those providing products or services to others.

Contributory negligence Used in legal defenses of claims or suits when the plaintiff's negligence was contributory to the act in dispute.

Coronary artery disease (CAD) Sometimes referred to as coronary heart disease (CHD). Almost always a result of atherosclerosis. Includes hypertension, stroke, congestive heart failure, peripheral vascular disease and valvular heart disease.

Creatine phosphate (CP) A high-energy phosphate molecule that is stored in cells and used to resynthesize ATP immediately.

Criminal law A system of law whereby certain defined conduct is statutorily prohibited under threat of criminal prosecution of those violating such laws. The unauthorized practice of medicine and other allied healthcare professional practices falls under this system.

Dehydrated Containing a less-than-optimal level of body water.

Densitometry Determination of variations in density by comparison with that of another material or standard. See *Hydrostatic weighing* for relation to body composition.

Diabetes mellitus A disease of carbohydrate metabolism in which an absolute or relative deficiency of insulin results in an inability to metabolize carbohydrates normally.

Diastolic blood pressure The pressure exerted by the blood on the blood vessel walls when the heart relaxes between contractions.

Dietary-induced thermogenesis A phenomenon sometimes referred to as the thermogenic response to food, which occurs when the body increases its metabolic rate with periods of overeating.

Distal Farthest from the midline of the body or the point of attachment.

Diuretics Medications that produce an increase in urine volume and sodium excretion.

Dyslipidemia Higher-than-normal levels of total cholesterol and triglycerides in the blood; associated with an increased risk of atherosclerosis.

Dyspnea Difficult or labored breathing. A feeling of "air hunger."

Eccentric movement A muscle action in which the muscle lengthens against a resistance while producing force.

Edema Swelling as a result of the collection of fluids within the body tissues.

Elasticity The level of ability of connective tissue to elongate and recover.

Electrolytes The minerals sodium, potassium and chlorine, which are dissolved in the body as electrically charged particles called ions.

Energy Relates to the ability to perform work. In this text, it is measured in calories derived from carbohydrates, protein or fat.

Energy balance The principle that body weight will stay the same when caloric intake equals caloric expenditure, and that a positive or negative energy balance will cause weight gain or weight loss, respectively.

Enzymes Proteins necessary to bring about biochemical reactions.

Essential amino acids Eight to 10 of the 23 different amino acids needed to make proteins. Called essential because the body cannot manufacture them; they must be obtained from the diet.

Essential fat Fat that cannot be produced by the body and must be supplied by the diet. Linoleic acid is the only essential fat.

Essential fatty acids See *Essential fat.*

Estrogen Generic term for estrus-producing steroid compounds; the female sex hormones.

Excess post-exercise oxygen consumption (EPOC) Increased oxygen requirement above RMR following a bout of exercise. Historically referred to as oxygen debt.

Fat An essential nutrient that provides energy, energy storage, insulation and contour to the body. 1 gram fat equals 9 kcals.

Fat-free mass That part of the body composition that represents everything but fat — blood, bones, connective tissue, organs and muscle. Also called lean body mass.

Fat soluble Susceptible to being dissolved in fat. Relating to vitamins, those that are stored in body fat, principally in the liver.

Fatty acids Clusters of carbon-chained atoms, which are the building blocks of dietary fat.

Flexibility The range of motion of a joint.

Food guide pyramid A guide, published in 1992 by the U.S. Dept. of Agriculture and the U.S. Dept. of Health & Human Services, to assist the public with daily food choices that will accomplish dietary goals.

Food model Plastic replica of a food serving size that gives a visual portion estimate for foods from the Food Guide Pyramid.

Forced vital capacity (FVC) The total volume of air that can be voluntarily moved in one breath, from full inspiration to maximum expiration, or vice versa.

Formative evaluation Ongoing tracking of a client's progress throughout a program.

Functional aerobic capacity The maximum physical performance of an individual, represented by maximal oxygen consumption, that is possible before reaching the anaerobic threshold.

Genetic predisposition A latent susceptibility to a disease or condition that is genetically determined.

Gluconeogenesis The process of forming carbohydrates from molecules such as amino acids and fatty acids.

Glucose A simple sugar; the simplest form in which all carbohydrates are used by the body for energy production.

Glycogen The chief carbohydrate storage material. It is formed by the liver and stored in the liver and muscle.

Health belief model A model to explain health-related behaviors that suggests that an individual's decision to adopt healthy behaviors is based largely upon their perception of susceptibility to an illness and the probable severity of the illness. The person's view of the benefits and costs of the change also are considered.

Health history questionnaire A form for obtaining important medical history or current conditions that may affect the safety of a physical activity program or indicate the need for referral to a medical professional for further evaluation.

Heat exhaustion A reaction to heat, marked by weakness and collapse, resulting from water or salt depletion. Characterized by profuse sweating, a drop in blood pressure, light-headedness, nausea, vomiting, decreased coordination and fainting.

Heat stroke A medical emergency, normally manifested by cessation of sweating and a dangerously high body temperature. An altered level of consciousness, seizures, coma and even death can result.

Hemoglobin The protein molecule in red blood cells specifically adapted to carry (by bonding with) oxygen molecules.

Heterogeneous population A population consisting of many diverse traits; not similar or uniform.

High-density lipoproteins (HDLs) A plasma complex of lipids and proteins that contain relatively more protein and less cholesterol and triglycerides. High HDL levels are associated with a low risk of coronary heart disease.

Hydrostatic weighing   An underwater test used to measure percentage of body fat and lean body mass, based on density principles of fat and lean tissue.

Hypercholesterolemia   An excess of cholesterol in the blood.

Hyperglycemia   An abnormally high content of glucose in the blood.

Hyperlipidemia   An excess of lipids in the blood.

Hypertension   High blood pressure, or the elevation of resting blood pressure above 140/90 mmHg.

Hypertrophy   An increase in the cross-sectional size of a muscle, usually in response to resistance training.

Hyperventilation   A condition of higher-than-normal volumes of breathing resulting in an abnormal loss of carbon dioxide from the blood. Dizziness may occur.

Hypoglycemia   A deficiency of glucose in the blood commonly caused by too much insulin, too little glucose or too much exercise. Most commonly found in the insulin-dependent diabetic and characterized by symptoms such as fatigue, dizziness, confusion, headache, nausea or anxiety.

Incomplete proteins   Foods that contain less than the nine to 10 essential amino acids.

Informed consent document   A written statement signed by a client prior to testing and/or programming that informs the client of the purpose(s), processes and all potential risks and discomforts of the testing or programming procedures.

Insoluble   Not able to be dissolved.

Insomnia   Inability to sleep; abnormal wakefulness.

Interval training   Short, high-intensity exercise periods alternated with periods of rest or lower intensity exercise.

Isokinetic   Of or pertaining to muscle contraction through a range of motion at a constant muscle tension and velocity.

Isometric   Of or pertaining to muscle contraction in which there is no change in the angle of the joint(s) involved, and little or no change in the length of the contracting muscle.

Isotonic   Of or pertaining to muscle contraction in which a constant load (resistance) is moved through the range of motion of the involved joint(s).

Jurisprudence   A system or body of law; the science or philosophy of law.

Kegel exercises   Exercises designed to tone the pelvic floor muscles by controlled isometric contraction and relaxation of the muscles surrounding the vagina.

Ketosis   A condition characterized by an abnormally elevated level of ketones in body fluids and tissues. A complication of diabetes mellitus and starvation.

Kilocalorie (kcal)   The amount of heat needed to increase the temperature of 1 kilogram of water 1 degree Celsius. Kcal is the appropriate term to express energy intake and energy expenditure. Also called Calorie.

Kinesiology   The study of the principles of biomechanics, anatomy and physiology combined to make the science of body movement.

Lapses   The expected slips or mistakes that are usually discreet events and are a normal part of the behavior-change process.

Laxatives   Drugs that loosen the bowels.

Lean body mass   See *Fat-free mass*.

Licensure   The granting of licenses to practice a profession. Usually granted at a state level.

Lifestyle behaviors   Actions and responses to stimulation in day-to-day life that affect a person's health (e.g., diet, physical activity, habits such as smoking).

Lipids   Fats.

Lipid profile   Levels of total cholesterol, HDLs, LDLs and triglycerides in the blood as measured in a laboratory.

Lipoprotein lipase The catalyst for the hydrolysis of triglycerides and their transport into the adipocyte (fat cell).

Liposuction The surgical removal of body fat.

Low-density lipoproteins (LDLs) A plasma complex of lipids and proteins that contains relatively more cholesterol and triglycerides and less protein. High LDL levels are associated with an increased risk of coronary heart disease.

Macronutrients The three categories of nutrients (fats, carbohydrates and protein) that supply energy to sustain life.

Medical clearance Written indication from a physician that a client may safely engage in a specific physical activity and/or weight-management program. This clearance may include specific recommendations from the physician concerning programming.

Menopause Cessation of menstruation in the human female, usually occurring between the ages of 48 and 50.

Metabolic functions See *Metabolism*.

Metabolism The chemical and physical processes in the body that provide energy for the maintenance of life.

Minerals Inorganic compounds that serve a variety of important functions in the body.

Mitochondria Specialized cell structures that contain oxidative enzymes needed by the cell to utilize oxygen for metabolism.

Modeling The process of learning by observing and imitating the behavior of others.

Monounsaturated fat A type of unsaturated fat (liquid at room temperature) that has one spot on the fatty acid for the addition of a hydrogen atom (e.g. oleic acid in olive oil).

Mortality The death rate, or ratio of actual deaths to expected deaths.

Myocardial infarction Death of a portion of the heart muscle as a result of interruption of the blood supply to the area. Commonly called a heart attack.

Myoglobin A compound similar to hemoglobin, which aids in the storage and transport of oxygen in the muscle cells.

Neuropathy A general term denoting functional disturbances in the peripheral nervous system. In diabetics it results in a decreased ability to sense pain or discomfort in the extremities, especially the feet.

Nutrients Components of food needed by the body. There are six classes of nutrients: water, minerals, vitamins, fats, carbohydrates and protein.

Nutrition The study of nutrients in foods and of their digestion, absorption, metabolism, storage and excretion.

Obesity The accumulation and storage of excess body fat. Usually defined as at least 20 percent above ideal weight, or more than 30 percent body fat for women and more than 23 percent body fat for men.

One repetition maximum (1RM) The amount of resistance that can be moved through the range of motion one time before the muscle is temporarily fatigued.

Osteoarthritis Degenerative joint disease occurring chiefly in older persons, characterized by degeneration of the articular cartilage, hypertrophy of the bones and changes in the synovial membrane.

Osteoporosis A disorder, primarily affecting postmenopausal women, in which bone density decreases and susceptibility to fractures increases.

Overload principle One of the Master Principles of human performance that states that beneficial adaptations occur in response to demands applied to the body at levels beyond a certain threshold (overload), but within the limits of tolerance and safety.

Palpitations Unduly rapid action of the heart that may be regular or irregular.

PAR-Q The Physical Activity Readiness Questionnaire. A form designed to identify the small number of adults for whom physical activity might be inappropriate, or those who should seek medical advice concerning physical activity. Considered a minimal standard for entry into low-to-moderate intensity exercise programs.

Percent Daily Value A replacement for the percent USRDA on the newer food labels. Gives information on whether a food item has a significant amount of a particular nutrient based on a 2,000-calorie diet.

Phytochemicals The chemicals found in plants that are sometimes used as dietary supplements.

Polyunsaturated fat A type of unsaturated fat (liquid at room temperature) that has two or more positions on the fatty acid available for hydrogen atoms, e.g., corn, safflower and soybean oils.

Post-exercise oxygen consumption See *Excess post-exercise oxygen consumption.*

Postmenopausal Refers to the period of time after menopause.

Prescription A written direction for the administration of a remedy.

Protein A compound composed of 22 to 23 amino acids that is the major structural component of all body tissue.

Proximal Nearest to the midline of the body or point of attachment.

Psychotropic medications Drugs that affect the mental state; capable of modifying mental activity.

Rating of perceived exertion (RPE) A scale, originally developed by Borg, that provides a standard means for evaluating a participant's perception of exercise effort. The original scale ranged from 6 to 20; a revised scale ranges from 0 to 10.

Recommended Dietary Allowance (RDA) The recommended daily amount of a nutrient needed to maintain optimal health.

Registration A state-imposed process by which those who have met established requirements register with a state

agency prior to delivering services.

Relapse In behavior change, the return of an original problem after many lapses (slips, mistakes) have occurred.

Residual air Also called residual lung volume. The amount of air remaining in the lungs following maximal exhalation.

Residual lung volume See *Residual air.*

Resting metabolic rate (RMR) The number of calories expended per unit of time at rest. Often used to approximate BMR. It is measured early in the morning in a lab after an overnight fast and at least eight hours of sleep at home.

Saturated fat Fatty acids carrying the maximal number of hydrogen atoms. These fats are solid at room temperature.

Scope of practice The range and limit of responsibilities normally associated with a specific job or profession.

Sedentary Doing or requiring much sitting; not active.

Self-efficacy One's perception of their ability to change or perform specific behaviors (e.g., exercise).

Serotonin A vasoconstrictor found in serum and many body tissues.

Serum cholesterol The levels of the fat-like sterol cholesterol that are measured in the blood.

Set-point theory The weight-control theory that states that each person has an established and "preferred" body weight. Metabolic adjustments are necessary to return to this established weight after a deviation from the set-point.

Shaping The reinforcement of successive approximations of a goal until the result is reached.

Sleep apnea Cessation of breathing while lying in the horizontal position, as during sleep.

Specificity principle One of the Master Principles of human performance that states that a specific demand (e.g., exercise) made on the body will result in a specific response by the body.

Spot reduction Unsubstantiated theory that contracting muscles will selectively reduce locally stored fat in the area where the exercise is performed.

Stages-of-change model A lifestyle modification model that suggests that people go through distinct, predictable stages when making lifestyle changes; precontemplation, contemplation, preparation, action and maintenance. The process is not always linear.

Standard of care Standards derived from respected authorities and/or professional associations used to evaluate provider conduct to determine if the care provided was appropriate.

Stepped-care model A model of treatment for obesity based on the premise that treatment can be cumulative or incremental.

Stimulus control methods In behavioral science, sometimes called "cue extinction," a means to break the connection between events or other stimuli and a behavior.

Stroke A sudden, and often severe attack due to blockage of an artery into the brain.

Stroke volume The volume of blood pumped from the left ventricle in one cycle of a heart beat.

Subcutaneous Beneath the skin.

Submaximal graded exercise test A test to evaluate cardiorespiratory fitness, performed at less than maximal effort and terminated before exhaustion.

Summative evaluation The evaluation process that occurs at the end of a program and during follow-up.

Sympathetic nervous system A division of the autonomic nervous system that activates the body to cope with some stressor (i.e., fight or flight response).

Sympathomimetic effect An effect similar to those impulses conveyed by fibers of the sympathetic nervous system.

Systolic blood pressure The pressure exerted by the blood on the vessel walls during ventricular contraction.

Talk test A subjective method for measuring exercise intensity by observing respiratory effort and the ability to talk while exercising.

Target heart rate (THR) The number of heartbeats per minute that indicate appropriate exercise intensity levels for an individual. Also called training heart rate.

Thermic effect of a meal An increase in energy expenditure due to digestive processes (digestion, absorption, metabolism of food). Also called thermic effect of food.

Tort law A system of law that governs the management and disposition of personal injury and wrongful death lawsuits.

Triglycerides The storage form of fat consisting of three molecules of fatty acid and a glycerol molecule.

Valsalva maneuver Forced exhalation against the narrowest part of the larynx through which air passes into and out of the trachea. Causes an increase in intrathoracic pressure that reduces venous return.

Vasodilators Medications that cause a relaxation of the smooth muscles cells of the walls of blood vessels and result in a widening of the lumen (opening) of the vessels.

Venous return Return of the circulatory fluids to the heart by way of the veins.

Very-low-calorie diets (VLCDs) A weight-loss program that consists only of liquid meals, and a calorie content that usually ranges between 420 and 800 kcal/day. VLCDs can only be used when under the care and supervision of a physician.

Viscera The large interior organs in any one of the three great cavities of the body, especially the abdomen.

Vitamins Organic substances that occur in small amounts in many foods and are necessary for normal metabolic functioning of the body.

VO₂ max   The point at which oxygen consumption reaches a period of little or no change with an additional workload.

Waist-to-hip ratio   A useful measure for determining health risk due to the site of fat storage. Calculated by dividing the ratio of abdominal girth (waist measurement) by the hip measurement.

Waiver   Voluntary abandonment of a right to file suit; not always legally binding.

Water soluble   Dissolvable in water. Refers to those vitamins that require adequate daily intake since the body excretes excesses in the urine.

Weight cycling   A pattern of periodic weight reduction followed by weight gain. Also called yo-yo dieting.

Index

Please check the ACE® certification you would like
to receive information on.

☐ Lifestyle & Weight Management Consultant
☐ Personal Trainer
☐ Aerobics Instructor

Name _____

Address _____

City _____

State _____

Zip _____

Home Phone ( ) _____

Work Phone ( ) _____

P97-023 9/96

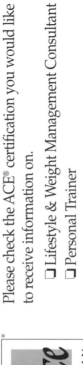

Please check the ACE® certification you would like
to receive information on.

☐ Lifestyle & Weight Management Consultant
☐ Personal Trainer
☐ Aerobics Instructor

Name _____

Address _____

City _____

State _____

Zip _____

Home Phone ( ) _____

Work Phone ( ) _____

P97-023 9/96

Please check the ACE® certification you would like
to receive information on.

☐ Lifestyle & Weight Management Consultant
☐ Personal Trainer
☐ Aerobics Instructor

Name _____

Address _____

City _____

State _____

Zip _____

Home Phone ( ) _____

Work Phone ( ) _____

P97-023 9/96

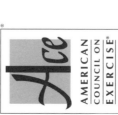

ACE
AMERICAN
COUNCIL ON
EXERCISE®

Please check the ACE® certification you would like
to receive information on.

☐ Lifestyle & Weight Management Consultant
☐ Personal Trainer
☐ Aerobics Instructor

Name _____

Address _____

City _____

State _____

Zip _____

Home Phone ( ) _____

Work Phone ( ) _____

P97-023 9/96

ACE
AMERICAN
COUNCIL ON
EXERCISE®

BUSINESS REPLY MAIL
FIRST-CLASS MAIL   PERMIT NO. 202113   SAN DIEGO CA

POSTAGE WILL BE PAID BY ADDRESSEE

AMERICAN COUNCIL ON EXERCISE®
PO BOX 910449
SAN DIEGO CA 92191-9961

NO POSTAGE
NECESSARY
IF MAILED
IN THE
UNITED STATES

BUSINESS REPLY MAIL
FIRST-CLASS MAIL   PERMIT NO. 202113   SAN DIEGO CA

POSTAGE WILL BE PAID BY ADDRESSEE

AMERICAN COUNCIL ON EXERCISE®
PO BOX 910449
SAN DIEGO CA 92191-9961

NO POSTAGE
NECESSARY
IF MAILED
IN THE
UNITED STATES

BUSINESS REPLY MAIL
FIRST-CLASS MAIL   PERMIT NO. 202113   SAN DIEGO CA

POSTAGE WILL BE PAID BY ADDRESSEE

AMERICAN COUNCIL ON EXERCISE®
PO BOX 910449
SAN DIEGO CA 92191-9961

NO POSTAGE
NECESSARY
IF MAILED
IN THE
UNITED STATES